US Foreign Policy and the War on Drugs

This book explores how US foreign policy has exacerbated the global drug problem. It analyses a crucial side effect of coercive US strategies on farmers, traffickers and governments: the geographic displacement of the cocaine and heroin industry. This volume thus offers an original explanation of the adaptability of drug markets to state pressure. Using IR theory, the book highlights the negative consequences of policies that rely on coercion.

To explain displacement, a causal mechanism is developed and applied to three cases. These case studies examine US anti-drug regimes at different times and in various regions: the destruction of the "French Connection" in the 1970s and its impact on Southeast Asia and Mexico; the shooting-down of suspected trafficking planes over Peru in the 1990s; and the current US-sponsored war in Colombia. While the link between foreign policy and displacement should not be oversimplified, Cornelius Friesendorf argues that US initiatives have been a major cause behind the global spread of cocaine and heroin. He thus calls for a revision of US policy.

The book will be of much interest to students of US foreign policy, security studies and International Relations.

Cornelius Friesendorf holds a Ph.D in International Relations from the University of Zurich and is currently a postdoctoral fellow at the University of Munich.

CSS studies in security and international relations
Series Editors: Andreas Wenger and Victor Mauer
Center for Security Studies, Swiss Federal Institute of Technology (ETH), Zurich

War Plans and Alliances in the Cold War
Threat perceptions in the East and West
Edited by Vojtech Mastny, Sven Holtsmark and Andreas Wenger

Transforming NATO in the Cold War
Challenges beyond deterrence in the 1960s
Edited by Andreas Wenger, Christian Nuenlist and Anna Locher

US Foreign Policy and the War on Drugs
Displacing the cocaine and heroin industry
Cornelius Friesendorf

US Foreign Policy and the War on Drugs

Displacing the cocaine and heroin industry

Cornelius Friesendorf

Routledge
Taylor & Francis Group
LONDON AND NEW YORK

First published 2007
by Routledge
2 Park Square, Milton Park, Abingdon, Oxfordshire OX14 4RN

Simultaneously published in the USA and Canada
by Routledge
711 Third Avenue, New York, NY 10017

First issued in paperback 2014

Routledge is an imprint of the Taylor & Francis Group, an informa business

Typeset in Times by Wearset Ltd, Boldon, Tyne and Wear

British Library Cataloguing in Publication Data
A catalogue record for this book is available from the British Library

Library of Congress Cataloging in Publication Data
Friesendorf, Cornelius.
US foreign policy and the war on drugs: displacing the cocaine and heroin industry/Cornelius Friesendorf.
p. cm. – (CSS studies in security and international relations)
Includes bibliographical references and index.
1. Drug control–United States–History. 2. Cocaine industry–Government policy–United States. 3. Heroin industry–Government policy–United States. 4. United States–Foreign relations–20th century. 5. United States–Foreign relations–21st century. I. Title. II. Title: United States foreign policy and the war on drugs.
HV5825.F756 2007
363.450973-dc22

2006025478

ISBN13: 978-1-138-88187-7 (pbk)
ISBN13: 978-0-415-41375-6 (hbk)

For Nedd

Contents

List of illustrations viii
Preface ix
List of abbreviations xi

Introduction 1

1 US drug policy and drug industry displacement 5

2 Targeting Turkey and the French Connection: the early 1970s 37

3 Targeting smugglers flying over the Andes: the 1990s 79

4 Targeting the Colombian drug industry: the early twenty-first centur 122

5 Drug industry displacement and side effects of foreign policy 166

6 Alternatives to the US war on drugs 179

Annex I: maps 190
Annex II: charts 198
Notes 200
Bibliography 205
Index 223

Illustrations

Figure

1 Explaining the displacement of the drug industry 33

Maps

1 Case studies 190
2 The Mediterranean Basin 191
3 Southeast Asia 192
4 Mexico 193
5 South America 194
6 Colombia 195
7 Peru 196
8 Bolivia 197

Charts

1 Andean coca cultivation, 1988–2005 198
2 Colombian coca cultivation and fumigation, and retail cocaine prices in the US, 1993–2003 199
3 US aid to Colombia, 1997–2005 199

Tables

1 Strategies against cocaine and heroin 8
2 Why US international drug policies are ineffective 19
3 Andean coca cultivation, 1988–2005 98

Preface

Writing this book has been a rewarding experience. It has helped me to better understand the ambiguities of international relations and human action. Drug policies show that humans can cope with danger in responsible and humane ways, but that their behavior can also be selfish and parochial. Writing the book has also reminded me of the importance of theory for bringing order into a very complex world (although only on paper), and of the need to leave the ivory tower for fieldwork (in a literal sense) to see whether reality corresponds with theory. Finally, I have been privileged to meet and interview some fascinating people during my research trips around Europe, the US, Asia, North Africa, and Latin America.

Talking to people about drugs and US foreign policy has been a crucial motivating factor during the five years of research and writing. I especially thank Andreas Wenger, my *Doktorvater*, who supported this project from its rocky start as a vague idea for a Ph.D. thesis to the finishing line, and who read drafts on holidays and weekends. His optimism has been inspiring. Moreover, working for him at the Center for Security Studies at the Swiss Federal Institute of Technology Zurich (ETH), has not only allowed me to finance my research, but also to acquire new skills. Many thanks also go to Christopher Daase, who convinced me that looking at a rather obscure topic of international relations was the right thing to do. Further support came from Peter Andreas, Thomas Biersteker, and James Der Derian, who invited me to the Watson Institute for International Studies, Brown University, where I spent a wonderful and very productive spring of 2005.

Chapters of this book were presented at the ETH Zurich, the German Political Science Association, the Midwest Political Science Association, American University, George Washington University, the Geneva School of Diplomacy and International Relations, the University of Geneva, the Friedrich-Ebert Foundation Berlin, and the Swiss Federal Police Office. For their help and comments, I thank Jan Bittner, Stefan Brem, James Der Derian, Jörg Friedrichs, Daniele Ganser, Andreas Goldthau, J. Michael Greig, Sylvie Guichard, Adam Isacson, Martin Jelsma, Florian Kohstall, Cynthia McClintock, Alfred W. McCoy, Robert Orttung, James Robinson, Theo Roncken, Regine Schönenberg, Holger Stritzel, Marie-Therese Tinnefeld, Coletta Youngers, and many others who had something to say about drugs and foreign policy, whether by e-mail, in conference halls, embassies, or on the coca fields (all errors and shortcomings are my responsibility). I am also grateful to Victor Mauer and Andreas Wenger for considering my manuscript as a contribution to this Routledge series, Marjorie François and Andrew Humphrys at Routledge, and the anonymous reviewers.

Special thanks go to the Guichards and to Poppy Willard for all the moments spent together in Geneva, the Canton de Vaud, and La Haute Savoie; Peter Andreas and Daniel Möckli for their advice; my parents for teaching me to appreciate words; Christopher Findlay for editing the manuscript; John Yates for correcting my English a long time ago; Bertrand Lefebvre for the maps; Ajaib Kochar for picking the right fruits in Delhi; and the courageous Milton Lérida in Bolivia.

But without Nedd Willard, this book would have never been completed. It is therefore dedicated to you.

Abbreviations

ABDP	Air Bridge Denial Program
AD	alternative development
AIDS	Acquired Immune Deficiency Syndrom
AUC	Autodefensas Unidas de Colombia (United Self-Defense Forces of Colombia)
AWACS	Airborne Warning and Control System
BNDD	Bureau of Narcotics and Dangerous Drugs
CIA	Central Intelligence Agency
CNP	Colombian National Police
DEA	Drug Enforcement Administration
DoD	Department of Defense
ELN	Ejército de Liberación Nacional (National Liberation Army)
EU	European Union
FARC	Fuerzas Armadas Revolucionarias de Colombia (Revolutionary Armed Forces of Colombia)
FBI	Federal Bureau of Investigation
FBN	Federal Bureau of Narcotics
FOL	Forward Operating Location
FPA	Foreign Policy Analysis
GAO	General Accounting Offic
GDP	Gross Domestic Product
GTZ	Deutsche Gesellschaft für Technische Zusammenarbeit (German Society for Technical Cooperation)
HIV	Human Immunodeficiency Viru
IDA	Institute for Defense Analyses
INCB	International Narcotics Control Board
INLEA	Bureau for International Narcotics and Law Enforcement Affairs
IPE	International Political Economy
IR	International Relations
IRA	Irish Republican Army
JAOC	Joint Air Operations Center
KMT	Kuomintang

NAFTA	North American Free Trade Association
NAS	Narcotics Affairs Section
NATO	North Atlantic Treaty Organisation
NDCS	National Drug Control Strategy
NGO	Nongovernmental Organization
NLF	National Liberation Front
OAS	Organization of American States
ODALE	Office of Drug Abuse Law Enforcemen
ONDCP	Office of National Drug Control Polic
SIVAM	Sistema de Vigilância da Amazônia (System for the Vigilance of the Amazon)
SOUTHCOM	Southern Command
TAT	Tactical Analysis Team
UMOPAR	Unidades Móviles de Patrullaje Rural (Mobile Rural Patrol Units)
UN	United Nations
UNFDAC	United Nations Fund for Drug Abuse Control
US	United States of America
USAID	US Agency for International Development
WOLA	Washington Office on Latin Americ

Introduction

Since the early 1970s, the cocaine and heroin industry has changed significantly Coca cultivation, coca paste production, and cocaine processing have increased (cocaine is made from coca paste, which is derived from the coca plant). Poppy cultivation, opium production, and heroin processing have also increased (heroin is made from opium, which comes from the opium poppy plant). More countries have been integrated into what has become a global illicit drug market. Drug traffickers have murdered policy-makers, judges, soldiers, policemen, and bystanders. They have also used corruption to facilitate their business activities. Moreover, illicit crop cultivation and drug production have destroyed sensitive natural habitats. On the drug consumption side, an increasing number of people have begun consuming cocaine and heroin, not least because many users of illicit drugs have switched from more harmless substances, especially cannabis and opium, to harder substances. Increasing drug consumption has led, among other problems, to a virtual explosion of AIDS in drug-consuming regions and along trafficking routes (for descriptions of these developments see Labrousse 2003; McCoy 2003; Stares 1996).

Governments have several options to try and reduce the illicit production, trafficking, and consumption of drugs. They can coerce suppliers and consumers to stop producing or consuming drugs; offer them alternatives to drug production and consumption; launch multilateral initiatives to prohibit specifi substances and improve law enforcement cooperation; arrest money launderers; or even invade countries that play a prominent role in drug production and trafficking

This book looks at coercive international initiatives against cocaine and heroin undertaken by the United States (US). Since the beginning of the twentieth century, and particularly since the early 1970s, the US has been trying to reduce drug supplies. As shown in the first chapter, the US federal government has trained and equipped security forces from numerous cocaine- and heroin-producing and transit countries. US policy-makers have put economic, political, and military pressure on countries whose anti-drug efforts they regarded as insufficient. US airplanes and helicopters have sprayed coca and poppy field with herbicides, and US satellites and reconnaissance aircraft have surveyed the moves of traffickers (Carpenter 2003; Chepesiuk 1999a). At the United Nations, the US has been strengthening the international drug control framework (Bewley-Taylor 1999; McAllister 1999).

It is puzzling that drug problems have been getting worse at the same time that the US has increased its anti-drug efforts. This simultaneity leads to the question of whether US governments are simply trying to keep apace with drug problems, or whether these problems are also a consequence of US policies. Would drug problems be worse were it not for US attempts to improve the situation, or would there be fewer problems if the US had not embarked on an anti-drug campaign? Many US policy-makers stress the first explanation. They argue that although US anti-drug policies have not solved drug problems, they have nevertheless prevented higher levels of drug consumption and drug-related problems. However, most drug policy researchers, many journalists, and some policy-makers favor the second explanation. They argue that US coercive drug policies have made matters worse, since the implementation of drug prohibition creates side effects such as human rights abuses, a weaker control of armed forces, violent conflict, environmental destruction, and corruption (Youngers and Rosin 2005).

This book shares the view that coercive drug policies can cause damage. However, instead of treating the side effects of these policies as given, it focuses on one of these assumed side effects: the displacement of drug production and trafficking. As shown in more detail below, critics of US drug policy argue that US initiatives against drugs have not reduced coca and poppy cultivation, cocaine and heroin production, and cocaine and heroin trafficking, but that the US has merely pushed the drug industry from one place to another. The aim of this book is to explain the link between the displacement of the illicit cocaine and heroin industry, on the one hand, and US international efforts to reduce the supply of cocaine and heroin, on the other.

By offering a heuristic explanation of displacement, the present work helps to solve the puzzle of why drug problems have become worse in a period during which the US has undertaken significant efforts against drugs. After all, whenever the drug industry moves to a new place, problems such as violence, corruption, and AIDS move along with it. Hence, by revealing the process of drug industry displacement, this book sheds light on worsening drug problems in general. If US anti-drug initiatives have contributed to a geographical displacement of the illicit drug industry, one can say that the US has made a bad situation worse.

Researchers have illuminated various aspects of the drug industry. As shown in the first chapter, some authors discuss the domestic motives behind US coercive drug policies, referring to prejudice, bureaucratic interests, and real or perceived drug problems (Baum 1997; Connolly 1999; Gordon 1994). Others show that policies against drug supplies have failed. Despite considerable efforts, drug prices in the US are relatively low, purity is high, and drugs are more or less freely available. Further, scholars explain policy ineffectiveness. Various obstacles impede progress against the illicit supply of cocaine and heroin, including the profitability of coca and poppy, under-funded security forces, the dependence of producing states on drug revenues, antagonistic US foreign policy interests, and economic transformation.

Some authors also look at the issue of drug industry displacement. However, existing analyses of this important aspect of the illicit drug industry and counter-drug policies have theoretical, methodological, and empirical shortcomings. First, scholars regard displacement as a tool for explaining policy ineffectiveness, and not as a research topic in its own right. Second, analyses based on single cases leave open the question of whether the findings can be generalized. Third, several works treat the displacement of drug production and traffickin unsystematically by simply listing, but not analyzing, instances of displacement, or by arbitrarily singling out presumed causal factors. Forth, explanations that focus on displacement as a result of US collusion with drug entrepreneurs neglect cases in which the US did not fully subordinate drug control to other interests. Last, some authors try to predict future displacement patterns, yet arrive at rather vague conclusions. Before predicting the future, one has to know what happened in the past.

This book is embedded in the discipline of International Relations (IR) and security studies. Although drugs and drug policies are key issues of international security, IR research on the topic is still relatively marginal. Moreover, IR says little about side effects of foreign policy. One finds many descriptions of side effects, but few explanations informed by a theoretical approach. IR theories help explain foreign policy decisions, state behavior, and problems of foreign policy implementation, but the *effects* of foreign policies are treated on the margins, despite their significant impact on humans and states. This shortcoming results not least from the fact that most scholars search for laws governing social life. However, the contingency, complexity, and dynamic nature of foreign policy side effects mean that searching for laws and engaging in variable-based theorizing is inappropriate when explaining side effects.

This book contributes to the drug policy debate by focusing on the causation of side effects in its own right, treating the question of policy effectiveness as a secondary issue. Moreover, by looking at three cases of drug industry displacement, the book goes beyond single-case analyses, revealing a general process of drug industry displacement independent of time, type of drug, and region. In addition, by looking at three prominent US initiatives against drugs, this book corrects the bias of drug policy scholars to focus on cases in which the US government subordinated drug control to other foreign-policy interests. Last, by looking at history, the book counterbalances the scholarly tendency to predict the future without first understanding the past

This book contributes to IR as well. It focuses on illicit activities and thus broadens the disciplinary spectrum. Moreover, by looking at side effects of foreign policy, it goes beyond the academic fixation on the genesis and implementation of foreign policy. Further, the book underlines the need to move toward a conception of causality that takes into account change, contingency, and complexity.

Causal mechanisms are alternatives to social laws. A causal mechanism provides an account of how presumed causes and effects are related (George and

Bennett 2005; Hedström and Swedberg 1998). To explain drug industry displacement, the first chapter develops a causal mechanism according to which US coercive international initiatives against cocaine and heroin lead to the displacement of drug production and trafficking because pressure is applied inconsistently, because the illicit drug industry responds flexibly to coercion, and because law enforcement in drug producing and transit states is weak. Moreover, contingent conditions that cannot be deduced from theories or common sense influence foreign policy outcomes

The plausibility of this causal mechanism is assessed in three case studies (see the maps in Annex I). The first examines US attempts in the early 1970s to reduce US heroin problems by putting pressure on Turkey, where opium was diverted into illegal channels, and on the Corsican French Connection, which supplied the bulk of the US heroin market. This case study analyzes the impact of the Nixon initiative on the drug industries in Southeast Asia and Mexico. The second case study analyses the Air Bridge Denial Program, an attempt by the US and the Andean states in the 1990s to prevent traffickers from flying drugs from Bolivia and Peru to Colombia. This case illuminates the initiative's impact on the Andean cocaine industry. The third case study examines US drug policies in Colombia since the late 1990s and their impact on drug industry displacement within Colombia and to other countries.

Two caveats must be mentioned here. First, it is difficult to generalize about displacement. The lack of reliable information on drugs and drug policies (Reuter and Greenfield 2001; Thoumi 2002a), and the complexity of displacement, are formidable methodological obstacles. But if it can be shown that the initial causal mechanism applies in three different cases, this would provide a clue that a general causal mechanism is at work. Second, this book acknowledges that displacement can result from many factors. The worsening of drug problems since the early 1970s coincides, for example, with an increase in people and goods crossing international borders, economic transformation processes, and changing social attitudes toward drug consumption.

The case studies do examine alternative explanations according to which factors other than US anti-drug policies led to the displacement of the drug industry. Examining alternative explanations helps to avoid exaggerating the ability of the US to shape international developments. However, one should not underestimate it either. Referring to the preponderance of the US in international affairs in general, Joseph Nye (2002/2003: 545) writes that "[n]ot since Rome has one nation loomed so large above the others." In international drug control, this certainly holds true.

1 US drug policy and drug industry displacement

This chapter first discusses drug problems and counter-strategies. Subsequently, it describes the US role in international drug control and the drug policy debate. It shows that researchers have answered many important questions, but that the displacement of the drug industry merits further discussion. The chapter then argues that scholars of IR have not paid enough attention to the illicit political economy, the effects of foreign policies, and contingency and complexity. Following this, a causal mechanism is developed that helps to explain the displacement of the illicit cocaine and heroin industry. The chapter ends with a discussion of methodology.

Changes in the cocaine and heroin industry

Over recent decades, the illicit cocaine and heroin economy has changed significantly. Poppy, opium, and heroin supplies have increased. Between 1971 and 1999, the annual global amount of illicit opium is estimated to have risen fivefold, from 1,200 to 6,100 metric tons (McCoy 2003: 20). Coca, coca paste, and cocaine supplies have increased as well. In 1983, potential coca production was 90,000 metric tons, but in 1999, it stood at 613,400 tons (Basov *et al.* 2001: 139). Between 1995 and 2001 alone, potential coca production increased by 62 percent (Lee 2002: 538).

Whereas illicit crop cultivation and drug production used to be confined to a limited number of countries, the drug industry is now spread around the world.[1] Poppy production has shifted from the Golden Triangle (Thailand, Burma, Laos) to the Golden Crescent (Iran, Afghanistan, Pakistan), as well as to Colombia and Central Asia. Coca, traditionally grown almost exclusively in Peru and Bolivia, is now cultivated mainly in Colombia. Similarly, drug trafficking routes have multiplied. Nowadays, there is hardly a country that does not serve as a transit or destination point of what has become a global illicit drug industry (Labrousse 2003; Stares 1996). Traffickers have also become more sophisticated and have struck mutual alliances (Williams 1995).

The effects of increased drug supplies can be dramatic. To take the example of Colombia, the number of people killed in the country during the 1990s is estimated at 250,000 (Zinecker 2002: 1). In 2005, the country had up to 3.7 million internally displaced persons, the world's second highest number after Sudan (Norwegian Refugee Council 2006: 10). This humanitarian catastrophe is partially a result of the drug trade.

The dynamics of drug demand are also staggering. In some countries, drug consumption has assumed appalling proportions. Pakistan had an estimated 1.5 million heroin addicts in 2000. Twenty years earlier, Pakistan had counted relatively few addicts (United Nations Office for Drug Control and Crime Prevention 2000: 4). Since the 1980s, the slums of Latin America have seen an increase in the numbers of people smoking *bazuco*, a mixture of coca paste and tobacco whose consumption can lead to severe brain damage. Industrialized countries have also experienced more drug consumption. The US counted 600,000 heroin users in 1993, a tenfold increase since 1967 (Bertram *et al.* 1996: 10).

The increase in cocaine and heroin consumption can partially be attributed to the fact that many drug consumers have switched from cannabis and opium to cocaine and heroin consumption. In addition, and related to this switch to harder drugs, methods of drug consumption have become more dangerous. The sharing of contaminated needles by heroin users has sped up the AIDS epidemic that has had a devastating impact on many communities and countries since the 1980s.

To be sure, drug problems are not new. In the nineteenth century, the British "Opium Wars" forced China to open its market to British opium produced in India. As a consequence, in 1906, an estimated 27 percent of the Chinese adult male population was addicted to opium, a level of addiction never reached before or since (McCoy 1996: 253). In Europe and North America, cocaine and heroin products were popular drugs, and their consumption was hardly regulated. Moreover, Western governments defended the interests of large drug-producing companies. It is thus not surprising that the drug trade expanded. Heroin and cocaine products from Europe and the US were shipped through Japan and Russia into China and elsewhere (Friman 1996; Gootenberg 1999; Walker 1991). Over time, however, drug consumption, production, and trade were criminalized and multilateral control mechanisms established. As a result, a thriving illicit trade developed that has seen unprecedented growth from the 1970s onwards.

What is the link between drugs on the one hand and IR and security on the other? Drugs are a prime topic of IR and security. Drug smuggling can trigger military interventions, as seen in 1989, when the US invaded Panama to arrest President Manuel Noriega, who was wanted in the US for drug trafficking Moreover, drugs can fuel violent domestic conflict. In Colombia, trafficker have mounted numerous attacks against the state, at times bringing it to near collapse. The Colombian conflict has become even more intractable since left-wing insurgents and right-wing paramilitaries began receiving revenues from the drug trade in the mid-1990s. In Afghanistan, both the Taliban and the Northern Alliance benefited from the industry, either by taxing poppy fields or by involving themselves directly in the traffic. In Peru, the Maoist Shining Path has induced peasants to grow coca and has protected traffickers from the Peruvian security forces.

The drug industry can undermine democratic stability as well. Trafficker bribe politicians, judges, and the police, and thereby undermine state accountability and legitimacy. Moreover, when drug entrepreneurs attack competitors or the state, they question a state's monopoly over the legitimate use of force. In Colombia, the government's inability to stop the violence has weakened the state. In Bolivia, peasant protests against coca eradication have led to numerous deaths and political turmoil.

With regard to the impact of drugs on economic security, the true size of the drug economy is unknown. In 1997, the United Nations (UN) estimated the annual value of the illicit drug economy at $400 billion, or around 8 percent of the global trade at the time (United Nations Drug Control Programme 1997).[2] While this figure is exaggerated (Reuter and Greenfield 2001; Thoumi 2002a), it is obvious that drugs generate much capital. The placement, layering, and reintegration of drug revenues distort national economies and may erode the stability of international financial markets. Further, the drug economy is a burden on public finances through property theft, lost earnings, or costs imposed by drugs on the criminal justice and health systems.

Last, the drug industry destroys the environment. Cocaine and heroin processing requires chemical products whose leftovers pollute soil and water. In addition, many hectares of pristine forests, which are important for both the local and the global ecosystem, have been cleared and replaced by coca and poppy fields

Strategies against drugs

States have undertaken significant efforts against drugs. Most obviously, they have prohibited the production, trafficking, distribution, and consumption of specific substances except for medical and scientific purposes. During the twentieth century, an ever-tighter global drug prohibition regime was created (Nadelmann 1990; Andreas and Nadelmann 2006). With regard to efforts of implementing prohibition, we can distinguish between coercion versus positive incentives, domestic versus international strategies, and demand-reduction versus supply-reduction strategies.[3] Table 1 summarizes these anti-drug strategies.

Coercive, supply-oriented strategies implemented *domestically* include the eradication of illicit coca and poppy; the arrest of peasants, traffickers, money launderers, chemists, and others involved in the drug trade; the social stigmatization of suppliers; the confiscation of drugs; the forfeiture of assets of suspected drug suppliers; the control of precursor chemicals diverted from legal trade flows; and action against money laundering. Coercive, supply-oriented strategies implemented on the *international* level encompass bilateral law enforcement support; drug interdiction close to borders; military and law enforcement operations; military invasion of other countries; political, economic, and normative pressure on foreign governments to induce them to reduce illicit drug supplies; and initiatives against money laundering and the diversion of precursor chemicals from the legal market.

Table 1 Strategies against cocaine and heroin*

	Supply		*Demand*	
	Coercion	*Positive incentives*	*Coercion*	*Positive incentives*
Domestic	Eradication of coca and poppy Arrest of suppliers Stigmatization of suppliers Confiscation of drug Asset forfeiture Control of precursor chemicals Anti-money laundering action	Crop substitution Alternative development Social integration of suppliers	Arrest of consumers Stigmatization of consumers Harm reduction	Prevention Treatment Research
International	Law enforcement support for other states Interdiction Military and law enforcement operations Military invasion Pressure on other states Control of precursor chemicals Initiatives against money laundering	Support for crop substitution Support for alternative development Support for integration of suppliers Support for harm reduction	Support for arrest of consumers Stigmatization of consumers	Support for prevention Support for treatment Support for research Support for harm reduction

Note

* These are ideal types. In reality, strategies overlap. Arresting drug consumers, for example, can reduce drug supplies, since consumers sometimes sell drugs to finance their habit

States can also provide positive incentives. *Domestic* strategies include crop substitution and alternative development (AD). AD aims to improve living conditions in coca and poppy cultivation zones by building schools and hospitals, guaranteeing peasants access to domestic and international markets, and introducing sustainable economic reforms (Deutsche Gesellschaft für Technische Zusammenarbeit 2001). Similarly, the strategy of harm reduction supports peasants and drug consumers through long-term measures and (re-)integrates them into society. *International*, supply-oriented policies that provide positive incentives may focus on crop substitution, AD, and the (re-)integration of drug suppliers into society.

States also have several options for reducing drug demand. On a *domestic* level, policy-makers who trust in coercive means to reduce drug problems can pass laws that lead to the arrest of drug consumers and ensure they receive high prison sentences. Politicians can also try to foster a climate against drug use that portrays users as reckless individuals and as a burden to society. Demand-oriented, coercive, *international* policies do the same, yet more indirectly. A state may support law enforcement directed at consumers or shape international norms against drug consumption.

In addition, a government can offer positive incentives to persuade users to give up drugs. *Domestically*, it may inform people about the dangers of drug consumption (prevention) or help someone give up the habit (treatment). It can also finance research on the causes of drug use and abuse. Moreover, a government may opt for harm reduction measures, including the decriminalization of drug consumption and controlled drug distribution to users. *Internationally*, governments can support prevention, treatment, research, and harm reduction bilaterally or multilaterally.

This book looks at policies of a net consuming state directed at net drug producing and transit states.[4] More specifically, it examines the international, supply-oriented, coercive drug policies of the US.[5]

The US and international drug control

The US has dominated international drug control from the beginnings of such efforts in the early twentieth century (Bewley-Taylor 1999; McAllister 1999). Concerned, among others, about opium consumption in the newly acquired Philippines, the US initiated a conference in Shanghai in 1909 at which 12 other states participated. Although the US did not reach its objective of a global opium ban, participants adopted several drug control resolutions. Three years later, at The Hague, governments again agreed on measures to regulate the opium trade, as well as the production of heroin and cocaine. After World War I, the US sponsored drug control initiatives in the League of Nations. Although the US was not a member of the League, US initiatives contributed to the collection of statistics, the dissemination of information, and the creation of a drug licensing system.

After World War II, the US lobbied successfully for a prohibition regime in the framework of the UN. The international drug control system is based on three conventions: the 1961 Single Convention on Narcotic Drugs and its 1972 amendment; the 1971 Convention on Psychotropic Substances; and the 1988 Convention against the Illicit Traffic in Narcotic Drugs and Psychotropic Substances. The US has played a prominent role both in the creation and implementation of these UN conventions.

Besides multilateralism, the US pursues bilateral and unilateral agendas. This aspect dominates over multilateralism, as it allows US policy-makers to better leverage the military, political, and economic capabilities of the US. During Operation Intercept in 1969, intensified inspections of individuals and vehicles on the US side of the US–Mexican border brought trans-border flows to a virtual standstill. Few drugs were confiscated, since smugglers simply awaited the end of the operation. Instead, Intercept had repercussions on the economy of the border region and worsened relations with Mexico (Gooberman 1974).

In the early 1970s, the Nixon administration and the US public were concerned about reports that substantial numbers of GIs stationed in Vietnam were consuming heroin, as well as widespread heroin consumption in the US. Most of the heroin sold on US streets was imported by the Marseille-based Corsican French Connection and originated from Turkish poppy fields. These supplies dried up when Turkey, threatened by a suspension of US aid, banned the cultivation of poppy, and when police forces from around the world eliminated the French Connection. When more drug imports from Southeast Asia and Mexico stifled this success, Washington conducted a herbicide spraying program with Mexico, and supplied Burma and other countries with equipment in order to reduce poppy cultivation in drug production zones often controlled by hill tribes and Communist insurgents. Thus, during the 1970s, the US steadily internationalized its law enforcement presence by supporting and equipping foreign security forces and by sending its own "cops across borders" (Nadelmann 1993).

In the 1980s, US foreign drug policies shifted into even higher gear. Concerned about a rise in the consumption of cocaine, and particularly crack cocaine, the US sent more personnel, money, and supplies to drug producing and transit countries. Republican Congressman Clay Shaw (FL), in 1988, expressed his concern about drugs and his demands for more resolute US attempts to control drugs as follows:

> [W]e have not yet begun to fight [. . .] We will not be able to take credit for a war against drugs until we bring the war to the fields where marijuana, cocaine, and poppies are grown [. . .] I believe the drugs grown in those fields are a greater threat to the future of this country than all the Russian missiles. If we can go in and take out a Soviet landing strip in Grenada, I believe we can go in and take out the crops that are hurting our children.
>
> (Quoted in Bertram *et al.* 1996: 155)

As part of its anti-drug efforts, the US began to make use of its armed forces. Many within the US military did not want to be drawn into drug control, which they saw as a police task. It was also feared that the "war on drugs" would expose soldiers to corruption, and that the drug war was a low-intensity conflic that could not be won and for which there was no exit strategy (Mabry 1989). Yet despite these reservations, military involvement in the "war on drugs" expanded. In 1986, President Ronald Reagan signed National Security Decision Directive 221, which declared the drug trade a threat to US national security.[6] In operations such as Blast Furnace and Snowcap, the US military helped South American security forces to destroy cocaine laboratories and coca fields, arrest drug traffickers, and confiscate drug

In 1989, the Pentagon became the lead agency for the detection and monitoring of aerial and maritime drug smuggling. The same year, the US invaded Panama with 24,000 troops, showing that conventional warfare was not excluded as a strategy option against drugs. The aim of the invasion was to capture Panama's president, Manuel Noriega, who was wanted in the US on drug trafficking charges. Noriega was taken to the US, where a Florida court sentenced him to 40 years in prison. By that time, the military had already begun to regard drug control as a way of mitigating the effects of budget cuts resulting from the end of the East–West conflict (Naylor 1995). Indeed, the Defense Department's drug control budget increased from around $5 million in 1982 to more than $1 billion at the beginning of the 1990s (Bertram *et al.* 1996: 112). The greater involvement of the US armed forces in drug control was enabled by repeated revisions of the *Posse Comitatus* Act in the 1980s and early 1990s. The act was passed after the Civil War and prevented the military from participating in law enforcement.

From 1986 onwards, the US government has also had an important economic means for coercing other states to implement drug control measures: certifica tion. Every year, the US president must present Congress with a list of countries that fail to cooperate with the US on drug control matters. Uncooperative states face economic sanctions, which may include a US veto in multilateral lending institutions against credits for the country in question as well as a suspension of US trade agreements. Certification has been a powerful means for influencin the policies and politics of states such as Bolivia, whose economy is highly dependent on US aid.[7]

In the 1990s, the US augmented supply reduction efforts. The Drug Enforcement Administration (DEA), the Federal Bureau of Investigation (FBI), the Central Intelligence Agency (CIA), and other agencies conducted operations around the globe, often together with military forces. US personnel trained European police officers at the International Law Enforcement Academy in Hungary, provided support to Thai troops in the jungles close to China, conducted operations against traffickers in Nigeria and Afghanistan, and passed on intelligence about suspects to Andean governments. Moreover, Washington has woven a net of bilateral legal assistance treaties providing for the extradition of suspects, among other measures.

The US engagement has varied from country to country. Morocco, for example, has traditionally supplied Western Europe with large quantities of hashish produced in the Northern Rif mountains, and its extensive coastline has long attracted cocaine smugglers. Nevertheless, France and the EU, and not the US, have been the most important external actors in Morocco's drug policy in the early twenty-first century.[8] And in Asia, the US has often distributed its funds via the UN.

It is in Latin America where the effects of coercive US drug control have been the most visible. Together with Peruvian security forces, the US intercepted smugglers who transported coca paste to Colombia by boat and light aircraft. Together with Bolivian security forces, the US has eradicated coca despite the resistance of well-organized farmers who consider coca an element of their culture and their only viable source of income (Ledebur 2005). In Colombia, US forces helped to dismantle large trafficking networks based in Medellín and Cali during the early and mid-1990s.

In 2000, Colombian President Andres Pastrana began to implement Plan Colombia, which was intended to end a protracted civil war and reduce drug supplies. As shown in Chapter 4, the US donated billions of dollars to Plan Colombia and subsequent programs, with most of the funding spent on military and police hardware and training. During this time, US aid was also used against insurgents as part of the US "war on terror."

It could be argued that US drug control is not overly coercive since AD, human rights programs, and judicial reforms are part of the US policy spectrum. While this is true, most US funds have been invested into coercive programs. Moreover, US aid payments are often conditional upon the destruction of coca and poppy. European development specialists criticize this, arguing that AD should not aim at short-term eradication goals, but forge a cooperative relationship with peasants (Deutsche Gesellschaft für Technische Zusammenarbeit 2001). One could also argue that US drug policy has a strong multilateral component, since the US strengthens UN and regional drug control programs to garner support from other countries. However, multilateral initiatives have been largely overshadowed by bilateralism and unilateralism. This is reflected in the fact that international organizations receive relatively little US funding, at least when compared to the overall size of the US anti-drug budget.

Finally, one could argue that US international drug control efforts are not that impressive, since domestic programs receive much more funding. From 1981 to 1995, interdiction and source country programs made up 21 percent of the federal drug budget, with source country programs receiving a mere 4 percent. However, Plan Colombia has significantly increased this share, despite earlier predictions by two prominent drug policy scholars that large increases in international programs were unlikely (Clawson and Lee 1998: ix). Since the 1980s, and particularly during the 1990s, the US federal drug control budget increased significantly. In 2001, it was at \$19.2 billion, up from \$3.6 billion in 1988 (Office of National Drug Control Policy 2001).[9] Even though domestic programs receive the most funding, enough money remains to guarantee US dominance internationally. According to John Walsh (2004: 8), in 1981 "the United States spent about \$375 million on source-country drug control and interdiction. In

2004, the United States spent $3.6 billion for these same purposes, making a total of nearly $45 billion over the quarter century since 1980, more than one-third of which has been spent during the last five years (2000–2004).

Other actors have had much less money at their disposal. The UN annual anti-drug budget has been at around $100 million, with donors earmarking up to 90 percent of the budget for particular programs. The European Union (EU) drug control funds are small as well, although AD projects and preferential trade agreements have been providing the EU with some leverage over the direction of international drug control (Joyce 1997).

This section showed that the US has undertaken significant international efforts to reduce illicit drug supplies, that it has preferred coercive over non-coercive strategies, and that it has a preference for bilateral and unilateral, instead of multilateral, action. What are the consequences of US drug policies?

Consequences of US drug policies

Drug policy researchers face a puzzle. Drug problems have become worse simultaneously with US attempts to curtail the illicit industry. To solve this conundrum, one could say that US policies reflect increasing drug problems, and that US policies have prevented a bad situation from getting worse. This is the (publicized) view of a majority of policy-makers and a minority of drug policy analysts. But one could also turn the argument around and say that drug problems partly result from US drug policies. This is the view of a minority of policy-makers and a majority of drug policy analysts.

Although this book is based on the premise that coercion can lead to negative effects, it does not assume a priori that all drug problems are simply side effects of coercive policies. Rather, it examines the question whether this is the case. To this end, the analysis focuses on the displacement of the illicit drug industry. In the past, coca and poppy cultivation, cocaine and heroin production, and cocaine and heroin smuggling have shifted from one location to another. The displacement process is highly complex and the result of various forces, including economic transformation, wars, and social attitudes toward drugs. Coercive drug policies also play a role.

But instead of taking for granted that the US has pushed drugs around the globe, the focus of this analysis is on the link between US drug policies and the displacement of the drug industry. The aim is to explain the displacement of the cocaine and heroin industries under state pressure. Shedding light on the displacement process helps to explain the coincidence of US anti-drug efforts and worsening drug problems. After all, displacement is a catalyst for other problems. When drugs move, violence, corruption, AIDS, and other problems move along with them.

The motives behind coercive US drug policies vary. Coercion can result, for example, from opportunistic behavior. Many politicians try to attract voters by promising to be "tough on drugs," thus forcing their political opponents to advocate even more repression. Similarly, the separation of the executive from the legislative branch in the US governmental system has often resulted in one branch accusing the other of not doing enough against drugs. As a consequence, Congress and the White House have proposed and implemented ever-tougher policies (Bertram *et al.* 1996: chapter 7).

Bureaucratic interests also matter. Numerous US federal agencies and departments are engaged in international drug control activities. They often derive large shares of their budgets from this involvement, which leads them to block drug control reforms that might cause their funds to be cut back. Agencies and departments seeking budget increases frequently try to extend their turf vis-à-vis bureaucratic rivals, and argue in favor of policy continuity, even for policies that have proven ineffective or counterproductive. As a former White House staffer who worked in the Carter administration said in a different context: "There isn't any government down there to manage. There is a series of subgovernments pursuing single interests of one kind or another" (Lloyd Cutler, quoted in Gillon 2000: 35).

In addition, US perceptions of drug problems help explain the penchant for coercive strategies. In US history, illicit drugs have often been perceived as a foreign problem and linked to unpopular immigrant groups. Many citizens feared that Mexicans would commit horrific crimes after having smoked marijuana, that blacks would rise up against whites under the influence of cocaine, and that Chinese would seduce white women under the influence of opium (Musto 1999). Moreover, drugs were seen as incompatible with US norms and values such as hard work and individual accountability. This sentiment was, and still is, reinforced by a popular conviction that heroin, cocaine, and cannabis are more alien to US culture than alcohol and tobacco.

Political opportunities, bureaucratic interests, and public perceptions thus help explain why US policy-makers and the general public often present drug problems as driven by drug supply and not by drug demand, and why drug supply is seen as a criminal phenomenon and not as resulting from social ills within in the US, or from poverty or weak institutions in drug producing and transit countries.

But more visible interests play a role as well: the blend of violent conflict and anti-Americanism that prevails particularly in Latin American drug producing and exporting countries deprives US businesses of market opportunities or may threaten their assets, although there are exceptions, such as the armaments industry. More directly, drugs are a burden on the US economy. In 2000, illegal drug use may have cost the US up to $160 billion (ONDCP 2002). This figur reflects indirect costs, such as losses in productivity and earnings, as well as direct costs such as healthcare, welfare, and the criminal justice system. Moreover, US diplomats, military personnel, law enforcement agents, business executives, and tourists have sometimes become the targets of traffickers. Statistics for drug-induced deaths in the US are cited as a further indicator for the graveness of the problem. The Office of National Drug Control Policy (ONDCP) estimated that drugs caused the deaths of 19,102 people in 1999. High death rates are, to a considerable extent, the result of relatively high US drug prevalence rates. At the end of the 1990s, 2.2 out of a thousand people in Germany consumed illicit drugs regularly, as compared to 21.3 people in the US (United Nations Offic for Drug Control and Crime Prevention 2000: 93). All these factors are important for understanding why the US has been conducting a "hundred years' war" on drugs (Bagley 1988).

In addition to the motives behind US efforts, journalists and researchers have also analyzed its consequences. Stephen Young's (2000: 1) verdict reflects the opinion of many observers:

> American drug policy does not solve drug problems, it aggravates them. Instead of trying to reduce drug harm, policy-makers pretend they can eliminate illegal drugs by fighting with as much violence as possible. Taking aim at the symptoms with a sledgehammer might seem effective, until the hammer hits a target and the corrosive residue splatters around society. Such an experience might lead the rational person to reconsider his plan; instead drug warriors order more sledgehammers to attack the new mess.

For critics of US drug policies, the concept of side effects is crucial. Most drug policy scholars see drug prohibition and coercive attempts to implement prohibition not only as being ineffective against drugs, but as creating various side effects (see MacCoun and Reuter 2001: chapter 6). With regard to prohibition, authors argue that prohibition has created a black market for psychoactive substances. This black market has evolved similarly to the black market created by alcohol prohibition in the 1920s, when bootleggers killed competitors, corrupted or killed policemen, switched from selling beer to selling whisky, and sold alcohol of poor quality that killed many drinkers (Zimring and Hawkins 1992: chapter 3). Authors argue that instead of spending billions of dollars on prohibition, governments should treat cocaine, heroin, marijuana, and synthetic substances like tobacco and alcohol. This would allow them to introduce quality controls and collect taxes on the trade, which can be used to cover health costs resulting from drug consumption.

Many problems result not from prohibition alone, but from a coercive implementation of prohibition. Traffickers only make a lot of money because prohibition is enforced. They pass the risks of their business activities on to consumers in the form of a "crime tax." Consumers have to pay a higher price for the illicitly traded commodity than they would have to if states were not enforcing prohibition. Besides the inflation of drug prices, coercive drug policies can have various other side effects.[10]

- Drug policies can exacerbate violence. Military aid, for example, is problematic since soldiers are trained to kill enemies, not to arrest citizens who enjoy constitutional rights. In Colombia, the military has an appalling human rights record, and some elements have cooperated with brutal paramilitary groups, which makes US military aid all the more problematic (Stokes 2005). Moreover, uncompromising US demands on foreign governments to extradite suspects or destroy illicit crops have prompted traffickers to resort to violent attacks on US interests and have led to sometimes violent peasant protests (Tokatlián 1995).

- US pressure on drug producing and transit countries can exacerbate nationalism. In Mexico, for example, anti-US nationalism existed long before the beginning of drug diplomacy, but has been fueled by US policies such as certification (González and Tienda 1989)
- US military aid can be detrimental to the democratic control of armed forces. This danger is particularly imminent during periods of transition from military to democratic rule. US officials argue that military aid programs and US oversight help ensure a monopoly of state control over the national territory and even foster democracy, human rights, and military accountability. Reality, however, more often resembles a zero-sum game in which a stronger military means a weaker democracy.
- Corruption is virulent when salaries are low and distinctions between the licit and illicit economy blurred. The drug-corruption relationship is circular: corruption attracts the drug economy, and drugs foster corruption. US pressure on foreign governments to reduce drug supplies exposes these governments to corruption. Corruption is particularly troubling when it affects the military, because, as former Bolivian president Gonzalo Sanchez de Lozado said: "When you have a corrupt chief of police, you fire him. When you have a corrupt chief of the army, he fires you" (quoted in Zirnite 1998: 173).
- Due to its inter-departmental character, drug control draws in numerous actors that often compete for budgets and engage in bureaucratic turf wars. US pressure to reshuffle competencies and create or abolish agencies can improve policy effectiveness and efficiency, but can also exacerbate bureaucratic rivalries.
- Prohibition and its enforcement can change drug consumption habits. When Asian governments closed opium dens and imprisoned consumers under US and UN pressure, many drug users switched from opium to heroin and from smoking to injection (Westermeyer 1982). In the US, the 1969 Operation Intercept increased heroin use among drug consumers who could not purchase marijuana anymore (Gooberman 1974). Increased heroin use is problematic, not least because consumers often share syringes that may contain the deadly HIV virus. Coercive drug control thus speeds up the AIDS epidemic (Malinowska-Sempruch *et al.* 2003).
- A central element in the US anti-drug strategy is the aerial fumigation of coca and poppy fields with herbicides. However, defoliants not only destroy opium poppy and coca plants, but also harm other plants, as well as animals. Moreover, herbicides pollute rivers and soil in sensitive ecosystems (Jelsma 2001).

These policy side effects help explain policy ineffectiveness. International drug control is intended to increase drug prices and decrease availability and purity, and thus reduce domestic drug use. However, "[a]verage importation and retail prices per pure gram of cocaine decreased respectively from US$75 and 400 in 1981 to US$25 and 170 in 1998. The average retail price of heroin to injection drug users fell by 50 percent between 1981 and 1998 and, during the same period, importation price dropped from US$500 to US$200" (Poret 2003: 466). Moreover, drug purity increased. The mean purity level of heroin was around 6 percent in 1987 and around 37 percent ten years later. In New York, levels even reached 60 percent (Common Sense for Drug Policy 2001: 35). Drugs are relatively freely available as well, as indicated by the fact that between 1988 and 1993, for example, cocaine-related emergencies went up 22 percent and heroin-related emergencies 65 percent (Bertram *et al.* 1996: 10).

How do drug policy side effects contribute to the ineffectiveness of US drug policies? The displacement of production and trafficking renders supply reduction programs ineffective. Violence impedes drug control because security forces often have no access to domestic conflict zones or meet with fierce resistance from peasants and traffickers. Nationalism can impede the signing of anti-narcotics treaties, information exchange, and joint law enforcement operations. Bureaucratic rivalries challenge drug control because agencies work against each other instead of arresting traffickers. Lastly, corruption means that US agents sometimes have to invest as much effort into collecting information on state actors as on traffickers

In addition to these policy side effects, critics cite other reasons for the ineffectiveness of US drug policies. Since some of these reasons are related to the displacement of the drug industry, they shall be briefly described

- The drug trade is a "victimless crime" in the sense that transactions are based on agreements between consumers and suppliers. This renders law enforcement action difficult, since peasants, dealers, and consumers lack incentives to contact the police.
- Interdicting cocaine and heroin is cumbersome, since these drugs are odorless and not bulky. The advantageous ratio of commodity weight to value helps to explain why the anti-drug regime has been less successful than are measures against piracy or slavery (Nadelmann 1990).
- Growing coca and poppy yields higher revenues for peasants than growing alternative agricultural products. Often, precarious living conditions foster coca and poppy cultivation. Although poverty is not a sufficient explanation for cultivation (Thoumi 2002b: 99–102), it may be a necessary one.
- Peasants often find it easier to market coca and opium poppy than other products, since traffickers lend money, pay in advance, and pick up the raw products directly at the farm.
- Coca and poppy are productive and relatively undemanding plants. A new coca bush can be harvested after one year, and then several times a year for up to 30 years.
- Many countries offer the right climatic conditions for coca and poppy cultivation. This enables a shift in cultivation from one place to another.

- Traffickers often have a technological edge over state security forces whose weapons, transport facilities, and communication equipment are inferior to their own.
- The drug industry lacks representatives with whom governments could negotiate. While the state can discuss regulations with leaders of trade unions or employers' organizations, the illegality of the drug trade largely forbids such negotiations.
- Anti-drug norms are often weak. Traffickers are not concerned about the health of consumers, and peasants often grow coca and poppy due to a lack of economic alternatives.
- Traditional cultivation and consumption of coca and opium products makes eradication politically risky. Coca and poppy have been consumed for centuries, for purposes ranging from the medical to the spiritual, and are integrated into the lives of rural populations. In their resistance to eradication, peasants are supported by international coalitions of activists sympathetic to their concerns.
- Governments have little control over some drug-producing regions. The Moroccan government has to be circumspect in its dealing with peasants in the Rif. In Colombia, rebel groups control large territories. And Pakistani security forces trying to enter tribal areas have often encountered fierc resistance.
- Governments of drug producing and transit countries are often more concerned about political stability or insurgency than about drugs, and even believe that there is a trade-off between drug control and counter-insurgency operations, as they fear that eradication and other drug control measures increase peasant support for rebels.
- Producing and transit states can be financially dependent on the drug economy. "[D]uring the 1990s, cocaine exports accounted for 30 percent of Peru's total exports and [. . .] the drug industry in Bolivia provided up to 20 percent of the country's GDP and approximately 20 percent of the adult employment" (Carpenter 2003: 92).
- Due to the risk of confiscation and arrest in the drugs trade, most of the added value is created in close proximity to consumers. This limits the impact of source-country programs on prices. To compensate for lost crops, traffickers can easily pay more to peasants, since drug prices in countries of origin are low. The RAND Corporation estimates that to reduce US cocaine consumption by 1 percent, the US would have to spend $34 million on domestic drug treatment and $783 million on coca eradication in source countries (Rydell and Everingham 1994).
- Some policies are incompatible with drug supply reduction. The US has frequently sacrificed drug control to other foreign policy interests, such as the fight against Communism and the securing of oil supplies. Moreover, there is a contradiction between free trade and drug control. The North American Free Trade Association (NAFTA), which has increased the flow of people and goods, makes drug interdiction more cumbersome (Andreas 1999: 127).

- Structural adjustment programs lead to cuts in public spending that can have dramatic economic consequences in poor countries. Poverty is also aggravated by protectionism. It is debatable, for example, whether the EU and US should demand a reduction of coca and poppy while closing their markets to agricultural imports.
- During the Cold War, tight border controls and low levels of economic interaction between East and West prevented drug trafficking. The lifting of these restrictions has offered opportunities to transnational organized crime. The end of proxy wars has also been conducive to trafficking. Some groups no longer supported by the US or the former USSR have become involved in trafficking to offset financial losses (Labrousse and Koutouzis 1996: 313).
- In North Africa, Eastern Europe, the former Yugoslavia, Latin America, or China, changes in traditional modes of economic interaction and political representation attract the illicit economy. Drug policies can do little to counteract these transformation processes.
- Sovereignty can undermine anti-drug efforts. Of course, despite Panama's sovereign status, the US invaded the country, and despite Bolivia's sovereignty, US pressure can lead to the dismissal of senior Bolivian official from office (Carpenter 2003: 142–143). Nevertheless, the US is usually obliged to coordinate drug control efforts with host states. These countries can constrain US policy options.

Table 2 summarizes the reasons for the ineffectiveness of coercive drug policies. By analyzing these factors, drug policy scholars have shed light on policy failure and drug policy side effects. However, research gaps remain.

Table 2 Why US international drug policies are ineffective

Side effects of coercive drug policy	*Characteristics of the cocaine and heroin economy*	*Foreign policies and changes in world politics*
Nationalism	Victimless crime	Antagonistic foreign policy interests
Violence	Drugs odorless, not bulky	Structure of international political economy
Corruption	Profitability of coca/popp	End of East–West conflic
Agency rivalries	Easy marketing	Transformation processes
Changes in production and traffickin	Coca undemanding and resilient	State sovereignty
	Coca/poppy grow at many places	
	Traffickers' technological edg	
	Trafficking not negotiabl	
	Limited access to producing regions	
	Weak anti-drug norms	
	Traditional consumption	
	Drugs not main concern of states	
	States dependent on revenues	
	Value-adding processes	

Research on the displacement of the drug industry

Scholars generally agree that states sometimes succeed in reducing drug production and trafficking, but that success is temporary as drug production moves to new areas, smuggling routes change, and new traffickers enter the market. Due to this displacement process, drugs continue to find their way to traditional and new drug consumption markets. To illustrate the effect of state pressure on the drug industry, observers use the image of a balloon. If a balloon filled with water or air is squeezed on one side, the air or water goes somewhere else. Thus, the displacement of the illicit drug industry is also known as the "balloon effect."

Writings on this "balloon effect" have several shortcomings. Some authors examine one case only. Ralph Seccombe (1995: 312) argues that drug control programs implemented in Pakistan's North West Frontier Province in the 1980s and early 1990s led to the displacement of opium poppy cultivation within this region. Single-case analyses leave open the question of whether the case is unique, i.e. whether an observed phenomenon is the result of a historically singular causal chain, or whether the same causal chain has led to similar outcomes elsewhere. Of course, the complexity of the drug economy hampers the generalization of causal processes. But it is not necessary to present a full-blown theory. One could start by finding similarities in an explorative manner, which is the approach adopted in the present book. This requires analyzing several cases. Andrew Bennett and Alexander George's (1997a: 3) critique of single-case studies apply to drug policy research as well:

> [I]ntensive single case studies in the past [. . .] did not contribute to an orderly, cumulative development of knowledge and theory about the phenomenon in question. Instead, as conducted in the past, each case study tended to go its own way, reflecting the special interests of each investigator and often being unduly shaped by such historical data as was readily available. As a result, idiosyncratic features of each case tended to shape the research questions differently. It is not surprising that single case studies, lacking "scientific consciousness," did not cumulate

Another problem is that scholars do not analyze the displacement process in sufficient empirical depth. Rensselaer Lee (2002) argues that US drug policies in South America have led to a proliferation of trafficking groups in Colombia, made traffickers switch from dealing in cocaine to dealing in heroin, and contributed to an increase in Colombian coca production. He further argues that these changes fuelled Colombian civil war. The relationship between assumed causes and effects, however, is not detailed enough, mainly because Lee treats the displacement of the drug industry merely as one negative consequence of US drug policies among many others. Ron Chepesiuk (1999a) refers to empirical examples of drug industry displacement to explain the ineffectiveness of US drug policies and to illustrate the negative impact of these policies on other countries. Displacement is treated rather superficially, however. Similarly, Ted

Galen Carpenter (2003) describes displacement and discusses reasons for its occurrence. But his focus is also on social conflict, human rights abuses, corruption, and nationalism. Side effects of foreign policy figure prominently in his book, but the causation of side effects does not.

> When the United States pressured Turkey in the 1970s to eradicate the cultivation of opium poppies, which were being used to make heroin, Mexico soon replaced Turkey as the leading supplier of heroin to the United States. [. . .] Shooting down suspected drug planes over Peru and other measures taken to disrupt the "air bridge" of coca shipments to processing labs in Colombia merely impelled the drug-trafficking organizations to subsidize the growing of coca in Colombia, thus minimizing the transportation problem.
>
> (Carpenter 2003: 115–117)

Eva Bertram, Morris Blachman, Kenneth Sharpe, and Peter Andreas (1996) provide an extremely valuable contribution to the drug policy debate. They examine domestic motives behind US drug policies and also look at changes in production and trafficking, arguing that peasants and traffickers can be replaced, destroyed crops replanted, laboratories built elsewhere, and smuggling routes and methods changed. As a State Department official, quoted by the authors, put it: "It's like hitting mercury with a hammer" (Bertram *et al.* 1996: 18). The authors cite some examples that show that the illicit drug industry adapts to law enforcement pressure. Moreover, they explain displacement processes by pointing, among others, to the profitability of drugs, different stages of value addition, and corruption. However, the discussion of displacement processes is arguably too brief to reveal how individual historical instances of displacement came about. The authors write, for example, that "[d]rug control campaigns against Turkish heroin production in the early 1970s helped stimulate the growth of the Mexican heroin industry" (Bertram *et al.* 1996: 19). While this may be true, the claim could have been supported by more empirical data.

Paul Stares (1996) provides another excellent overview of drug problems and drug policy problems. He describes the globalization of the industry, develops a taxonomy of drug policies, looks at the effects of drug production, trafficking and consumption, and discusses the problems of drug control. He does not treat displacement systematically, however, but rather forces the reader to excavate explanatory factors from an array of arguments. Although displacement is a result of many factors, all of which are interconnected, it must be shown *how* these factors are connected.

Other authors opt for a similarly cursory analysis of drug industry displacement. Looking at the effects of the destruction of the Turkish and French heroin pipeline on the US heroin market in the early 1970s, LaMond Tullis (1991: 2) writes that the "resulting shortage of heroin enabled Asian, Mexican and Pakistani traffickers to penetrate the American market as well as increase production to cover supply shortages elsewhere." In an analysis of a US aerial interdiction program in South America implemented during the 1990s, researchers at The International Institute for Strategic Studies (2000: 2) write rather superficiall that the "result was a dramatic reduction in the number of [trafficking] flights. Betsy Marsh's (2004: 8) analysis of drug industry displacement is similarly unsatisfactory.

> Studies have repeatedly shown that forced eradication programs stimulate farmers to move elsewhere and replant, induce growers to plant larger areas of illicit crops in anticipation of eradication, and cause illegal drug production to shift abroad in the classic balloon effect. [. . .] Just as attempting to flatten an inflated balloon will cause the air to spread out in all directions, successful eradication in one area temporarily lowers the supply, thereby raising the price for the illicit crop and stimulating production elsewhere. For example, when Mexico suppressed marijuana production it blossomed in Colombia. When Turkey suppressed opium production, it sprang up in Mexico. [. . .] When Bolivia and Peru suppressed coca cultivation, production migrated north to Colombia.

Even works that deal exclusively with the displacement of the drug industry and that analyze several cases have shortcomings. Frank Mora (1996) offers an insightful analysis of the impact of US drug policies on Brazil and South America's Southern Cone countries. He looks at the coincidence of spillover processes and US anti-drug initiatives during 1984–1986 and 1989–1991, showing that conditions such as weak law enforcement in new production and trafficking zones, as well as inadequate and slow US responses to border spillover, were present in both phases. However, the analysis is arguably too short to deduce insights about displacement processes in general. Moreover, Mora does not explicitly integrate explanatory factors into his research design.

Besides not paying enough attention to causality, the literature on drug industry displacement suffers from another shortcoming: case selection bias. This shortcoming affects not only minor works, but also a *magnum opus* on US drug policies, Alfred McCoy's *The Politics of Heroin*.[11] McCoy argues convincingly that a combination of US protection and coercion has led to shifts in heroin production and trafficking, and ultimately to a globalization of heroin-related problems. He shows that CIA agents have cooperated with traffickers against Communists in various countries, and that traffickers have used US pressure on competing producing regions and trafficking groups to their advantage

There is ample evidence that CIA activities are crucial for explaining changes in the structure of the drug industry. As a former senior DEA official said: "[I]n my 30-year history in the Drug Enforcement Administration and related agencies, the major targets of my investigations almost invariably turned out to be working for the CIA" (quoted in Scott 2003: 186). But although official collusion with drug entrepreneurs is of academic interest and politically troubling, observers accord too much importance to collusion when explaining the globalization of drug problems. After all, the CIA and other agencies have at times also formed part of the coercive apparatus. This factor is not sufficiently appreciated by McCoy and others, who focus much more on collusion than on "real" anti-drug initiatives.

While most works look at past instances of displacement, Shona Morrison (1997) deals with the future. She identifies countries that might experience an increase in illicit drug production. The way production shifts depends on countries' economic, political, and social conditions, including law enforcement, economic development, climatic conditions, and the availability of specialized skills. After looking at each of these factors, Morrison publishes a long list of potential drug producing states. Her article is innovative and policy-relevant, since it fosters awareness that poverty and other issues must be addressed to avoid displacement. However, her approach reveals the problem of predicting complex phenomena. Morrison discusses numerous conditions enabling displacement. To theorize about displacement, however, means showing which combination of factors lead to spillover processes, and discussing whether each instance of drug industry displacement is unique or whether there are regularities. Researchers examining regularities must compare past, and not future, instances of drug industry displacement. Explaining the past yields more specific insights of displacement than looking at hypothetical future cases of displacement.

Three other authors adopt an approach similar to that of Morrison (Calvani *et al.* 1997). They demonstrate the conditions that make countries attractive to the drug economy, and they examine strategies for reducing vulnerabilities. To this end, they offer an index for measuring states' drug resistance, which includes variables pertaining to countries' cultural, political, geographic, demographic, and economic conditions. The authors justify their comprehensive list of 24 variables by arguing that "drug trafficking is a highly complex global phenomenon which proliferates depending on specific mixes of converging stimuli rather than on a few discrete factors" (Calvani *et al.* 1997: 662). But if 24 variables influ ence the displacement of the illicit drug industry, the number of possible developments is enormous. Thus, predictive efforts result in a meaningless proliferation of possible causal pathways.

Hence, authors who examine the displacement of the drug industry look at too few cases, treat the causality of displacement in a superficial manner, favor instances of US collusion with drug entrepreneurs over cases of US coercion, and attempt to predict the future instead of first explaining the past. The present book adds value to the debate on displacement by developing a causal mechanism of displacement and assessing it in three case studies. Before outlining this mechanism, the next section discusses shortcomings of research on side effects of foreign policy.

Research on side effects of foreign policy

This book uses the term "side effect." A side effect can be defined as a peripheral or secondary effect of purposive human action. Many authors prefer the terms "unintended consequence," "perverse effect," or "unanticipated consequence." The latter terms underline that the outcomes of human action can be unplanned. But identifying intended or unintended consequences is a delicate undertaking, since one cannot look into the minds of decision-makers. Certainly the question of whether policy outcomes are intended can be pertinent for explaining side effects.[12] The first case study of this book, for example, asks whether policy-makers might have planned the displacement of the drug industry, since assessing this question sheds light on the actors behind displacement and makes the explanation richer. However, intentions will be interpreted on a case-by-case basis and as impartially as possible in this book.

Side effects are everywhere. One only needs to think of modern offices where more paper is used than in older ones, "light" cigarettes that make people smoke more and inhale deeper, and antibiotics that breed new bacteria (Tenner 1996). In the social sciences, the notion of side effects is popular as well. Adam Smith's "invisible hand" metaphor invokes the potentially positive social effect of egotistic individual action (Smith 1976 [1776]). Similarly, Friedrich von Hayek, Karl Popper, and other liberals opposed to state regulation have emphasized the benefits of unfettered economic activity [13]

These are arguably positive side effects, but generally the notion has a negative connotation. This becomes clear when looking at IR and security. Military intervention, even when undertaken for humanitarian purposes, can cause "collateral damage." Economic sanctions can harm civilian populations as well. Moreover, they can also help authoritarian rulers consolidate domestic support by allowing them to portray sanctions as acts of external aggression, and they can contribute to the criminalization of states and societies (Andreas 2005; Byman and Waxman 2002: 105–114). Supporting another state's government or one of its domestic groups can backfire when the government or group suddenly turns against its supporter. But non-coercive strategies can also have problematic consequences. For instance, NGOs that attempt to strengthen civil society in developing countries can become engaged in conflict with other civil-society actors (Stiles 2002). In addition, humanitarian aid can reinforce relations of domination and exploitation and even support the war aims of combatants (Loane and Moyroud 2001: 49; Anderson 1999).

The social science literature deals with hundreds of side effects. However, most authors describe; they do not explain.[14] Jon Elster's distinction between description and explanation is illuminating: "It *is* inherently satisfactory for the mind to discover that good sometimes leads to evil and evil to good; that less can be more and more can be less; or that individual rationality can bring about collective irrationality and vice versa. And it *is* easy to mistake the thrill of discovery for the thrill of explanation" (Elster 1990: 131 (italics in the original)).

The thrill of discovery is reflected in the terminological efforts of IR scholars. Authors write about "the retreat of the state," reflecting an increase in criminalized activities; the rise of a multi-centric world in which states and non-state actors compete for authority; and the limited steering capacities of governments in a globalized world (Strange 1996; Rosenau 1990). Scholars observe an increasing incongruence of political, economic, and societal spaces, describe transnational organized crime as the dark side of globalization, and speak of Courtesan states and the corruption of civil society (Brock and Albert 1995; Mittelman and Johnston 1999). Although these are interesting insights, the problem with new terms and taxonomies is that they are more descriptive than explanatory. Terminological innovation does not replace theorizing, but merely reveals the inability of traditional theory to explain important aspects of international life – such as side effects of foreign policy.

Foreign Policy Analysis (FPA) examines resources, capabilities, instruments, and actors. It studies the making of foreign policies by looking at policy-makers' perceptions, the impact of perceptions on political outcomes, and group dynamics in decision-making (Hill 2003). But FPA stops short of explaining the *consequences* of decisions. A main preoccupation of FPA is to explain foreign policy decisions. To the extent that FPA does refer to foreign policy consequences, it merely considers these consequences in terms of feedback for subsequent decisions (see, for example, Dawisha 1977). It is equally important to treat these decisions as "independent variables" in order to explain their consequences, i.e. to shift foreign policy consequences to the center of analysis.

Authors who look at the implementation of foreign policies take FPA one step further (Smith and Clarke 1985; Hill 2003: chapter 6). They focus on the way a decision is implemented as the main determinant of foreign policy success or failure. In many cases, implementation is the crucial link between decisions and outcomes, since implementation problems can lead to undesirable outcomes. It is important, however, to go beyond implementation and look at the policies themselves. After all, as Robert Merton (1936: 894) wrote a long time ago, the consequences of purposive action "result from the interplay of the action and the objective situation." A flawed policy, even if it is smoothly implemented, can fail to achieve its objective. The US might force country A to reduce drug production, but if no simultaneous pressure is exerted on country B, the drug industry might shift to that country. Hence, looking only at implementation means missing part of the picture.

Similar to FPA, IR theories are ill equipped to accommodate side effects of foreign policy. Many authors go beyond FPA by not only explaining foreign policy decisions but, more generally, strategies and preferences. Constructivists have (re-)introduced ideational factors to the study of international politics and have thereby challenged rationalist approaches that emphasize material capabilities. Other authors derive expectations about state behavior from neorealism or liberalism. While these approaches are marked by ontological and epistemological differences, they all neglect the consequences of foreign policies.

Why has IR scholarship neglected side effects of foreign policy? This shortcoming results predominantly from the search for laws of social life – a search that leads nowhere when analyzing side effects of foreign policy.

Laws and mechanisms in IR

Many IR scholars espouse the search for social laws. This indicates the continuing popularity of Carl Hempel's (1942; 1965) notion of "covering laws." The debate on covering laws has become rather convoluted and shall not be repeated here. It shall merely be noted that covering law research is about the discovery of relationships between causes and effects that are generally applicable, i.e. independently of temporal and spatial constellations. At the core of the search for laws is a belief in prediction and determinism. Theorists who aim at discovering laws of social life want to predict phenomena in the past, present, and future.[15]

The quest for covering laws reveals the dominance of positivism in IR. Stated simply, positivists believe that scholarship should objectively reveal verifiabl facts or regularities through scientific methods. Positivists argue that in order to explain a phenomenon, researchers must subsume the issue under if–then statements. Moreover, positivists have a strong preference for parsimonious explanations. Ideally, a research design should allow the researcher to explain as much as possible with as few independent or intervening variables as possible (King *et al.* 1994: chapter 3). Positivists "emphasize causal theory as a 'means' of control, revealing surprising similarities with 'manipulability' thinking" (Kurki 2002: 17). To test covering laws against reality, these laws, as well as the hypotheses derived from the laws, must be couched into variables that can be operationalized.

One should not overstate the predictive, deterministic nature of law-based theorizing. Indeed, one could argue that laws, as correlations, are probabilistic. If a statistician shows that Cause A leads to Effect B in 99 percent of the cases analyzed, he has constructed a probabilistic theory. Moreover, most IR scholars searching for laws would not claim to be able to predict specific events. Structural theorists, for example, aim at predicting broad trends that can occur at one point or another, but not specific events and their timing (Lebow and Risse-Kappen 1996: 2). Still, positivist IR theory does not take specific temporal and spatial constellations seriously and continues to espouse the ideal of the social law.

The search for social laws is problematic because many important international phenomena are temporally and spatially contingent. War, for example, is the dynamic interaction of combatants, and the outcome of war depends on contingent factors and – indeed – chance. Carl von Clausewitz therefore emphasized that the outcome of war is unpredictable (Beyerchen 1992/1993). Similarly, the outcomes of a foreign policy initiative against drugs can vary significantly. Laws predicting the effect of the initiative in sufficient detail to be able to speak meaningfully of a law are thus unlikely to pass the reality test. This does not mean that social science research should no longer generalize. But generalization must leave room for contingency. The outcome of war, the intensity of terrorism, or the displacement of the drug industry are likely to be influence by geography, surprising technological developments, the mental state of key players, and a host of other factors, all of which make the search for predictive laws futile.

The intolerance toward contingency helps to explain why most IR theorists have neglected crucial international phenomena and left them to the devices of area specialists or other disciplines (on the neglect of terrorism research by IR scholars, see Leheny 2002). Searching for laws leads to method-driven research and pushes many issues to the disciplinary margins. Much more problem-driven research is needed to move IR closer to reality. The illicit international political economy and state counter-strategies have received little attention from scholars of security studies, despite the impact of the illicit economy on security. Even International Political Economy (IPE), a major sub-field of IR, has had relatively little to say about illicit activities (Andreas 2004), despite the growth of black and grey markets. The difficulty of IPE in coming to terms with illicit activities is underlined by Richard Friman's (2003) critique of the work of Susan Strange and her conception of what she called "the mafias." Friman shows that Strange relies on state-centric concepts that lead her to overstate the threat posed by crime to state power and to understate the social construction of crime as a threat.

To be sure, IR scholars no longer ignore non-state actors, as the literature on Nongovernmental Organizations (NGOs), epistemic communities, or private companies testifies. But these actors pursue licit activities. When examining illicit activities, researchers are confronted with a much higher degree of complexity, which makes the search for deterministic "if–then" laws futile – or will only return "laws" of the most banal sort, such as the notion that drug demand will always find a source of supply. Complexity increases because illicit economic sectors are constituted by a seemingly unlimited number of actors. Moreover, these actors interact in ways that are difficult to model. The clandestine nature of their operations poses further difficulties for the observer. It is thus not surprising that the literature on war economies, a promising research agenda that brings together security studies, IPE, and the study of the illicit, is still rather descriptive (see, for example, Kaldor 1999: chapter 5).

Showing how criminalized activities change in response to state policies – the aim of the present book – is even more difficult than "only" analyzing criminalized activities. It is neither certain nor impossible that a particular foreign policy will lead to a particular side effect. Moreover, different causal paths can lead to the same outcome. A deterministic conception of causality is therefore inappropriate for the study of foreign policy side effects. There may be a "law of side effects," but someone who invokes this law merely says that human activity always yields unforeseen results. When explaining a specific class of events, complexity and contingency quickly reveal the limits of predictive, law-based theorizing. Drug production and trafficking might shift from country A to country B after US pressure on country A. Without considering contingent conditions such as domestic turmoil in country B that attracted the drug industry, one cannot explain why the drug industry moved to country B.

In addition to the neglect of contingency, there is another reason why IR researchers say little about side effects of foreign policy: the under-appreciation of change, particularly complex change. During the Cold War, IR scholars focused on stasis. Change was seen as dangerous, since it might have upset the nuclear balance. The end of the Cold War and globalization, which have led to calls for a reorientation of IR (Grande and Risse 2000), have improved the discipline's track record. Scholars have analyzed, for example, how institutions adapt to a new environment by changing their forms and functions (Haftendorn *et al.* 1999). Nevertheless, change remains enigmatic. Sociologist Gary Itzkowitz (1996: 230) writes that the "record of describing and explaining social change by social theorists and scientists is embarrassingly small." The lack of attention paid to change goes hand in hand with a neglect of foreign policy side effects. After all, side effects imply change. Things are different after the implementation of a foreign policy than they were before.

The neglect of change reflects the continuing dominance of positivist law-based theorizing in IR. Such research does not acknowledge the complexity of change. Moreover, it does not provide sufficiently fine-grained explanations. Law-based theorizing tries to discover regularities. If one discovers regularities between foreign policies and the explanandum, one still needs to know *why* the outcome occurred. There may be regularities between changes in the weather and barometer readings, but without referring to the functioning of barometers, one cannot properly explain these regularities.

Fortunately, there is an alternative to law-based theorizing: mechanism-based theorizing. Explaining with mechanisms means specifying the conditions intervening between an initial impetus and an outcome. Causal mechanisms offer non-deterministic accounts of links between causes and effects. Mechanism-based theorizing implies that diverse causal forces, such as technological innovations or the evolution of sovereignty, have an impact on observed phenomena; that it is important to identify these forces, or social "cogs and wheels" (Elster 1989: 3), linking causes and effects; and that causation is probabilistic instead of deterministic. A phenomenon is explained when its underlying causal forces are shown to be necessary (albeit not always sufficient) to bring about the observed phenomenon (Daase 1999: 80). It must be shown that without the forces constituting the causal mechanism, the phenomenon would not have occurred, or would have occurred along different spatial and temporal lines.

Although some political scientists have elaborated on mechanisms (Yee 1996; Dessler 1991; Byman and Waxman 2002: 52–57), mechanism-based theorizing remains relatively obscure. This is not least because mechanisms "involve physical, social, or psychological causal processes that ultimately cannot be directly observed. We can only hypothesize about underlying causal mechanisms and make imperfect inferences about them on the basis of observed data" (Bennett and George 2001: 139). It is probably this obscure nature of many causal mechanisms that leads some scholars to combine mechanism-based theorizing with established elements of causal research. Gary King, Robert Keohane, and Sidney Verba (1994: 86–87), for instance, push mechanisms into the realm of positivism by arguing that including dependent and independent variables into mechanisms is a prerequisite for causal inference.

But what if numerous explanatory factors interact in complex and dynamic ways, if causes do not precede effects, and if factors cannot be operationalized due to a lack of data? Drug researchers face all these problems. Hence, this book does not adopt a narrow and positivist conception of causation and causal mechanisms, but a more hermeneutic one. Instead of speaking of variables, the terms "explanatory factor," "enabling condition," and "background condition" are used. Variables imply that an assumed cause X and an assumed effect Y are independent from one another and that X precedes Y in time (Wendt 1999: 84 and 88). Moreover, variables must vary.

These conditions for causal inference are a straightjacket for drug policy scholars. It would be misleading to conceive of the inability or unwillingness of a government to prevent the spillover of drug trafficking onto the national territory as an independent variable for displacement. It is rather an enabling condition for displacement. Similarly, the ability of drug entrepreneurs to adapt to law enforcement pressure does not precede industry displacement, but is a characteristic of the drug industry, reflecting the network structure of traffickin groups (see below). Neither should adaptation be considered a variable, because although the adaptive capacities of trafficking groups vary, adaptation is a permanent feature of the drug industry.

Not introducing variables into mechanism-based theories is a virtue rather than a vice, because this approach provides more fine-grained explanations. Variable-based works often do not look at the structure between assumed causes and effects, particularly when this structure cannot be directly observed. By focusing on the structure that gives the link between "variables" meaning, explanations become more plausible. Andrew Bennett and Alexander George (1997b: 2–3) argue that "whether the causal powers inherent in a variable are activated in a particular case depends on the presence of contingent conditions. [. . .] Such contingent conditions and counteracting forces can enable, conceal, or override the causal powers of a variable."

Thus, causal mechanisms, in their non-variable based variant, allow the researcher to provide a meaningful interpretation of links between causal factors. Mechanism-based theorizing espouses a soft concept of causality; it helps both to understand and explain side effects of foreign policy (see Hollis and Smith 1990). Explaining social processes forces researchers to describe the environment that allowed the process to happen. To explain why a chess player has made a specifi move, one has to refer to the rules of chess allowing the player to make this move. The rules of chess did not "cause" the move. Rather, they enable the player to make this move and, together with other factors, help explain it (Wendt 1998: 113). With regard to drugs, industry displacement is enabled by the rules of the game, such as price mechanisms, which in turn result from the interplay of demand and supply. Milja Kurki (2002: 30 and 34) writes that rules

> are causal in the sense that they constrain action and make action possible. [N]ot only are rules produced by other causes but rules themselves constrain and enable behaviour to take a certain path (they "tip balance of

> events") and thus they should be considered causal in nature. [. . .] We need causal theories that instead of generalizing about "observed" effects explain the mechanisms, or rather complexes (even if unobservable) that generate effects.

The flexible business structure of drug entrepreneurs, state collusion in illicit activities, or the tendency of the US government to apply foreign policy pressure selectively are not variables that determine industry displacement, but background conditions that make displacement possible. The role of these factors is causal, although not in a positivist sense.

A causal mechanism of displacement

Further above, it was shown that existing accounts of drug industry displacement under state pressure have shortcomings. Due to the lack of testable theories and hypotheses, a tentative explanation of displacement must be developed from scratch. The present section develops a causal mechanism that comprises several elements. First, the mechanism must include an initial impetus that sets in motion a chain of events. A US international initiative against drugs is the starting point for analyzing the initiative's consequences. To speak of a foreign policy side effect, it must be shown that a foreign policy caused, or significantl contributed, to an outcome.

Moreover, a causal mechanism must address the question of whether foreign policies are implemented holistically. The US often applies selective pressure on peasants, traffickers, and governments. Policy selectivity is multi-faceted and can result from the subordination of drug policy concerns to other interests, or from a failure to respond quickly to new developments. Moreover, the sovereignty of drug producing and transit states, although varying significantly, can constrain the US freedom of maneuver. Inconsistent coercion as a consequence of contravening interests, inertia, and state sovereignty are likely to influence the displacement of the drug industry.

Further, a causal mechanism must take into account the "nature of a problematic situation" (George 2000: 75). Two characteristics of the drug industry are relevant here. The first is the innate flexibility of the industry and its capacity to adapt to pressure. Coca and poppy cultivation, cocaine and heroin production, and drug smuggling are not monopolistic activities. Coca and poppy can be cultivated in many countries, drug laboratories are moveable, new traffickin routes and methods are discovered every day, and numerous actors compete for market shares. The potential consequences for drug control efforts are obvious. Less coca and poppy cultivation in one country, for example, can allow another country to fill the gap. Displacement is enabled by the fact that the land needed to cultivate coca and poppy is relatively small, as described in a UN report:

> Together, the total areas under opium poppy or coca bush are, for example, just a quarter of the size of Puerto Rico, and two or three times the size of

> cities such as New York or Berlin. Even in the main drug producing countries, the total areas under opium poppy or coca bush represent only about 1 per cent of arable land. Yet if just 1 per cent of arable land in a few medium-sized countries is needed to guarantee global supply of heroin and cocaine, there remains a constant danger of displacement: production shifting to other areas in response to eradication.
>
> (United Nations Office for Drug Control and Crime Prevention 2000: 25

The illicit drug economy is a self-reproducing system that lacks a center of gravity. Price mechanisms illustrate the drug trade's reproductive capacity. When coca and poppy fields are destroyed in one area, the price for these crops goes up (as long as the demand for cocaine and heroin remains stable). Higher prices are incentives for peasants elsewhere to engage in cultivation. Drug prices can also increase when states immobilize a trafficking group with a large market share. The resulting price rise then attracts new entrepreneurs. As former Colombian president Virgilio Barco said: "The only law that the narcoterrorists don't break is the law of supply and demand" (quoted in Chepesiuk 1999a: 67). Sometimes a government cannot even dismantle a specific group, since the group responds innovatively to pressure. Researchers at the RAND Corporation have developed complex models for explaining the ways traffickers adapt to law enforcement (Crawford and Reuter 1988). A former head of the Mexican police put it more simply: "Stop the traffic on the ground and they take it to the air. Control the air and they go by sea. It's a battle with no end" (quoted in Chepesiuk 1999a: 257). The network structure of drug trafficking partly accounts for traffickers' capacity to resist law enforcement pressure, as Phil Williams (1998: 159; see also Arquilla and Ronfeldt 2001) argues:

> Networks are a highly efficient and effective organizational structure for drug traffickers. Network organizations are fast, flexible, and forward looking. They put function over form and are far less concerned with neat organizational charts and jurisdictional niceties than with their overall effectiveness in reaching their goals. In contrast, governments are composed of and rely on large, bureaucratic hierarchies that operate according to standard operational procedures, are bound by budgetary constraints, and are, for the most part, cumbersome.

This quote alludes to the second set of drug industry characteristics that helps explain displacement: the limited capacities of states to enforce laws against drugs. The US General Accounting Office acknowledges this problem: "Although U.S. heroin control programs [. . .] have had some limited success, U.S. efforts have not reduced the flow of heroin from the region because producers and traffickers shift transportation routes and growing areas into countries with inadequate law enforcement capacity or political will" (quoted in Chepesiuk 1999a: 123). Patrick Clawson and Rensselaer Lee (1998: x–xi) write:

> [W]hat happens in the Andean countries depends much more on the locals than on the Americans. And while the United States can influence what the locals do, the basic factor determining their actions is and will remain local conditions. The adage that all politics is local applies in the Andes as well as in the United States. Andean politicians may listen carefully to what U.S. envoys say, but the politicians will decide what to do, based on the sociology, economics, and politics of their own countries, not primarily because of U.S. pressure.

Bruce Bagley (1988) argues that US policy-makers make wrong assumptions about the drug industry. They look at it from the perspective of realism and its notion of states as the central actors in international politics. By putting other governments under pressure, the US hopes to reduce drug supplies. However, law enforcement tends to be weak in producing and transit countries due to (a) weak government control over parts of the national territory; (b) a tendency among producing and transit states to subordinate drug control to other interests, such as counter-insurgency operations; (c) corruption; (d) insufficient financia resources; and (e) bureaucratic rivalries. These (and possibly other) factors presumably influence the displacement of the drug industry

In addition to (a) selective pressure, (b) industry flexibility, and (c) weak law enforcement, US anti-drug initiatives are likely to coincide with contingent conditions that contribute to displacement. For example, US military aid for a drug producing country can come at the same time as a military coup that forces some traffickers to leave the country. In this case, displacement would not only result from US military aid, but also from domestic political changes in a drug producing country. Similarly, if a recession leads to a dramatic rise in rural poverty, farmers may resort to illicit coca and poppy cultivation. In this case, the displacement of the drug industry to the country in recession would not only be a result of US diplomatic pressure on another country. Such contingent conditions cannot be deduced from any theory, but have to be discovered in the course of the empirical research, as emphasized by Gary Itzkowitz (1996: 145): "Contingency demands [. . .] that theory be constructed as a useful tool for uncovering contingent relationships, not a decree for empirical reality." Contingencies are crucial for examining side effects. When they influence an observed outcome, but occur independently of the action taken by a policy initiator, the outcome is not only a side effect of foreign policy, but also a consequence of other causes.

The causal mechanism that serves as a tentative heuristic explanation for the displacement of drug production and trafficking under US pressure can be formulated as follows: *US international initiatives against cocaine and heroin lead to displacement because the US applies pressure selectively, because the illicit drug industry responds flexibly to coercion, and because law enforcement in producing and transit states is weak. Moreover, contingent factors influence the displacement process.*

One could argue that this is no mechanism in the sense of a linear, consecu-

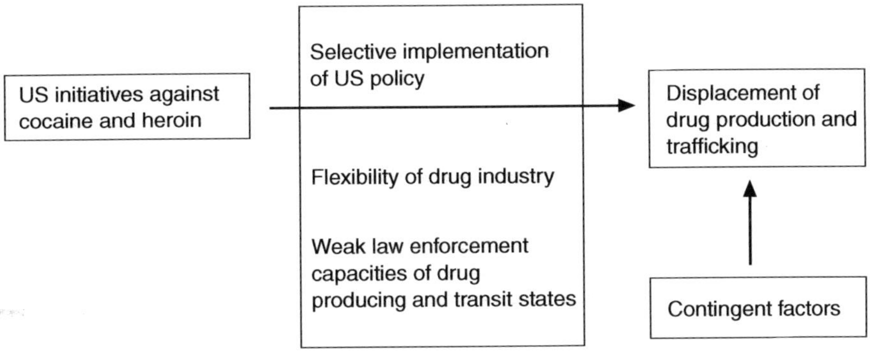

Figure 1 Explaining the displacement of the drug industry.

tive causal path. An ideal causal mechanism is one whose elements follow one another chronologically. However, in the drug trade, various rules of the game, background factors, and contingent conditions operate simultaneously or randomly. Moreover, they interact with one another and sometimes reinforce each other. Hence, the causal mechanism proposed here does not posit a chronology. While one can look at displacement as a chronological sequence of events, the causal process underlying this sequence of events is not chronological, but should rather be regarded as an interactive set of factors. The mechanism described in this book is thus more complicated than the predictable workings of a technical device, as epitomized by the wheels and springs of a watch. The apparatus inside a watch moves in a non-random fashion. There is no such precise mechanism for displacement. This makes it challenging to analyze displacement empirically. However, a two-step methodology that distinguishes the sequence of events from the causal factors underlying this sequence helps to shed light on displacement.

Methodology and structure of the book

Establishing causal relationships is particularly difficult when discussing drugs – not least because of a lack of data. Since traffickers do not publish business reports, researchers often have to resort to unconventional methods of obtaining information in a difficult environment, sometimes taking high personal risks, including kidnapping and assassination (Goldsmith 2003; Yawnghwe 1993: 307). Using information provided by governments is tricky as well. Figures for coca and poppy cultivation are unreliable, among other reasons, because peasants hide coca and poppy among licit crops or plant illicit crops at high altitudes with frequent cloud coverage to reduce the likelihood of their fields being detected by reconnaissance planes or satellites. Moreover, governments can inflate the quantities of seizures to create the impression that law enforcement is working. John Walsh (2004: 9) writes:

> Traditional drug war indicators – even when they are properly understood as measures of activities or operations – are ambiguous and open to conflicting interpretations. Indeed, the very figures typically trumpeted as evidence of supply-side drug control progress can just as easily be read as evidence of a stalemate or a worsening situation. For example, larger and more frequent drug seizures are often presented as evidence of policy success, and lauded as a testament to more vigorous enforcement, but they may simply reflect increased drug production and trafficking. Or they may be the result of both more enforcement and more drugs in circulation – the seizure statistics themselves provide no clue.

Similarly, governments can publish overly optimistic figures of coca and poppy eradication, manipulate anti-drug budgets, or reduce the number of drug addicts on paper. To make matters worse for the analyst, little is known about the forces involved in some anti-drug operations and their activities. Due to these data problems, the available information must be treated carefully, and information from different sources must be compared. The complexity of drug problems is an additional impediment for establishing causality. Is cannabis a "gateway drug" that inevitably leads to the consumption of harder drugs? Does drug consumption per se lead to theft, robbery, and murder, or is crime rather a consequence of law enforcement (Inciardi 1981)? Do coercive drug policies reduce the number of drug users? These uncertainties underline the need for cautious causal claims.

In this book, process tracing is used to assess the plausibility of the causal mechanism. This method helps to "identify the intervening causal process – the causal chain and causal mechanism" between assumed causes and effects (George and Bennett 2005: 206). Process tracing transforms researchers into detectives who pursue "several suspects and clues, constructing possible chronologies and causal paths backward from the crime scene and forward from the last known whereabouts of the suspects" (George and Bennett 2005: 218). The method is similar to historical analysis, which requires analyzing a lot of data and inferring from multiple weak elements rather than single instances of strong evidence (Elman and Elman 2001: 29–30). To provide a convincing account of how US drug policies and displacement are linked, process tracing must discuss empirical black boxes. As mentioned further above, explaining a phenomenon means showing which causal forces are necessary for creating it.

The present book analyzes three cases, each of which has a similar structure. The first section puts a specific US anti-drug initiative into context by examining US perceptions of drug problems and US domestic politics related to the initiative. The chapter then presents a chronological analysis of the initiative. Through process tracing, the section discusses whether the initiative coincided with displacement. This provides a first clue for explaining the link between the initiative and displacement. If displacement occurred *before* or *simultaneously with* the implementation of the US initiative in the country, the initiative did not *cause* displacement, but may have merely accelerated it.

To better explain displacement, a subsequent section discusses each element of the causal mechanism, as well as black boxes and alternative explanations. Hence, while the first step focuses on chronology, the second step focuses on analytical categories. Process tracing is used for both steps. Process tracing is a more obvious methodological choice for analyzing a chronological sequence of events, but it can also be fruitful for studying explanatory categories such as "policy selectivity" or "weak law enforcement." After all, these explanatory elements are empirically part and parcel of the chronological account, although they do not follow one another, but occur simultaneously or randomly during the chain of events. Hence, the analysis proceeds in two steps, one of which is chronological and the other analytical.

The first case examines the initiative of the Nixon administration against Turkish poppy cultivation and the French Connection in the early 1970s, which may have led to an increase in poppy production and heroin trafficking in Southeast Asia and Mexico. The second case study looks at the Air Bridge Denial Program. From the later 1980s on, the US cooperated with Peru and Bolivia against traffickers who transported coca paste to laboratories in Colombia on small aircraft. The program was suspended in 2001 after the Peruvian Air Force shot down a plane carrying a US missionary family. This chapter examines whether the program has led to an increase in Colombian coca production and whether it has changed drug trafficking patterns in South America. The third case study analyzes whether Plan Colombia and its successor program shifted drug production and trafficking within Colombia and from Colombia to neighboring states in the early twenty-first century. US support to the Colombian government merits a closer look due to the historically unprecedented scale of US involvement.

The present research design may not go unchallenged. One could argue that theorizing displacement, i.e. finding general patterns in the causation of displacement, requires a comparative case study design that includes control cases and a limited number of controlled variables (see King *et al.* 1994: 43–46). This would mean, for example, to compare a case in which the US applied pressure selectively with one in which it adopted a holistic approach (if such a case exists), or to look at an anti-drug initiative in which a producing state possesses weak law enforcement capabilities with an initiative untroubled by this problem (if such a case exists). Hence, one would try to control the explanatory factors (US anti-drug initiatives, policy inconsistency, industry flexibility, weak law-enforcement capacities, and contingent factors) and the explanandum (displacement).

However, as discussed above, variable-based theorizing is often inappropriate for examining the illicit political economy. Factors such as "industry flexibility are not variables. Moreover, for using controlled variation, one needs to have a vague idea of possible causal processes. The poor state of displacement theorizing means that displacement must first be studied in a hermeneutic, explorative manner. The case studies do not "test" the causal mechanism, but rather provide a plausibility probe, and are thus part of an early stage of theorizing. This approach imposes limits on generalization. But if the causal mechanism provides a plausible explanation of displacement in the three cases analyzed, this would be a clue that a general mechanism is at work. After all, the three cases look at different regions, periods, and drugs.

The lack of variation in this book is a virtue rather than a vice. The case studies not only verify processes, i.e. assess the plausibility of the causal mechanism, but also serve as a means of process induction (Bennett and George 1997b: 5). Process tracing may show that the same causal mechanism operates in all three cases, but along different "causal paths" (Daase 1999: 268). This would add value to IR theorizing. Due to their focus on letting "dependent variables" and "independent variables" vary, IR scholars neglect variation in causal processes, not least because equifinality (when different conditions, factors, and chains of events lead to the same result) is perceived as a methodological problem. However, similarities and variations in causal processes are not obstacles to theorizing, but essential characteristics of foreign policy side effects. Revealing similarities and variations through inductive empirical research contributes to theory building.

Three caveats are noteworthy. First, it is not argued that all instances of drug industry displacement are a consequence of US anti-drug initiatives. Displacement results from numerous factors and can occur independently of US policies. Second, the US is not the only country that implements foreign drug policies selectively. French intelligence services, for instance, have also colluded with drug entrepreneurs (Labrousse 2000). Third, this book does not deny the detrimental impact of synthetic substances and cannabis on security. This work focuses on cocaine and heroin since these drugs have raised the greatest concern in the US, and since cocaine and heroin contribute more to pitting the US against other states than cannabis and synthetic drugs, which are produced domestically as well.

The following three chapters form the empirical core of this book. Chapter 5 first summarizes the empirical results and then discusses their implications for the theorization of drug displacement and foreign policy side effects. It argues that IR scholars should strike a balance between parsimonious explanations and those that give due credit to complexity, be more skeptical about law-based theorizing, and espouse contingent generalizations.

The last chapter examines alternatives to US coercive drug policies. It shows that harm reduction is better suited for dealing with drug problems than coercive drug policies at home and abroad. Harm reduction does not solve drug problems, but it leads to fewer and less damaging side effects than coercion. However, instituting harm reduction on an international level is hampered by many factors. Most importantly, US domestic politics are conducive to the continuing pursuit of ineffective and harmful drug policies.

2 Targeting Turkey and the French Connection

The early 1970s

Introduction

This case study focuses on an important period in the globalization of drug problems: the early 1970s. The aim is to understand and explain the increase in poppy cultivation, heroin production, and drug trafficking in Southeast Asia and Mexico during that period. The chapter describes US domestic politics in the late 1960s and early 1970s that gave rise to an initiative against drug supplies from Turkey and France. It then provides a chronological discussion of the initiative, examining whether the initiative was accompanied by a shift of the drug industry from the Mediterranean to Southeast Asia and Mexico. As a second step for analyzing displacement, the discussion refers to the causal mechanism developed in the first chapter. Finally, empirical black boxes and alternative explanations are examined.

US perceptions and politics

In 1968, US psychologist Timothy Leary advised his compatriots to take LSD and "turn on, tune in, and drop out" (quoted in McWilliams 1990: 44). This is what many did, consuming a variety of other drugs as well. The US became a mass market for illicit drugs in the 1960s for several reasons, as Paul Stares (1996: 24) writes:

> the passage of the baby boom generation through ages 15–24, resulting in a 50 per cent increase in this cohort by the end of the decade; the widespread rejection of the values, norms, and socializing institutions of the 1950s, which came to be seen as conformist, constraining, and hypocritical; a concomitant shift toward the celebration of feelings, spontaneity, and intuitiveness that drugs were seen to promote; a surge in discretionary income (U.S. GNP doubled in the 1960s), leading to the rise of consumerism and with it rising expectations for continual stimulation and instant gratification; and widespread political alienation along generational lines, exacerbated by the Vietnam War.

The most popular drug was cannabis, but many drug consumers also took synthetic substances, and some used heroin. Heroin consumption patterns changed significantly, particularly at the end of the decade. Until around 1969, young blacks and Hispanics constituted the main user groups. They were subsequently joined by members of the white suburban middle-class (Courtwright 2001: 165–183; Phares 1973). Parallel to this trend, the number of heroin users increased considerably. One indicator of this trend is the higher incidence of narcotics-related hepatitis cases, which rose from around 4,000 in 1966 to around 36,000 in 1971 (Musto 1999: 248). Moreover, the number of heroin users, as well as heroin addicts (not all users are addicts), seems to have increased as well, although the extent of the increase is unclear. David Musto (1999: 248) writes that the number of heroin users increased from about 50,000 in 1960 to about half a million in 1970. But the US Bureau of Narcotics and Dangerous Drugs (BNDD), which replaced the Federal Bureau of Narcotics (FBN) in 1968, announced more staggering figures. It alleged that the number of *addicted* users had increased from 68,000 in 1969 to 315,000 in 1970, and then to 559,000 in 1971 (see Epstein 1977: 172). Officials consequently spoke of a tenfold increase in the addict population.

Edward Epstein (1977: 109–110, 174–177) warns, however, that the BNDD estimates are based on dubious calculations. Instead of discovering new addicts, the Bureau used the 1969 data and arrived at higher numbers for the subsequent years by changing the statistical formulas. Peter Reuter concurs with this critique. Writing about "mythical numbers," he argues that there is "a strong interest in keeping the number high and none in keeping it correct" (Reuter 1984: 136). Officials engaged in creative bookkeeping not only in Washington, but also at the state level. From the mid-1960s to the mid-1970s, New York State Governor Nelson Rockefeller persistently argued that drug addicts were responsible for half of the crimes committed in New York City and that addicts stole goods worth several billion dollars every year. He did not provide reliable sources for these allegations. Moreover, political opportunities dictated the way he expanded the number of addicts in New York City and then contracted them to cite evidence for the success of his tough law enforcement stance (Epstein 1977: chapter 2; Durlacher 2000: 63).

Yet no matter how significant the increase in drug consumption and crime really was, many US citizens felt that drug consumption and drug-related crime had gotten out of hand. The headlines were increasingly dominated by burglaries and robberies supposedly committed by addicts, as well as widespread police corruption resulting from a thriving illicit drug economy. The concern that heroin addiction was no longer a class issue but that it cut across societal strata, entailing a wave of crime, had helped Richard Nixon to become US president in November 1968. His promise to reduce drug consumption and crime made him popular at a time when even liberals such as *Washington Post* publisher Katherine Graham asked if it would not be a good idea to deploy troops onto the streets of Washington, DC (Musto and Korsmeyer 2002: 41). The close connection in the public perception between drugs and crime was shown in a 1971 poll on the nation's most pressing problems, when US citizens listed heroin addiction third after Vietnam and the state of the US economy (Courtwright 2001: 170).

Yet while drugs and crime were interrelated, there also was a link between drugs and Vietnam. In the late 1960s, heroin use among US service personnel in Southeast Asia appeared to increase. Heroin was first made available to US troops on a large scale in 1968 when a group of soldiers coming from Thailand to South Vietnam brought the drug with them (Bresler 1980: 12). From then on, the US government as well as the general public feared that soldiers under the influence of drugs would not be able to perform their military duties. Moreover, the US public feared that addicted soldiers, once they had returned to the United States, might apply their military skills to the drug business and thereby increase domestic levels of violence.

To observe the situation on the ground, White House member Egil Krogh visited Vietnam in August 1970 and reported back to Nixon that heroin and other drugs were freely available there. Soon after, in October 1970, the US military command reported an increase of drug-related deaths among soldiers from 16 in 1969 to 25 in 1970 (Musto and Korsmeyer 2002: 50). More bad news came from two Congressmen, Morgan Murphy (D-IL) and Robert Steele (R-CT), who visited South Vietnam in April 1971 to find out how serious the drug situation was. On April 29, Steele presented the White House with information he had gathered by speaking to US personnel in Vietnam, which indicated that 10–15 percent of all GIs stationed in Vietnam were addicted to heroin. In some units, the rate reached even 25 percent (Massing 2000: 107; King 1972: 332; Simmons and Said 1974: 22).

Although these figures were probably exaggerated and quickly dismissed by White House officials (King 1972: 332), the media now focused on drug problems in Vietnam, which were not only imaginary. As one writer (Booth 1998: 271) vividly describes the situation in Vietnam: "Heroin was available at roadside stalls on every highway out of Saigon, and on the route to the main US army base at Long Binh, as well as from itinerant peddlers, newspaper and ice-cream vendors, restaurant owners, brothel keepers and their whores and domestic servants employed on US bases. No barracks was without a resident dealer."

To reduce drug demand, the White House largely adopted a medical stance and put prevention and treatment over coercion. In 1969, Nixon proposed the Comprehensive Drug Abuse Prevention and Control Act, which passed Congress the following year. The act restructured US federal drug legislation and created different categories of drugs. This law and other laws provided for lighter and more flexible prison sentences for drug users than earlier laws such as the 1956 Narcotic Control Act. A crucial element in the administration's demand reduction strategy was methadone maintenance, which gained momentum when the Vietnam heroin problem became more visible. Nixon's drug policy advisor and addiction expert Jerome Jaffe argued that it was easy to neglect and stigmatize heroin addicts from disadvantaged minority groups, but that it was "a lot harder to do that with people you've sent as part of the military to fight your battles on foreign soil and say that, you know, you're not worthy of special consideration" (quoted in Courtwright 2001: 171). The Nixon administration, although conservative in other policy fields, pursued non-coercive drug policies informed by medical insights whose disappearance many regret even 30 years later (Jaffe 2002).

> The budget for federal drug law enforcement, $43 million in fiscal 1970, rose to $292 million in fiscal year 1974. But the prevention budget, which included research, education, and training as well as treatment, rose from $59 million to $462 million during the same period. [. . .] Over 60 per cent of federal funds went toward demand reduction. By September 1972 Jaffe and Nixon could boast that SAODAP [the Special Action Office for Drug Abuse Prevention] had expanded federally funded treatment capacity more in the past year than in the previous 50. [. . .] Though Nixon drew the line at heroin maintenance, the number of methadone patients shot up from 9,000 in 1971 to 73,000 at the end of 1973.
>
> (Courtwright 2001: 172)

To alleviate the Vietnam drug problem, the administration implemented a scheme whereby soldiers had to have their urine tested before being allowed to return to the US. Those tested positive for heroin consumption were detoxifie or treated. Since this prolonged their stay in Vietnam, the strategy made many soldiers give up heroin, as most servicemen could not wait to leave Southeast Asia. Implementation of the urine-testing scheme began on June 18, 1971 and may have helped to avert the prospect of tens of thousands of drug-using veterans roaming the streets of the US. Yet heroin consumption also decreased, since access to the drug was more difficult in the US than in Vietnam, which corroborated the theory that drug supply feeds drug demand. But drug consumption presumably also declined because veterans no longer oscillated between boredom, danger, and a lack of purpose, as many had done in Vietnam. For all these reasons, less than 1 percent of soldiers who had used heroin in Southeast Asia continued to do so two years after leaving the US Army (Epstein 1977: 32, 188; DuPont 1978: 184).

Besides reducing drug demand, the US also attempted to reduce drug supplies. As shown further below, Cold War policies imposed limits on US supply reduction efforts in Southeast Asia. The White House thus focused its efforts on Turkey and France. In Turkey, opium poppy had been planted for thousands of years. Turkish peasants made cooking oil from poppy seeds and salad of the leaves, burned the stalks in winter as heating material, fed the husks to their animals, and used the juice for medical purposes. Most plants grew on the Western Anatolian plains with the Afyon province (afyon stands for opium in Turkish) at its center (see Annex I, Map 2). Some of the opium paste extracted from poppy was used for medical morphine production and other licit purposes. Since the late 1940s, however, significant amounts of opium were diverted into illicit channels. Peasants sold opium paste to middlemen, who converted it into morphine base in Turkey, Syria, and Lebanon. From there, the morphine base was transported to Marseille by sea or via Bulgaria, Yugoslavia, and Munich (Krüger 1980: 87). In and around Marseille, the Corsican French Connection employed chemists who transformed the morphine base into heroin of the highest quality (No. 4 heroin). Subsequently, the drug was smuggled to the US, mainly to New York, either directly or via Latin America or Canada. In 1966, the head of the BNDD, John Cusack, claimed that that 80 percent of the heroin consumed in the US came from Turkish poppy fields and was smuggled into the US by the French Connection (Lamberti and Lamour 1973: 237; Epstein 1977: 89).

After Nixon had won the presidential election, he emphasized, on September 22, 1969, "that we have to tackle the heroin problem regardless of the foreign policy consequences. I understand that the major problem is with Turkey and to a lesser extent with France and Italy" (quoted in Musto and Korsmeyer 2002: 44). Suddenly, drugs were a prime concern of US foreign policy. In a nationally televised speech on June 1, 1971, Nixon promised quick progress on the drug issue. On June 17, the White House conveyed new anti-drug legislation to Congress, which included a message in which Nixon reiterated his ambition to cut off foreign drug supply, arguing that "the problem has assumed the dimension of a national emergency. If we cannot destroy the drug menace in America, then it will surely in time destroy us" (quoted in Simmons and Said 1974: 23). On June 18, Nixon reiterated this message before media executives: "Drug traffic is public enemy number one domestically in the United States today and we must wage a total offensive, worldwide, nationwide, government-wide, and, if I might say so, media-wide" (quoted in Epstein 1977: 178).

There were several motives behind Nixon's foreign drug policies. Most obviously, he had to show progress in the drug field to bolster domestic support among a conservative electorate concerned about drugs, the drugs-crime nexus, and the drugs-crime-Vietnam link. Moreover, the White House was under pressure from Congress. From 1969, proposals for ultimatums to be presented to Turkey to end poppy cultivation began to pile up in the Senate and the House (Brouet 1991: 120). On May 27, 1971, Murphy and Steele submitted a report to a House committee that urged the administration to increase pressure on producing states in general and Turkey in particular, even though the report acknowledged that Southeast Asia produced much more opium than Turkey (Murphy and Steel 1971). This report, as well as numerous bills introduced by various Congressional bodies, put tremendous pressure on Nixon to reduce drug supplies.

Some authors suggest more sinister motives. Epstein argues that the administration manufactured a drug scare to create powerful federal drug enforcement agencies needed to impose order on an unruly federal bureaucracy consisting of semi-independent fiefdoms. In 1972, the Office of Drug Abuse Law Enforcement (ODALE) was created, which quickly became notorious through its use of "no-knock" legal provisions that led to assaults on innocent individuals and families. A year later, federal drug control agencies were integrated into the DEA. According to Epstein (1977; see also McWilliams 1991: 373), drug control thus provided the White House with a convenient pretext to extend its domestic power base. This claim should not be dismissed lightly. The Watergate investigations revealed that some of the government operatives involved in the bugging scandal (the "plumbers") were part of the new drug enforcement system. The lengths to which the administration would go to achieve its objectives were further indicated by attempts to establish clandestine anti-drug units that were authorized, among other tasks, to assassinate traffickers (Epstein 1977: 142, 161; McWilliams 1991: 374; Krüger 1980: 161; Marshall 1993: 172–173). In 1974, a former high-level official said to Epstein (1977: 241): "If not for Watergate, can you imagine what [the White House] would have done with the Drug Enforcement Agency?"

Danish journalist Henrik Krüger (1980) takes these thoughts a step further. He argues that the White House dismantled the French Connection to allow a multilateral right-wing conglomerate composed of Cuban criminals, the US–Italian *Cosa Nostra*, and reactionary intelligence services to fill the gap. Although some of Krüger's assertions are questionable, he makes a convincing case that there are similarities in the way criminal organizations and secret services function. After all, both are specialists in what a former CIA agent called the "clandestine arts" (Lucien Conein, quoted in McCoy 1991: 15).

At this point, the domestic motives behind the Nixon initiative shall not be discussed further. What matters here is that during the late 1960s and early 1970s, the Nixon administration was under significant domestic pressure to reduce illicit heroin supplies smuggled into the US from abroad, and mainly from Turkey and France. The following section discusses the Nixon initiative against Turkish opium and French heroin.

The Nixon initiative

To examine the way in which drug markets responded to the Nixon initiative, one must look at events prior to the initiative. Historians rightly argue that in order to give meaning to an event, one must show how the event is related to prior developments. The present book heeds this advice. The chronological narrative can be started at the time of World War II.

The Mediterranean

Marseille had already been a thriving location for drug production and traffickin before World War II (Block 1989). However, the French Connection only rose to international prominence after the war, and not least due to US interference in French politics. Having won the war against the Axis powers, the US and the Soviet Union soon found themselves pitched against each other. The US was concerned about communism in France, and particularly in Marseille. There, labor unions and the French Communist party attracted workers, many of which were employed in the harbor, which was strategically important since US goods, delivered in the framework of the Marshall Plan, arrived in Marseille. A blockade of the harbor could have upset the US design for the economic reconstruction of Europe. Moreover, the harbor was militarily important since it was the hub for the deployment of troops and equipment to Indochina, where the French Expeditionary Corps was fighting a war against Ho Chi Min's Communists

Hence, the Truman administration was haunted by the fear of Marseille becoming a Communist city, and this fear was fed by general unrest and strikes of dockworkers in 1947 and 1950 (the French Communist Party supported these only half-heartedly, but this did not lead to more differentiated US views). To contain Communism, US agents needed local allies. In Marseille, the staunchest anti-Communists were criminals of Corsican origin, many of which had collaborated with the German Gestapo during World War II. Pragmatically, US agents struck alliances with Marseille criminals, which broke up strikes and assaulted Communists (McCoy 1991: 60–61). In return for these services, US agents turned a blind eye on the criminal activities of the Corsicans, who gradually strengthened their control over the waterfront and also began to produce and sell drugs on a major scale. According to the French police, the first heroin laboratories in Marseille became operational in 1951 (McCoy 1991: 63). By the early 1950s, the danger of Communism in Marseille had receded, and the US had won a Cold War battle in Europe. However, the US paid dearly for this victory in the form of heroin imports from Marseille, which increased steadily.

Although the French Connection controlled heroin production facilities and a trafficking network, it needed partners to purchase opium, transform it into morphine, bring it to Marseille, smuggle it into the US, and distribute it there. The Connection found a natural ally in the US–Italian Mafia, which, similar to the Corsicans, benefited from US security strategies. During World War II, US military planners apparently contacted Charles "Lucky" Luciano, a *Cosa Nostra* (Our Cause) don serving a long prison term in New York.[1] This was the time when US strategists were preparing a major event: the invasion of Sicily. Since the Mafia partly controlled Western Sicily, where US forces were supposed to land, the US Navy needed Luciano's network to acquire intelligence and increase local support for the invasion. The Mafia, in turn, had an interest in ending fascist rule, since it had suffered great losses under Mussolini, who regarded the Mafia as a threat to his supremacy

The successful 1943 invasion paved the way for the liberation of Italy from fascism. Apparently in return for his services, Luciano was released from prison in 1946. He moved to Sicily and soon became engaged in the heroin business in cooperation with other Mafiosi, some of which had also been deported from the US (McCoy 1991: 38–41). Between 1948 and 1950, the Sicilian Mafia diverted an estimated 400 kilograms of legally produced heroin from an Italian pharmaceutical company for illicit purposes (Cusack 1974: 244). When the Italian government suspended the licensed manufacture of heroin in July 1951, Luciano and his collaborators had already established other sources. Most importantly, Turkish opium was transformed into morphine base in Lebanon and then into heroin in Luciano's laboratories in Sicily and in Marseille laboratories controlled by the French Connection.

There are several reasons why the Italian Mafia left heroin manufacturing in the hands of the French Connection from the early 1950s on. One was that the chemists of Marseille were among the best in the world. For many years, only they were able to produce high-grade No. 4 heroin. This type of heroin is 80 to 99 percent pure and thus much purer than No. 3 heroin, which made it more popular among some users, yet also more expensive. No. 4 heroin is soluble in water and can be injected. Its production is difficult and dangerous: several chemists died when their laboratories exploded during the tricky ether precipitation process. In addition to this comparative advantage in chemistry, Marseille offered a safe political environment (McCoy 1991: 44). Moreover, Marseille was close to the perfume-producing sites of Southern France, which provided the acetic anhydride needed for refining morphine into heroin (Stares 1996: 22)

Hence, Marseille was perfectly suited as a drug production and smuggling center. Although the US official estimate, according to which Marseille heroin accounted for 80 percent of US heroin imports, may have been exaggerated, Marseille laboratories did indeed supply the bulk of heroin on the US market for around 20 years, from the early 1950s until the demise of the French Connection in the early 1970s. Once the heroin had left the Marseille laboratories, Luciano and his Corsican partners exported it to the US. For this, and for the distribution of heroin in the US, Luciano relied on other criminals. The most important were Meyer Lansky, who organized the finances of the illegal empire mainly through banks in Zurich and Geneva, and the Trafficante family. Lansky and the Traffi cantes, who were based in Cuba and Florida, also had stakes in gambling and other businesses. As Alfred McCoy (1991: 40) writes, "for almost 20 years the Luciano–Lansky–Trafficante partnership remained a major feature of the international heroin traffic.

The US was understandably concerned about these developments, and the importance of drug control gradually grew. When the threat of Communism in Marseille had receded, the former proxy was no longer expedient for the US government, and an increase in US drug consumption and crime meant that US politicians and the general public became increasingly intolerant of the low importance France accorded to the Corsican criminals. Thus, when Nixon took office time was ripe for action against the French Connection. In May 1970, Nixon told the new US ambassador to France, Arthur Watson: "Your job is to clean up the heroin problem in France. . . . That is the most important priority today" (quoted in Epstein 1977: 93). Upon his arrival in France, Watson found that few French offi cials regarded heroin addiction and the traffickers as a menace, and that the number of French police assigned to anti-drug forces was negligible (Cusack 1974: 249).

To change this, the US embassy launched a public-relations campaign against drugs. This campaign, US diplomatic pressure, and signs that growing quantities of heroin were consumed within France slowly changed French views on heroin. Moreover, the new Pompidou administration, which had replaced the de Gaulle administration, was keen on eliminating the French Connection. This attempt may have been informed by the interest to restructure the French intelligence system, parts of which were apparently linked to the Corsican Mafia. Thus, abolishing the French Connection helped to bring in new people loyal to the new administration (Krüger 1980).

These developments led to an increase in the number of French police and prosecutors assigned to reducing drug supplies, and to an amelioration of US–French law enforcement cooperation. Whereas in 1969, only eight officer had worked for Marseille's anti-narcotics unit, their number grew to 77 in 1971 (McCoy 1991: 69). The increasing police presence was facilitated by a US–French police cooperation agreement for which negotiations had begun in autumn 1969 and which was signed in February 1971. The agreement intensifie bilateral law enforcement cooperation, among others through training courses for French police officers in the US [2]

From mid-1971 into 1973, unprecedented international law enforcement pressure ended the impunity of the French Connection. In October 1971, a prominent trafficker was arrested and 106 kilograms of No. 4 heroin seized in Paris following a joint DEA–French investigation. As a consequence of this operation, many other syndicate members received long prison sentences. In January 1972, the French police seized more than 400 kilograms of heroin on the fishing boat *Le Caprice des Temps*, which marked a new world record (McCoy 1991: 69). In March 1972, the French police made the last important seizure of Middle Eastern morphine when they arrested a Turkish senator with 321 pounds of morphine base (McCoy 1991: 73). The drying up of Turkish supplies as a consequence of the 1971 Turkish poppy ban (see below) compounded problems for the French Connection. Moreover, French agents destroyed important heroin laboratories in and around Marseille. In July 1972, they found three laboratories, one of which could have produced enough to supply one-fifth of the US annual demand for heroin (Massing 2000: 123). Police action was not confined to Europe; in Latin America, police confiscated significant amounts of heroin destined for the US market, and Latin American governments extradited prominent Corsican criminals to the US. All over the world, members of the French Connection were sentenced to long prison terms, committed suicide, were killed by government agents, or killed each other (Krüger 1980). In the first half of 1973, thirty Mafia members were murdered, primarily in Paris, Marseilles, and Lyon

The year 1973 marked the end of the French Connection. The Connection made a brief comeback at the end of the 1970s when police raided several laboratories supplied with morphine by the Italian Mafia (Kaplan 1983: 67; Booth 1998: 251). However, the Connection never was the same after having been dismantled from 1971 to 1973. In the later 1970s, opium production sources and trafficking groups were too diversified, and too many competitors were involved in the business to allow the Connection to come close to the position it had enjoyed in the 1950s and 1960s.

The Nixon administration not only put pressure on France and the French Connection, but also on Turkey, as mentioned above. In a way, Nixon only radicalized the Turkey policy of the Johnson administration, which had brought a mix of aid and pressure to bear on Turkey from 1965 onwards (Spain 1975: 297; Turner 1975). In 1968, the White House gave a $3 million loan to Turkey to help the country prevent the diversion of poppy into illicit channels and to find alternative crops. As a negative incentive, the US bought less opium for its pharmaceutical industry from Turkey and more from India, and it persuaded other members of the North Atlantic Treaty Organisation (NATO) to do the same (Epstein 1977: 90).

In early 1970, the US declared that it had come close to signing an agreement with Turkey that would end poppy cultivation. The *New York Times* (January 7, 1970, quoted in Musto and Korsmeyer 2002: 44) quoted sources as foreseeing a "drying up of a very large part of the heroin traffic into the United States in the next one to three years." Indeed, there were signs of hope. The Justice Party of Prime Minister Demirel reduced the number of provinces in which poppy could be cultivated from 18 in 1967 to seven in 1970, and from seven to only four in 1971, although these four provinces were still able to meet the US demand for heroin (Lamberti and Lamour 1973: 241, 244). Despite domestic opposition, the Turkish government responded to US pressure since the country depended on US economic support, as well as US military support within NATO. In his memoirs, former US law enforcement liaison officer Charles Siragusa explained how the US utilized its economic leverage over other countries: "The police overseas almost always worked willingly with us. It was their superiors in the Government who were sometimes unhappy that we had entered their countries. Most of the time though, I found that a casual mention of the possibility of shutting off our foreign-aid programs, dropped in the proper quarters, brought grudging permission for our operations almost immediately" (quoted in King 1972: 225).

The White House demanded that Turkey either prevent the diversion of opium into illicit channels or prohibit poppy cultivation. Most people in the US administration shared the view of Nixon's US ambassador to Turkey, William Handley, that the second option was preferable as they saw the Turkish government incapable of limiting poppy cultivation and opium production to licit purposes. This view was probably correct, since peasants preferred to sell their harvest to traffickers rather than the government, as the former paid more than the latter. The US made its wishes clear at the bilateral and multilateral levels. On March 12, 1971, Prime Minister Suleyman Demirel bowed to the pressure of the Turkish armed forces and stepped down. The Turkish military had issued an ultimatum saying that it would rule the country if the government did not take effective steps against a wave of terrorist attacks committed by radical right-wing and left-wing groups, and unless the government managed to reverse the economic decline, two problems that had plagued the country for several years.

Demirel was succeeded by Nihat Erim who was backed by the Turkish military and indicated, on April 5, the government's intention to ban poppy cultivation. Only a few days before, Handley had conveyed to Erim the strong views of the Nixon administration on the matter (Lamberti and Lamour 1973: 246). In June 1971, Nixon sent a personal note to the US embassy in Ankara in which he emphasized the need to make rapid and visible progress on the drug front. Upon receiving the telegram, the embassy increased its pressure on the Erim administration. Finally, on June 29, 1971, the latter announced that the 1971–1972 poppy harvest would be the last. Apart from US pressure, the decision was also prompted by the government's concerns about the image of Turkey abroad (Simmons and Said 1974: 43).

The decision provoked angry reactions among the Turkish elite and public, which accused the government of giving in to US pressure. In August 1971, 21 Turkish senators introduced a bill to reverse the ban, and a year later, 200 parliamentarians did likewise. Nevertheless, the government rigorously enforced the ban, to the detriment of roughly 600,000 Turks whose livelihood depended on poppy production (Lamberti and Lamour 1973: 250). To ease their plight and to regain domestic political ground, the Erim administration demanded compensation from the US. In order to extract a maximum amount of money from the US, Erim cunningly increased the price paid to peasants for their last opium harvest by 65 percent. This yielded the figure of $432 million, but at the end, Turkey had to be content with a mere $35.7 million following the intervention of a Greek Cypriot White House staff who had already prevented a pre-emptive US purchase of poppy in 1970 and who now objected to a higher compensation (Epstein 1977: 88). In November 1971, Congressman Seymour Halpern (R-NY) made this figure public. US politicians doubted the effectiveness of the ban, while Turkish politicians said that ten times more money would be needed to compensate for the economic losses resulting from the ban (Musto and Korsmeyer 2002: 46). Subsequently, Turkey saw several changes of governments, and in October 1973 returned to democratic rule, not least because the hugely unpopular poppy ban had discredited the military government.

In February 1974, Turkey informed the US that it would lift the ban. By that time, Washington had paid $23 million of the total $35.7 million (Reuter 1985: 90).[3] On July 1, 1974, cultivation was resumed in seven provinces, leading to bitter reactions among US policy-makers and the US public. As before, Congress wanted to cut all aid, and the *New York Post* even called the Turkish decision "an act of war" and demanded that the US Air Force bomb Turkish poppy fields (quoted in Spain 1975: 302). However, Turkey did not again become a prime US supplier of illicit drugs, mainly because the introduction of a new harvesting method and coercive measures allowed the government henceforth to prevent the illicit diversion of opium. Thirty years later, significan amounts of heroin are still smuggled through Turkey (Labrousse 2003: Turkey), but its licit opium industry, which is one of the world's largest, has been more or less under the firm control of the Turkish government since the 1971 poppy ban

The White House thus eventually managed to convince France and Turkey to end drug production and trafficking. The French Connection was suffocated under the pressure of multilateral law enforcement cooperation, the Turkish government banned the cultivation of opium poppy, and Nixon's popularity received a boost. However, Corsicans had no monopoly over international drug trafficking, and Turkey was not the only poppy-supplying country. Southeast Asian and Mexican suppliers, in particular, were ideally placed to fill any gap resulting from a disruption of the flow of heroin from the Mediterranean

Southeast Asia

Turkey may have supplied most of the opium for the US heroin market, but the country was a small producer compared to other sources. When the opium ban was announced, Turkish production made up a mere 7 percent of the global illicit opium production. Almost 70 percent was produced elsewhere, in the border region of Burma, Laos, and Thailand, known as the "Golden Triangle" (McCoy 2004: 47; Bruun *et al.* 1975: 232–233; see Annex I, Map 3). A combination of factors can account for this, including the 1955 Iranian opium ban, which forced Southeast Asian consumers to find new supplies; the implementation of drug prohibition by Southeast Asian governments, which made many consumers switch from smoking opium to injecting heroin; the end of Chinese opium production following the victory of Mao's Communist forces over the Nationalist Kuomintang army; and the expansion of drug production and trafficking under French colonial rule

Although these developments were important for the expansion of the Southeast Asian drug industry, the focus here is on the wars in Southeast Asia and the US role therein. Washington's fight against Communism increased Southeast Asian drug production in the 1950s and 1960s, and the withdrawal of US troops from Vietnam, which coincided with US pressure on Turkey and France, was conducive to the integration of Southeast Asia into the global drug market.

Fighting drug traffickers and Communists simultaneously is impossible when the former are necessary for fighting the latter. This was the case in Southeast Asia. While the US government, and particularly the shrewd FBN director Harry Anslinger, accused Communist states of masterminding drug trafficking operations to weaken Western societies (Walker 1991: 172–175, 195–198), the CIA struck alliances with anti-Communist, drug trafficking forces. Alfred McCoy analyzes the nexus between intelligence agencies and drug entrepreneurs in *The Politics of Heroin* (1991), a complex and authoritative book of more than 600 pages in small print, as well as in several articles. He underlines that the CIA did not participate directly in the drug traffic, as for example a branch of the French intelligence apparatus had done, and that the involvement of CIA agents in the drug business was not a result of corruption. CIA involvement was rather "an inadvertent but almost inevitable consequence of its cold war tactics" (McCoy 1991: 20). CIA covert warfare played a crucial role in creating the heroin-trafficking complex that continues to plague the Golden Triangle, and the world, today.

Among the CIA's first allies were remnants of Chiang Kai-Shek's Chinese Nationalist (Kuomintang, KMT) Party. After Mao's victory in the Chinese civil war, the Nationalist army fled across the border into Burma, from where it made seven attempts between 1950 and 1952 to invade the People's Republic and overthrow Mao. Although the KMT, which had around 14,000 troops at the time, received support from the CIA, it was beaten back every time by Mao's armies (Bresler 1980: 67; Lamberti and Lamour 1973: chapter 7). Following these failures, the CIA installed and sustained KMT troops along the border of

Burma and China to help deter a Chinese invasion of Southeast Asia. Soon, the KMT controlled the Shan states, Burma's prime opium-producing region (Booth 1998: 258–259).

While it can be doubted that the KMT presence was the main factor that prevented a Chinese communist invasion, it is certain that the Nationalist forces increased opium supplies, building upon a policy that Chiang Kai-Shek had already pursued in the 1930s (Walker 1991: 82). They forced tribal peasants in the Shan states to plant poppy, organized the transport of opium through the Golden Triangle's difficult terrain, and sent heroin to Bangkok. Due to these activities, the Shan Plateau experienced a drug boom, and so did the Golden Triangle as a whole. In the late 1950s, the region produced about 700 tons of raw opium per year, or roughly 50 percent of the global illicit supply. This was suffi cient to sustain its local consumer population and, more importantly in the present context, to supply other world regions with drugs (Booth 1998: chapter 24; Dupont 1999: 441; McCoy 1999: 306).

In 1961, in a joint military campaign, China and Burma evicted the KMT remnants from Burma. The KMT then established camps across the border in Thailand. Around 4,000 KMT troops were flown out of Thailand to Taiwan with support from the US State Department. Around 20,000 troops remained in Thailand. In 1969, a second airlift to Taiwan was organized. This second airlift greatly diminished the size of the Nationalist army, which henceforth became known as Chinese Irregular Forces (Bresler 1980: 68). Since the CIA no longer supported them, they became even more dependent on illicit revenues. They were involved in the Thai drug trade and, despite their eviction from Burma, continued to control the production and trade of opium in the Shan states until the early 1980s, sending missions into Burma to buy Burmese opium and transport it back to Thailand by armed mule trains (Booth 1998: 263). Some opium warlords, however, remained in Burma and organized the business from there. The most prominent was the opium warlord Khun Sa, who survived attacks by various factions and armies and maneuvered so skillfully between the KMT, Burmese Communist insurgents, and the Thai, Chinese, and Burmese armed forces, that by the early 1980s, his Shan United Army had deprived the KMT of much of its drug revenues (McCoy 1999; Booth 1998: 263–264).

US support was also extended to Thailand. From 1947 to 1973, Thailand was ruled by various military and police administrations that financially "survived on opium" (Booth 1998: 262). But since the Thai regimes were staunchly anti-Communist, they received US support. In their fight against Communism, in turn, the Thais – and particularly Police General Phao Sriyanonda, who dominated Thai politics from 1951 to 1957 – cooperated with the KMT. For instance, the Chinese Nationalists helped the Thai generals in the years between 1967 to 1971 when the Red Meo, a Hmong Communist organization, staged a revolt against the Thai government in North Thailand. The Nationalists readily responded to the Thai government's appeal to fight the insurgents (Bresler 1980: 69; McCoy 1991: 362–363). Only occasionally, when the KMT presence became too embarrassing, or when the Nationalists deprived the Thais of revenues from the drug trade, did the Thai government abandon its policy of tolerating Nationalist operations on Thai territory, resulting in the use of force against the Nationalists.

In its largest operation ever undertaken, the CIA also supported the government of Laos and, from 1960 to 1974, created and sustained a secret army of 30,000 Hmong tribesmen in northern Laos (McCoy 2004: 45–46). The Hmong army fought against Pathet Lao Communists near the border with North Vietnam, protected radar installations that were instrumental for bombing North Vietnam, and rescued US pilots whose planes had been shot down. The Hmong's cash crop was opium, and the CIA allowed the Hmong commanders to use planes and helicopters belonging to Air America, a CIA-operated airline, to collect opium from highland villages and fly it to opium markets and heroin laboratories in Laos and South Vietnam. Hmong cadres and opium brokers benefited from this Hmong–CIA link, but the main beneficiary was the head of the Laotian military government, General Ouane Rattikone, a valuable asset in the US fight against Communism. In 1965, he had emerged victorious from a Laotian feud and had pushed opium-transporting small charter airlines controlled by Corsicans, who had stayed in Southeast Asia following the French withdrawal from Indochina, out of business. In their place, Air America transported Hmong opium at least until 1971.

In 1967, Rattikone's attempts to control the drug industry received another boost. Having crossed the Mekong from Burma into Laos, his troops joined a battle between Khun Sa and the KMT that had been sparked by Khun Sa's refusal to pay the KMT opium tax. Rattikone ordered the indiscriminate bombing and subsequent sweeping of the battlefield with paratroopers, dispersing both the KMT and Khun Sa's forces who had to leave their mules and opium loads behind. This intervention allowed Rattikone and his aides to tax opium caravans entering Laos from Burma, hitherto a prerogative of the KMT. Moreover, the Laotian government could now better benefit from heroin manufacturing. At the time of the battle, only morphine and No. 3 heroin were manufactured in the region. Two years later, Chinese chemists from Hong Kong were already processing high-quality No. 4 heroin for US troops in Vietnam, but increasingly also for the world market. Hence, the 1967 Opium War was an event of global significance. Besides, it allowed Rattikone to retire in 1971 as a very rich man (see Lamberti and Lamour 1973: 121–122; McCoy 1991: 288–376).

The US failed to control the activities of its allies, not only in countries such as Laos and Burma, where it operated through proxy forces. In Vietnam, US combat troops were directly fighting the Communist National Liberation Front (NLF, also known colloquially as "Viet Cong"). Various South Vietnamese administrations were deeply involved in drug trafficking, a fact ignored by many US policy-makers and agents whose prime concern was to defeat Communism in cooperation with South Vietnamese regimes. Air America's 1965 take-over of the Corsican opium air link involved the South Vietnamese intelligence and military apparatus more directly in drug trafficking from Laos to Vietnam, although

Vietnamese officials continued to cooperate with the Corsican intelligence and drug distribution network. The opium arriving in Saigon was supplied by planes that took off from airstrips in northern Laos (Inglis 1975: 196; McCoy 1991: 196–222; Booth 1998: 267–268). Once in Saigon, the opium or morphine base was distributed in the city, taken to Hong Kong by Chinese drug entrepreneurs, or exported to Europe.

Despite these activities, Southeast Asia was not fully integrated into the world drug market until 1970, as indicated by a 1969 estimate of the BNDD according to which Southeast Asia supplied only 5 percent of the US heroin market (McCoy 2000: 204; Booth 1998: 255). It was Asian societies who consumed most of the Golden Triangle opium, which was converted into heroin in Hong Kong, Bangkok, and Singapore.[4] However, Southeast Asia was ready to be integrated into the global drug market. After all, the region counted close to a million drug users, poppy cultivation was thriving, and sophisticated traffickin organizations run or backed by governments transported opium from the poppy fields to the cities, with US authorities watching without intervening. Moreover, as shown in the following paragraphs, the US military presence in Vietnam fostered the production of high-quality heroin, and the eventual withdrawal of US troops from Vietnam meant that the Southeast Asian drug market expanded beyond the region.

Before the production of No. 4 heroin, chemists in Bangkok and the Golden Triangle had supplied the Asian market with low-grade No. 3 heroin. But in late 1969 and the early 1970s, a network of heroin laboratories in the Golden Triangle was opened, which was run mainly by Chinese chemists from Hong Kong and controlled by Nationalist Chinese generals in Thailand and the Royal Lao Army. These laboratories (of which there may have been 15 by 1971) soon began supplying US troops in Vietnam with No. 4 heroin. Within two years after the first heroin laboratories opened in the Golden Triangle, they produced an estimated 70 percent of global illicit heroin supplies (Renard 1996: 58–59; Brouet 1991: 131; McCoy 1991: 222, 253, 286). This showed that US government support for drug-dealing Cold War proxies had backfired and that US drug problems in Vietnam were partly of US making.

Yet Southeast Asian heroin production affected the US not only in Vietnam but also in the US proper. After Nixon was elected, he followed up on his promise to "vietnamize" the conflict. In 1969, Washington began a rapid withdrawal of US troops. Their number, once more than half a million, dwindled fast. In 1973, the year of the Vietnam peace accord, the last troops were withdrawn, leaving only a small number of US personnel behind. Chemists and traffickers in the Golden Triangle, watching their main customers disappear, had to expand their operations beyond the region if they did not want to go out of business. As a consequence, increasing quantities of No. 4 heroin found their way to the US, as well as to Europe and Australia.[5] The profitability of the drug trade as a consequence of increased exports is shown in the fact that wholesale prices of heroin at Southeast Asian laboratories increased considerably (by 44 percent between September 1970 and April 1971), at a period when the number of GIs dwindled by 30 percent. The regional price of raw opium went up as well, although this had already occurred between 1968 and early 1970 (McCoy 1991: 286).

No. 4 heroin laboratories only appeared in the Golden Triangle in the late 1960s, but chemists in Hong Kong had already been able to produce No. 4 heroin years before (on the Hong Kong drug trade see McCoy 1991: chapter 6). Almost all the chemists and traffickers in the Crown Colony were from the Chiu chau dialect group. The Chiu chau Triads, whose members had immigrated to Hong Kong from Shanghai in the late 1940s, were ruthless, efficient, and almost immune to police infiltration. Within a few years of their arrival in Hong Kong, the Chiu chau had defeated their main competitor, the Green Gang (Bresler 1980: 33). From the 1950s onward, the Chiu chau syndicates were firmly in control of the Crown Colony's drug trade. Their specialization in the narcotics trade guaranteed them significant revenues, not least because the colony had the highest per capita number of drug addicts in the world. In 1970, their number was estimated at 100,000 out of a population of four million. By 1972, the number had grown to 150,000, or 3.6 percent of the population, a level not matched by any other country (McCoy 1991: 389). Many addicts had switched from opium to heroin following the closure of opium dens and police harassment of opium users.

Almost all Hong Kong addicts smoked No. 3 heroin as they could not afford the more expensive No. 4 variety. The Chiu chau syndicates thus had to sell their No. 4 variety elsewhere. One obvious customer group were US soldiers in Vietnam, but Hong Kong traders were also looking beyond the region. It is not clear how much No. 4 heroin was produced and how much was exported to which countries, and when. What can be said is that from the late 1960s, police uncovered smuggling operations in many countries of the world that had been masterminded by Hong Kong criminals. In a coordinated raid in January 1967, the police in Australia and the US broke up a criminal group that had been smuggling heroin from Hong Kong to the US. Most ring members were Australians who had been hired by the Chiu chau (see McCoy 1991: 279, for this case and the one after). In 1970, US police put a stop to a significant drug conspiracy when they arrested several Filipino couriers who arrived in the US with heroin from Hong Kong that was to be delivered to Mafia distributors. From 1969 to 1970, the group had smuggled an estimated 1,000 kilograms of Hong Kong heroin into the US, which may have amounted to up to 20 percent of the US annual heroin consumption. Since the drug was processed from opium that came from poppy fields in Thailand and Burma, the arrests were a valuable indicator for the growth of Southeast Asia's share in the global drug economy. This reading is also supported by the fact that in 1971 and 1972, Chinese and Western sailors hired by Chiu chau syndicates smuggled around 1,000 pounds of heroin into New York City (McCoy 1991: 392).

The restructuring of the world heroin market was evident in Hong Kong, but also in Saigon, Bangkok, Manila, and other cities that became important transit points for Golden Triangle heroin to the US and Europe. Operating from Bangkok, for example, former US servicemen who owned bars in the bustling city smuggled large amounts of No. 4 heroin into the US until their arrest in 1976 (Bresler 1980: 74; McCoy 1991: 392). Laos, hitherto known for its poppy fields, became a more visible heroin supplier as well. On April 5, 1971, more than 7 kilograms of Laotian heroin were seized in New Jersey (McCoy 1991: 286, 377). On 25 April, French agents arrested the designated Laotian ambassador with 60 kilograms of heroin in Paris. The drugs came from northern Laos and were destined for the United States. In November 1971, a Filipino diplomat and a Chinese businessman, upon arriving from the Laotian capital Vientiane, were arrested in New York with more than 15 kilograms of heroin (McCoy 1991: 259, 284). As shown above, the victory of the Laotian military in the 1967 Opium War created perfect conditions for the country's graduation from opium supplier to heroin exporter. In addition, South America, where Corsican criminals had their stronghold, and the Caribbean, which was controlled by the Traffi cante family and other Mafiosi, served as important transit regions for Southeast Asian heroin. From 1968 to 1973, the Marseille-born Auguste Ricord supposedly smuggled heroin worth $2.5 billion from Argentina and Paraguay mainly through the Caribbean into the US.

The US authorities, and particularly the State Department, found it difficult to alter their long-held belief that the US heroin problem was made in Turkey and Marseille and that the French Connection held a near monopoly over the global heroin trade. Only in November 1972 did the BNDD issue a statement, according to which Southeast Asia supplied 30, and not 5, percent of the US heroin market, with Turkey holding 60 percent (Newsday 1973: xiv; McCoy 1991: 259). Someone observing the situation in early 1973 could reasonably fear that Asia would take over the position formerly held by Turkey and France.

This did not happen, however. By late 1975, only 8–9 percent of the heroin seized in US cities came from Southeast Asia (McCoy 1991: 392). Hence, one cannot simply say that Southeast Asia replaced Turkey and Marseille as the hub of drug production and that Asian trafficking replaced the French Connection. The drug industry did shift from the Mediterranean to Southeast Asia, but not entirely and only for a limited period. This interpretation is supported by figure indicating an improvement of US domestic drug problems. In August 1972, law enforcement officials announced a shortage in the New York metropolitan area, and on October 24, the BNDD reported a heroin shortage in the Eastern United States, which had developed over the previous months mainly in cities hitherto supplied by the French Connection (Newsday 1973: xiii; Massing 2000: 124). Less than a year later, on September 11, 1973, Nixon proclaimed that "we have turned the corner on drug addiction in the United States" (quoted in Musto 1999: 259). Following the 1971 peak of 559,000 heroin addicts, the administration cited a drop in the number of addicts by 400,000. The heroin shortage was still felt in 1974. On July 16, 1974, Congressman Lester Wolff (D-NY) said:

> From the peak of over half a million heroin addicts, 1973 saw for the firs time rates of overdose deaths, drug related hepatitis, and drug related property crimes decline throughout the United States. The quality and quantity

> of heroin have decreased, while the price has increased. One milligram of heroin in New York City cost 44 cents in 1972; by mid 1973 it had risen to $1.52. Street level purity of heroin sold to addicts decreased 52 per cent during the same period, from 7.7 per cent to 3.7 per cent. A heroin shortage has existed for almost 24 months.
>
> (Quoted in Congress 1974: 10)

Figures purportedly showing an improvement of US drug problems must be read cautiously. It is not clear whether there were really fewer addicts. As mentioned further above, it is well possible that the 1971 peak figure was inflated which would mean that addiction was reduced only statistically (Epstein 1977: 177). Mike Gray (1998: 95) describes the juggling of statistics that was to bolster Nixon's 1972 re-election campaign as follows:

> By 1972 [. . .], the appearance of a growing addict population was becoming an embarrassment. This huge jump had occurred, after all, on Nixon's watch, and this was an election year. So the White House called the head man at the Bureau of Narcotics and told him to cool it. The drug agency, responding instantly to this shift in the wind, arbitrarily cut the number of junkies to 150,000 in the next report, and the administration was able to take credit for the overnight cure of some 400,000 addicts.

But even if the heroin shortage was not as dramatic as the White House said, there probably was a shortage. Besides increasing heroin prices and decreasing quality, this shortage is also indicated by the fact that the US pharmaceutical industry and medical staff did not have sufficient morphine at their disposal, leading the government, from 1975 to 1977, to experiment with the domestic cultivation of poppy (Schroeder 1980: 128).

The heroin shortage affecting the US drug market between 1972 and 1974 is important for assessing the impact of Nixon's anti-drug policies on drug markets. It shows that Southeast Asia was unable to fill the gap left by Turkey and the French Connection. If it had filled the gap, the US would probably not have seen a heroin shortage.

Although Southeast Asia did not completely fill the gap left by France and Turkey, heroin imports from the region, and the public debate about CIA links to drug entrepreneurs, still proved embarrassing to the Nixon administration. The publication of McCoy's book in 1972 led to Congressional hearings in which McCoy repeated his research findings. He was even invited to testify before the powerful Senate Foreign Relations Committee chaired by Senator William Fulbright, who said that he had known about CIA involvement in drug trafficking for many years and then added that nobody could stop it (McCoy 2003: xx). These testimonies, CIA attempts to prevent the publication of McCoy's book, and evidence from other sources about the role of the CIA aroused the concerns of many US policy-makers as well as the public, which was already concerned about Nixon's secretive style of government.

To salvage its success in Turkey and France and to bolster its credibility, the White House increased its efforts against Southeast Asian heroin. On June 14, 1971, three days before elevating drugs to a prime foreign-policy issue, Nixon held consultation with the US ambassadors to several countries, including Southeast Asian countries (Wellmann 1974: 67, 75). Later in the year, and in the following years, the US signed several memoranda of understanding and bilateral drug control treaties with Southeast Asian governments. In September 1971, for example, a Thai–US Memorandum of Understanding to cooperate on narcotics matters was signed. Moreover, US personnel helped to destroy poppy fields, as in 1973 when Hmong fields were eradicated (Westermeyer 1982: 279). Representatives of the US government and of host governments also began to attend ceremonies at which drug bonfires were lit under great fanfare, although it was far from clear whether the material burned actually was opium.

In addition, the US forced states to introduce anti-drug laws. In August 1971, for example, Laos passed a prohibitive drug law and began implementing it in November, after the US had threatened a cut in aid. Lao officials were not too concerned about the law, since it mainly affected the lower echelons of the drug business. "The American aim was to starve the heroin refineries of stocks but they continued in business whilst the ordinary smoker was hit by the closure of opium dens and retailers" (Booth 1998: 269). Moreover, Lao official saw that "they would receive a few more jeeps, a few more boats, a few more helicopters, a few more guns, and a few more dollars" (Westermeyer 1982: 273).

First, these measures were ineffective, but then progress set in as Washington sent more agents to Southeast Asia and spent more money in the fight against drugs. In 1972, only two special narcotics agents had operated in the region. In late 1974, their number rose to 31 (McCoy 1991: 391).[6] In the early twenty-firs century, when hundreds of US agents roam the globe, 31 agents do not seem to constitute a major force. In the mid-1970s they did. Most agents were sent to Bangkok, taking with them $12 million in anti-drug aid (McCoy 2000: 205; McCoy 2004: 48). Their task was aided by a revolution in October 1973 that changed Thai politics. The new civilian government, which replaced the military until 1977, tried to distance itself from the shady activities of its predecessor. Although relations with the US were tense, in the field of drug control Thailand and the US now shared common ground.

In Burma, things were more difficult. It took until June 1974 for the US and the Burmese governments to sign a bilateral drug control agreement. Over the following years, the State Department delivered 25 helicopters and five transport aircraft to help the Burmese military destroy poppy fields, attack drug refineries and disrupt opium caravans. During 1975–1976, these helicopters reportedly helped to seize and destroy 17 heroin laboratories, intercept nine caravans, and destroy 18,000 acres of poppy fields (Wiant 1985: 138).[7] All across Southeast Asia, the US increased its law enforcement presence and funding. While most of the funds were disbursed through bilateral agreements, Washington also invested considerable sums into multilateral drug control efforts. Most of the multilateral funding was spent on crop substitution, which helped reduce poppy cultivation particularly in Thailand.[8]

By 1975, US and local agents had entrenched their position in Southeast Asia, and particularly in Bangkok. As a consequence, Southeast Asia only supplied 8–13 percent of the US heroin market in 1975 (McCoy 1991: 392; Van Wert 1982: 132). But since heroin laboratories continued to operate and poppies to grow, traffickers exported more drugs to Western Europe and Australia (Trebach 1993: 117–121; McCoy 2000: 205–206). In 1976, an estimated 30 tons of heroin were sent to the world market (Nations 1976). European police forces seized ever more drugs and arrested ever more traffickers, mainly of Chinese origin. Amsterdam became the hub of European heroin distribution due to its large Chinese immigrant community and the city's proximity to US soldiers stationed in West Germany whom the Chinese hoped to win as new customers. In early 1976, a Dutch official (Amsterdam's Police Commisaris, Gerard Toorenaar, quoted in Bresler 1980: 135) remarked that it was "raining heroin in Holland."[9] As a consequence of increasing drug imports, Western Europe and Australia experienced an upsurge in heroin addiction and drug-related deaths.

Alfred McCoy aptly (1991: 394) summarizes the process leading to a restructuring of the world drugs trade. He argues that US international policies in the early 1970s increased

> the complexity of world heroin trade by expanding the number of markets and sources, making eventual suppression even more difficult. In the mid-1960s Hong Kong and Marseille were the only major producers of heroin for the world market. A decade later, Mexico, Burma, Thailand, and Malaysia joined their ranks. In the mid-1960s the United States had the only major heroin market among the affluent nations, but a decade later major consumers included not only the United States, with still more addicts, but also Western Europe and Australia. With a larger number of markets and suppliers, the web of trafficking became far more complex and the capacity of syndicates to survive police suppression increased.

As noted in this quote, besides the Golden Triangle, the Nixon initiative against Turkish opium and the French Connection had an impact on other regions as well. These include Western Europe and Australia, but there are more. The discussion now turns to the effects of the Nixon initiative on a US neighbor: Mexico.

Mexico

A Mexican lament goes: "Poor Mexico. So far from God, so close to the United States." Mexicans citing it often refer to drugs as evidence for its truth. They argue that US drug policies have aggravated drug-related problems in Mexico, the most pressing of which are violence and corruption. The following part shows that Mexico became the most important US heroin supplier following the Turkish poppy ban and the elimination of the French Connection.

Opium production in Mexico seems to have taken off in the 1920s and 1930s. Responding to price incentives created by US drug prohibition, Chinese immigrants are believed to have grown poppy in the states of Sinaloa and Sonora (Toro 1995: 7). This aroused US concerns and led some US agents to illegally cross the border into Mexico to pursue smugglers. Gradually, Mexico tightened controls over opium, heroin, cocaine, and cannabis production and trade. Drug control was motivated by the concern that anti-government forces would use revenues from the drug trade to purchase weapons, the hope that controls would stop US incursions into Mexico, and the attempt to curtail the influence of unruly regional governors who benefited from the drug trade

World War II changed the US drug policy stance toward Mexico. Now the US asked the country to grow cannabis and poppy, although it continued to try and curb illicit cultivation and trafficking (Walker 1996: 120–130). Hemp was needed to manufacture ropes, and poppy was needed to produce medical morphine whose demand skyrocketed due to an increase in the number of wounded US soldiers. Washington's strategy to increase the Mexican opium output came at a cost. The need for medical morphine had been overestimated, and by 1944, production was out of control (Smith 2000: 134).

Incentives to stimulate Mexican drug production also came from drug traffickers who saw an opportunity to replace European and Asian sources disrupted by the war with opium from Mexico. With heroin prices reaching record levels by the end of the war, the American drug dealer Howard Meltzer tried to establish a Mexican Connection in 1945 (McCoy 1991: 42). For a couple of months it seemed that his scheme would succeed, but then things went wrong, and Meltzer was arrested. He had lacked the necessary contacts, territorial control, and finan cial resources, all of which the *Cosa Nostra* and the French Connection possessed. By the beginning of the 1950s, these two groups had built a Mediterranean heroin empire that ruled out serious competition from Mexico for many years. Despite Meltzer's failure to turn Mexico into a center of drug production and trafficking, poppy continued to grow in the country.

In the 1950s and 1960s, the issue of Mexican cannabis pitched the US against Mexico and attracted the wrath of the vociferous Harry Anslinger. Opium was produced as well, albeit on a small scale. To eradicate poppy fields, the Mexican government embarked on its first national campaign, *La Gran Campaña*, in 1948. Now, the military became involved in crop eradication, operating not only in the traditional northern producing states of Sinaloa, Durango, and Chihuahua (which in the 1970s became known as the *triángulo crítico*), but also in other states (see Annex I, Map 4) (Toro 1995: 13; Craig 1978). The operation went on for many years, with questionable results. Growers and traffickers often evaded law enforcement by bribing or killing officials and by relocating their activities. During this period, the US supported the Mexican effort, albeit sporadically. In 1960 and 1961, US and Mexican government officials held meetings to discuss how the US could help to eradicate poppies and cannabis. In 1962 and 1964, US

Presidents Kennedy and Johnson met with their Mexican counterparts to discuss drug issues. In 1964, increased drug trafficking along the US–Mexican border attracted the attention of a US Senate subcommittee. And in 1965 and 1966, both governments discussed an increase in US aviation support against drug suppliers (Van Wert 1982: 18–19, 244–252).

When Nixon assumed office in 1969, he accepted the reasoning of his shadowy advisor Gordon Liddy and embarked on a conflict with Mexico. On September 21, 1969, 2,000 US officials, to the surprise of Mexico and even the US State Department, began intense searches of persons and vehicles crossing the US border from Mexico. Operation Intercept lasted for 17 days, brought border flows to a near standstill, and damaged the economy on both sides of the border. Few drugs were confiscated, since traffickers simply stockpiled their supplies and waited for the operation to end, and Mexican nationalism received a major boost. The Nixon administration nevertheless called the operation a success, arguing that it had shown the US's determination to reduce drug supplies and had forced Mexico to commit itself to this goal.

Following Operation Intercept, opium and heroin, rather than marijuana, dominated US–Mexican drug diplomacy. As in Southeast Asia, it took Washington some time to understand market changes and respond to them. While the US focused on Turkey and the French Connection, and then on Southeast Asia, drug entrepreneurs in Mexico increased heroin production and exports.

It is not clear *how* Mexico became the US's main heroin supplier. But there is consensus among drug experts *that* Mexico filled the gap left by Turkey and the French Connection. Richard Craig (1978: 130) expresses the consensus in simple terms: "When illegal Turkish production was checked, Mexico filled the gap." Similarly, Peter Reuter (1985: 90) writes: "The immediate effect [of the Turkish poppy ban] was significant; purity declined and prices rose. However, it appears that this shortfall in supply was quickly offset by the development of Mexican heroin production. It is quite plausible that this was a simple coincidence, but most observers believe that it was a response to the opportunity provided by the Turkish ban." This is also Peter Lupsha and Kip Schlegel's (1980: 4) argument. They write that the dismantlement of the French Connection led to a fundamental restructuring of the heroin market and to substantial increases of Mexican poppy cultivation and drug trafficking

As shown above, the closure of the Mediterranean heroin pipeline was followed by a US heroin shortage, and Southeast Asia did not entirely fill the gap left by Turkey and France. US drug consumers had to pay more for drugs, and higher drug prices provided an incentive for drug entrepreneurs to tap Mexico's potential. Mexico's production was almost exclusively destined for export, as the country had no domestic market to speak of (Riley 1996: 255–256). Mexico's share of the global heroin production has always been small, even at peak production periods. But this did not prevent Mexico from becoming the prime US supplier of the "Mexican brown" heroin variety (a name that alludes to the drug's relatively low quality), although there is no consensus when exactly Mexico came to dominate the US heroin market.

In their budget hearings in 1970, the BNDD said that Mexican heroin supplies were relatively insignificant (Lupsha and Schlegel 1980: 3). María Toro (1995: 16) writes that Mexico supplied a mere 10–15 percent of US heroin in 1972. A CIA report of May 1972 estimated Mexico's share of the US heroin market at 20–25 percent (Lamberti and Lamour 1973: 75). Alfred McCoy (1991: 392) writes that Mexico's share of the US heroin market in 1972 was 39 percent. This figure is close to estimates by official sources, including the House Select Committee on Narcotics Abuse and Control (whose Chief Counsel in 1977 was Joseph Nellis), and the US International Narcotic Enforcement Officers Association (International Drug Report 1976). By 1973, it was relatively obvious that Mexico dominated the US heroin market, with an estimated share of 63 percent, and for 1974, estimates vary between 76 and 80 percent (International Drug Report 1976; Reuter 1985: 90; Craig 1978: 120). In 1975, the National Narcotics Intelligence Consumers Committee, representing different US federal agencies, estimated that 87 percent of US heroin supplies (or 6.5 metric tons) came from Mexico (Van Wert 1982: 131; Toro 1995: 16).

Hence, some variation notwithstanding, these figures show that increasing Mexican drug exports coincided with the closure of the Mediterranean heroin pipeline following US pressure on Turkey and the French Connection. This development had severe consequences for the US: it ended the heroin shortage of the years 1972 and 1973, which had resulted mainly from the Mediterranean supply cut. From 1974 onward, the number of US first-time heroin users rose again. For the first three months of 1974, the DEA reported an increase in heroin availability and purity, a decline in prices, and an increase in heroin-related deaths. David Musto and Pamela Korsmeyer (2002: 139), in the cautious manner that marks their book, write that "[p]art of this phenomenon was probably due to increasing amounts of Mexican heroin on the market." Thus, the heroin epidemic of 1967 to 1971 was followed by a second epidemic lasting from 1974 to 1976 (Courtwright 2001: 166).

The US response to the Mexican drug boom was slow, as shown further below. It took until 1975 to initiate an effective anti-drug program at whose core was the aerial spraying of poppy fields with herbicides, a more effective method than manual eradication. In 1976, spraying began on a large scale in the framework of Operation Condor, which soon reduced poppy cultivation considerably.[10] Mexican law enforcement agents, working alongside US staff, also arrested thousands of peasants and traffickers. US assistance increased from $1.3 million in 1973 to $15.6 million in 1975 to almost $18 million in 1978. Concomitantly with the increase in US funding, poppy eradication increased. In 1972, around 2,700 hectares of poppy plants were eradicated, in 1975 around 10,000, and in 1977 around 18,000 (Toro 1995: 20, 64; Tullis 1995: 104–105). Washington also deployed more US agents to Mexico. "During the 1970s, the critical decade of opium poppy and marijuana eradication, the INC [International Narcotics Control] program pumped more than $95 million into Mexico. Aid included 64 helicopters, 24 airplanes, submachine and shotguns, tear gas projectiles, and at least 30 full-time DEA agents working in conjunction with the Federal Police" (Marshall 1993: 153).

A detailed breakdown of the US–Mexican eradication campaign would go beyond the scope of this study. Suffice it to say that the campaign was temporarily successful. From March 1976 and March 1978, the average purity of heroin seized in the US decreased from 6.6 to 3.5 percent. In 1976, Mexico supplied an estimated 75 percent of US heroin, but in 1980 only 24 percent (Kaplan 1983: 74; Lupsha 1981: 96–97). Reduced supplies led to fewer overdose deaths, drug-related hospital emergencies, and drug treatment admissions. In the late 1970s and early 1980s, however, new problems arose. In Mexico, poppy cultivation shifted from the north to more isolated regions where fumigation was difficult Afghanistan and Pakistan became the world's largest opium and heroin producers, not least due to CIA protection of the anti-Communist Mujahideen who established a thriving drug industry (Emdad-ul Haq 2000; Labrousse 1992; Bellis 1981: 85–87). And the Golden Triangle, despite ups and downs in drug production resulting from varying climatic, military, and political conditions, continued to supply the US and other countries with high-grade heroin. The success in the Mediterranean had been temporary, and so was the success in Mexico (President's Commission on Organized Crime 1986: Consultant Paper, Part 1).

This section showed that one should not oversimplify and say that the Nixon initiative against Turkish opium and the French Connection was the only reason for displacement. US cooperation with drug-trafficking clients, as well as other factors unrelated to the Nixon initiative, had already positioned Southeast Asia as an alternative source. Moreover, although the Nixon initiative served as a catalyst for Southeast Asia's joining the world drug market, there were other catalysts as well, notably the US military presence in, and withdrawal from, Vietnam.

Furthermore, to say that Southeast Asia replaced France and Turkey is only half-true, since the former region had never dominated the US drug market as much as the Mediterranean pipeline had, as indicated by the shortage of heroin on the US market. In Mexico, on the contrary, the displacement effect is much more visible. While Mediterranean supplies dwindled, Mexico increased its share of the US market, establishing a near-monopoly in 1975. Why did the poppy/opium/heroin industry shift from the Mediterranean to Southeast Asia and Mexico?

Explaining displacement

As argued in the first chapter, to assess the effects of a foreign drug policy initiative, one must look at whether the initiative is implemented selectively, how traffickers respond to it, and whether governments implement drug control measures. Moreover, one must look at contingent conditions.

US selective pressure

Ideally, a government attacks a problem wherever it arises. In reality, foreign policy is often compromised by short-term thinking, conflicting interests, and flawed assumptions about the causes and consequences of the problem. The Nixon administration focused on Turkey and the French Connection, but failed to apply equal pressure on the drug industry in Southeast Asia and prevent the spillover of the drug industry to Mexico. Clinging to the belief that 80 percent of the drugs consumed in the US came from the Mediterranean, Washington operated "on a law-enforcement model of localized vice suppression [. . .] without considering the complex market dynamics of the illicit opium trade" (McCoy 2000: 206).

Several reasons account for the selectivity of US drug policies. One is that the Nixon administration had little knowledge about drugs, as Daniel Patrick Moynihan, a member of the Nixon cabinet, admits. Writing in 2002, he refers to a memorandum he had written for the Attorney General in 1969 shortly after Nixon's inauguration and in which he stated that "most of the heroin is grown in Turkey and Syria, and processed in France" (of course, heroin does not grow, only opium poppy does). Moynihan (2002: 27–28) acknowledges that "[w]e knew nothing much" about drugs. The notion that other producing regions could be attacked once the Mediterranean heroin pipeline had been destroyed was popular among US policy-makers. However, the notion was flawed since it was based on the false assumption that drug markets are static. US policy-makers failed to see that once drug production sites and trafficking routes had spread around the globe, the drug industry would be immune to control efforts.

Yet insufficient knowledge about the drug industry as a sign of policy selectivity is arguably dwarfed by a combination of political opportunism and Cold War interests. Turkey was the most logical target since pressure on the country promised the quick returns that Nixon needed at home (Brouet 1991: 119). Turkey was financially and militarily dependent on the US and therefore had to yield to Washington's demands. Moreover, Turkey's authoritarian political system and the government's firm control over the national territory helped to implement drug control measures. But perhaps more importantly, pressure on Turkey deflected attention from drug trafficking in Asia. As Rufus King (1972: 338) writes: "When the Administration in Washington began being increasingly embarrassed by stories of heroin in Saigon – which could not be traced to Turkey and some of which was clearly traceable through U.S. allies to Laos, Thailand, and Burma – diversionary publicity about Turkey was stepped up."

Nixon accepted a souring of diplomatic relations with France and Turkey to demonstrate progress on the drug front, but in Southeast Asia, the administration was unwilling to sacrifice its containment policy to drug control. William Walker (1991: 217) writes that US officials "accepted and even suborned opium and narcotics trafficking as the ironic cost of seeking security in a dangerous world that they had helped to create." A former DEA undercover agent who had left the agency in disappointment said in the late 1980s: "[W]e gave up the drug war in favor of a war against communism. In fact, we made a conscious choice . . . the war on drugs is a fraud, [. . .] full of mistakes, false promises, and ineptitude" (Michael Levine, quoted in Lintner 1999: 417). McCoy (1991: 130, 383) summarizes the blend of disregard for international norms and the promotion of

Cold War interests underlying US policies in Southeast Asia, as well as the consequences of these policies, as follows:

> [T]he embrace of the warlord and his opium trade was a perverse personal triumph, the act of a machismo warrior casting off the bureaucratic controls of his commanders half a world away. Whether a corrupt Thai police general, ruthless Hmong tribal commanders, or a cynical Chinese opium warlord, CIA agents embraced them all, reveling in their defiance of civil standards for politics and warfare. Since the CIA headquarters in Washington saw the field operatives as front-line troops in the cold war, agency officials did not ask questions about methods as long as they produced results. [. . .] American involvement [in the drug trade] had gone far beyond coincidental complicity; embassies had covered up involvement by client governments, CIA contract airlines had carried opium, and individual CIA agents had winked at the opium traffic. As an indirect consequence of American involvement in the Golden Triangle until 1972, opium production steadily increased, No. 4 heroin production flourished, and the area's poppy fields became linked to markets in Europe and the United States

The US policy to fight Communism through proxy armies inevitably led it to forge an alliance with drug traffickers. In the Golden Triangle, a rough and mountainous terrain, poor infrastructure, and war made opium the only lucrative and reliable cash crop. Since US financial aid to its regional allies was insufficient, the numerous armed groups in the region depended on revenues from the drug trade. In 1967, a KMT commander said: "Necessity knows no law. That is why we deal with opium. We have to continue to fight the evil of Communism, and to fight you must have an army, and an army must have guns, and to buy guns you must have money. In these mountains the only money is opium" (General Tuan Shi-wen, quoted in Bresler 1980: 68–69).

Yet US agents maintained silence not only about the activities of non-state armed groups in the region, but also about governmental involvement in the drug trade. In Laos, the State Department and CIA officials did everything to leave the BNDD in the dark about the trafficking activities of the Laotian government, going so far as to use legal arguments to prevent the drug control agency from installing an antenna in Vientiane (Brouet 1991: 142). In a US official publication on Laos, issued in the early 1970s, only three sentences of 349 pages were devoted to opium, one of which was historical and the last of which notes that "this form of trade has virtually ceased" (quoted in Kunnes 1972: 30).

In South Vietnam, Vice-President Nguyen Cao Ky used the country's air force to smuggle large amounts of opium from Laos to Vietnam. The US embassy in Saigon did nothing to put an end to this. Instead, it replaced councilors who had spoken out against the corruption of the US host government with less troublesome staff (Brouet 1991: 139–140). Similarly, when the authoritarian and US-installed South Vietnamese President Nguyen Van Thieu was accused of complicity in the drug trade, the White House did not investigate, despite the fact that in 1972 a US Senate subcommittee received information about pervasive corruption in Saigon (Booth 1998: 273–274). As shown below, not only the US Mafia, but also the Corsicans anticipated an eventual cessation of Turkish opium supplies and, as a consequence, tried to procure more opium from Southeast Asia. CIA agents stationed in Vietnam knew about the activities of the Corsicans and the involvement of Vietnamese officials, but did not pass their knowledge on to the BNDD since they did not want to embarrass their clients who had struck a cooperative relationship with the Corsicans. Embassy officials adopted a similar posture. As a consequence, US agencies put pressure on France to eliminate the Marseille branch of the French Connection, but the Connection's Southeast Asian wing was largely left untouched (McCoy 1991: 250–259).

Domestic pressure forced the Nixon administration to adopt a more coherent stance. When news spread about the number of US soldiers in Vietnam consuming heroin, when the criminal activities of US proxies became a big topic in public debate, and when it became apparent that Southeast Asia was supplying increasing amounts of heroin to the US, Congress and the American public challenged the administration's implicit Cold War reasoning that Communism came first and drugs second. Reluctantly, the administration adopted drug control measures in Southeast Asia. This rethinking was eased by the withdrawal of US troops from the region, which weakened the links between the US and some drug-dealing, anti-Communist host governments.

Still, in 1971 and 1972, the Nixon administration's anti-drug efforts in Southeast Asia continued to be rather symbolic and piece-meal, while the region's drug industry continued to thrive and its entrepreneurs prepared to smuggle large amounts of drugs into the United States. US policy in 1972 had a somewhat schizophrenic touch to it, as described in the *Far Eastern Economic Review*:

> Wide publicity attended recent visits to Asia by top American narcotics offi cials seeking new plans to stamp out illegal drug trade. But not much attention seems to have been paid to American collusion with corrupt high-level Southeast Asian government officials to maintain and expand this trade. The Indochina War has highlighted both Southeast Asia's growing importance as a center of heroin production and heavy American involvement in drug trafficking
>
> (Nussbaum 1972)

Slowly, however, US-sponsored law enforcement in the region gained momentum. Prohibition laws, poppy eradication, heroin seizures, the arrest of traffickers, and more US funding and personnel began to pay off for the US.[11] While increased law enforcement in Southeast Asia prevented the region from filling the gap left by France and Turkey, other countries and regions, and particularly Australia and Western Europe, felt the effects of Southeast Asian drug imports.

The Nixon administration also neglected Mexico, where it applied pressure too late and where drug control was initially ineffective. In March 1970, Nixon announced a US–Mexican agreement to reduce drug smuggling, including $1 million in technical assistance for the eradication of poppy and cannabis plants. The main thrust of the program was directed against Mexican marijuana (Gooberman 1974: 182). Over the following months and years, Washington increased the number of customs officers along the border. In 1972, Nixon ordered the US Air Force to install radar stations in Texas and New Mexico and maintain interceptors on alert status to deter smugglers who transported drugs into the US in light aircraft flying at "cactus level" (Time Magazine, quoted in Gooberman 1974: 184). In 1973, the two governments struck an agreement that committed Mexico to reducing poppy cultivation and the US to supplying funding and equipment. In the same year, crop eradication began in the Sierra Madre. Initially, thousands of Mexican troops, equipped with hoes and machetes, destroyed poppy fields manually. The US provided transportation and equipment. This effort had little impact, and in 1974, the US still had to urge Mexico to follow through on its promise to reduce drug production. By this time it was obvious that Mexico had become the primary source of the US heroin market.

Mexico offered the ideal geographical, climatic, economic, and political conditions for drug production and trafficking, and Washington's belated policies did not help. If Washington had supplied the Mexican government with the necessary means at an earlier stage, Mexico's conquest of the US heroin market might have been averted. But as it was, it took until 1974 for Mexico to act effectively against production and trafficking, and another year until the government began to arrest members of major drug rings and not just small growers and dealers. During the 1975–1976 campaign, 16 large drug trafficking operations were disrupted and their leaders indicted (Craig 1978: 120, 125). More importantly, the Mexican government ceded to the longstanding US wish that herbicidal defoliants be used, a decision it had procrastinated for many years.

The subsequent Mexican–US campaign against heroin marked the second success story in Washington's foreign drug policy after the success in France and Turkey. That the success in Mexico did not last is another story. For the purposes of this study, it is sufficient to state that the selectivity of the US anti-drug effort contributed to increasing drug production and trafficking in Southeast Asia and Mexico.

The flexibility of the drug industry

To understand and explain the displacement of the drug industry from the Mediterranean to Southeast Asia and Mexico, one must look at traffickers responses to state pressure as well. As many times before and after, drug entrepreneurs proved highly flexible and were thus able to continue their activities, or even to expand them when governments put pressure on competitors. The most prominent loser during the restructuring process analyzed in this chapter was the

French Connection, and the main winners were trafficking groups operating in Southeast Asia, Mexico, and the US.

To be sure, the Corsicans did try to evade state pressure. For a time, it seemed that these attempts would succeed. From the mid-1960s, that is several years before its elimination, the French Connection explored new sources of supply. Corsicans anticipated the eventual closure of the Turkish opium pipeline, correctly interpreting the decision of the Turkish government to reduce the number of opium producing provinces as a first step toward an eventual complete ban. The French Connection "saw the handwriting on the wall and began to shift their morphine base sources to Southeast Asia," a US narcotics official said in 1971 (John Warner, quoted in McCoy 1991: 73)

Corsicans were well entrenched in Laos and Vietnam. Indeed, one can speak of a "Southeast Asian branch of the French Connection" (Booth 1998: 266). Corsicans, many of whom had been part of the French intelligence network during the Indochina war, had stayed in the region after the withdrawal of the French colonial administration and smuggled opium from Laos to Vietnam until 1965. Working in tandem with the South Vietnamese government, they were involved in legal and illegal businesses in Saigon and Vientiane, and they smuggled drugs to European laboratories. In a 1971 interview, a high-level CIA offi cial told Alfred McCoy that in 1965/1966, people close to Premier Ky had informed Saigon-based Corsican criminals that they were free to export drugs to Europe for a hefty commission (McCoy 1991: 250). Indeed, in the second half of the 1960s significant amounts of Southeast Asian drugs seemed to have reached Europe, and especially Marseille. But under pressure from other criminals and governments, key Corsican players were arrested or killed, as described further above.

US criminals fared better. They probably aggrandized the Mexican drug industry, which soon dominated the US heroin market (although not much is known about the evolution of the Mexican heroin market in the early 1970s, as discussed further below). In doing so, traffickers learned from past experiences. Operation Intercept had demonstrated the US determination to reduce drug supplies and the need to become more sophisticated. Thus, in the wake of Operation Intercept, the smuggling of drugs from Mexico to the US by air increased substantially, as traffickers thought that this was a less risky and more lucrative method than smuggling drugs overland (Baum 1997: 24).

With regard to the *Cosa Nostra*, their flexibility is obvious when looking at Southeast Asia. Like their Corsican counterparts, US–Italian crime bosses probably anticipated a closure of the Mediterranean pipeline early on. Hence, they tapped the Southeast Asian opium market to reduce their dependence on that source of supply. The business talent of US Mafiosi is indicated by a business trip of Santo Trafficante Jr, a central crime figure. In 1968, he went to Saigon, Hong Kong, and Singapore to explore the possibility of procuring more drugs from Southeast Asia for delivery to the US. In Saigon, he might have met with Corsican criminals (McCoy 1991: 76, 250, 253; Carnwath and Smith 2002: 62). If this is true, it shows that relations between the Corsican and US Mafia were still fairly cordial at that time. However, Henrik Krüger's (1980: 149, 190) reading of the events is somewhat different:

> Trafficante liked what he saw in his Southeast Asian tour. With enough trained chemists, his Mob could be supplied with heroin at a fraction of what it was then paying out to the Corsicans. But first the smuggling networks had to be worked out and the Corsicans had to be eliminated. So Santo Trafficante began his war against the Corsicans. [. . .] In addition to motives he might have shared with the CIA, Trafficante had many other reasons to take part in the heroin coup. First, it meant cheaper heroin deliveries and therefore greater profits. Second, he wanted the Corsicans out because, behind his and the rest of the Syndicate's backs, they had began setting up their own U.S. distribution network. Finally, Trafficante's drug Mob did not want to see a repeat of BNDD Operation Eagle [a US raid against his network].

As all war zones, Vietnam offered numerous illegal income opportunities, including narcotics. Hence, the escalation of the Vietnam war was beneficial to Trafficante and other US Mafia bosses, who had been forced to look for new supply sources anyway in order to substitute Turkish opium supplies and to reduce their dependence on the French Connection: "The cutting of the supply of Turkish morphine base forced the American Mafia to find a new heroin source, for which they had in fact already been searching, appreciating the pressure being put on Turkey to stop production" (Booth 1998: 251). To be sure, we do not know how exactly the US Mafia reorganized the international heroin traffic. Krüger (1980: 122–123) writes that Mafia bosses held a criminal summit on July 4–16, 1970 at the Hotel Sole in Palermo, Sicily, where they decided to increase their investments in Southeast Asia to tap the region's resources for their global smuggling activities. Although this assessment may accord too much importance to one meeting, it is safe to say that *Cosa Nostra* entrepreneurs did not drag their heels.

Criminals from Eastern countries also proved able to exploit any business opportunity that would arise. Particularly the Chiu chau, utilizing their skills in smuggling and chemistry, helped to integrate the hitherto regional Southeast Asian drug market into the global drug market. Benefiting from the willingness of Asian officials to accept bribes, as well as the US position, according to which the fight against communism was more important than the fight against drugs, they produced large quantities of high-quality heroin. The drugs were firs sold to American soldiers in the region and later shipped to the US. When that became too difficult, Chinese traffickers redirected drug flows to Europe and Australia.

The response of governments to these developments was half-hearted. While US drug policy was implemented selectively and ineffectively, the governments of Southeast Asian countries and Mexico were largely unwilling or unable to implement drug control measures. Drug entrepreneurs profited from the resulting inertia and often circumvented state attempts to curb the illicit business. When governments introduced drug prohibition laws, traffickers diverted drugs from legal sources. When governments introduced control measures to prevent this diversion, traffickers found new sources. In 1969, the International Narcotics Control Board wrote that "[u]nfortunately, these sources are both extensive and prolific and they constitute an enormous reserve. Some of these sources are remote and even now are difficult to access" (quoted in Bruun *et al.* 1975: 232). This certainly was the case with Southeast Asia and Mexico.

Weak law enforcement

The selective implementation of foreign drug policies and the ability of drug entrepreneurs to adapt are two important elements for understanding and explaining the displacement of the illicit drug industry. Another factor to be taken into account is whether governments of drug-producing and transit states implement anti-drug measures. Drug control can be hampered, among other factors, by a lack of governmental control over the national territory, countervailing interests, corruption, insufficient resources, and bureaucratic rivalries.

In Southeast Asia, the drug industry was thriving because Southeast Asian governments and the US put other interests over drug control, and because some Southeast Asian officials and policy-makers actively participated in the business. In building up their narcotics empire, the Chiu chau of Hong Kong, for example, benefited from rampant corruption within the colony's Chinese and British police force. Officers acted against heroin consumers, small dealers, and independent dens, but not against the syndicates who paid the officers. Indeed, "the degree to which the Royal Hong Kong Police Force became involved in corruption – not only in accepting bribes from criminals but also in actually having major criminals in their ranks – must make it a group of law enforcement officers unique in the annals of crime" (Bresler 1980: 40)

But even if governments had wanted to reduce drug supplies, formidable obstacles would have remained. Laos exemplifies the challenge in enforcing drug laws:

> There were not enough police in Laos to enforce an antiopium law. Much of Laos at the time was a no-man's-land, under the control of neither the central government nor the communist Pathet Lao. Were it theoretically possible to cover the country with enough police to suppress opium, there was still the issue of police attitudes toward opium, which were [. . .] widely varying and ambivalent [. . .] Even among the police, known opium users and addicts continued in their jobs so long as they were able to maintain their responsibilities.
>
> (Westermeyer 1982: 273)

A lack of territorial control was one of the obstacles of drug control, and not only in Laos. In Thailand, the KMT controlled parts of the North, although sometimes in tacit agreement with the government. The Thai government had to take into account left-wing insurgency, which it did not want to fuel by eradicating poppy (Lamberti and Lamour 1973: 106–109). In Burma, various insurgent and trafficking groups roamed the country. Moreover, US relations with Burma were highly conflictive, precluding the exertion of effective US pressure on the country. Perhaps more importantly, Rangoon put its counterinsurgency campaign before drug control (McCoy 2004: 52). In an interview of September 25, 1972, Nelson G. Gross, the State Department's coordinator for drug control, describes the resulting problems:

> I have met with Chairman Ne Win of Burma, and so has Secretary Rogers. We have explored means by which we might help in their interdicting along the supply route and also at the point of heroin processing, which is now concentrated in Tachilek, Burma. Our experts have had follow-up discussions with Burmese officials as to how this might be accomplished. We are disappointed that thus far, Government officials in Burma have determined that they will go it alone – without any United States help. The result is that we are trying to compensate by energizing all the resources at our command at the transit points as the opium moves out from Burma – mainly in Thailand, Laos, Vietnam, but also in outer-lying points such as Hong Kong, Manila, Singapore, Indonesia and Malaysia.
>
> (Quoted in McCoy 1974: 151)

In Mexico, the state's inability to enforce drug laws was conducive to the growth of the heroin industry as well. One of the factors hampering drug control was geography. Mexico shares a 3,200-km-long, porous border with the US, and the high-density trade between the two countries allowed traffickers to conceal their illicit goods among the many items that legally crossed the border (Reuter 1985: 91; Schroeder 1980: 131–132). Moreover, producing drugs close to consumers helped traffickers to reduce transaction costs. In addition, regions such as the Sierra Madre in Mexico's north are rugged, difficult to access, and offer the right climate for poppy cultivation. The vastness and remoteness of producing regions provided traffickers with strategic depth and created problems for the relatively few soldiers and policemen ordered to reduce drug supplies. Even in the later 1970s, when Operation Condor was in full swing, the number of government troops was small. Often "no more than five hundred to one thousand men are responsible for up to one hundred square miles of *very* rough and often all-but inaccessible terrain" (Craig 1978: 116 (italics in the original)). A lack of equipment and funding also hampered drug control in Mexico, as illustrated in a 1972 *Washington Post* article:

> Earlier this week Mexican authorities were planning a major strike operation against members of drug trafficking gangs thought to be holed up in a group of ranches with their private army of some 70 pistoleros. Because of the absence of cars for the Mexican police, officials planning the strike had

> to rent 11 station wagons from the Hertz Co. as mobile strike vehicles. "The Hertz people insisted on $500 up front," one official explained. The Mexican government was unable to meet the demand.
>
> (Quoted in Simmons and Said 1974: 35–36)

Worse still, the Mexican military and police lacked helicopters, which were indispensable for gathering intelligence and transporting troops to poppy fields And often, security forces in Sonora, Sinaloa, or Guerrero found themselves outgunned by poppy growers and drug traffickers who had sufficient funds for buying automatic weapons since they could barter drugs for arms. In addition to a lack of equipment and funding, corruption proved a formidable challenge to drug control. There is no reliable data showing which Mexican officials were bribed, how much was paid by whom, and which officials actively participated in the business. But given the fact that corruption has been (and continues to be) an integral part of the Mexican political system and that Mexican officials had a habit, if not a duty, to take bribes, it is easy to infer that corruption fostered the growth of Mexican drug production and trafficking [12]

A further impediment to drug control was weak interagency coordination. The Mexican armed forces did not relish the task of drug control, regarding it as police work. Moreover, they were reluctant to cooperate with the Mexican Federal Police (Craig 1978: 117–118). To complicate matters further, many Mexican officials harbored resentments against the US and therefore refused to participate in the implementation of what they regarded as a US agenda, believing that Mexican drug production was exclusively a consequence of US drug consumption. Writing in the late 1990s, Cottam and Marenin (1999: 209–240) argue that "[c]ooperation between Mexican and United States law enforcement agencies is minimal, conflicted, and beset by reciprocal accusations of corruption, inefficiency, cultural arrogance, legal insensitivity, and professional jealousies." In the second half of the 1970s, relations were not quite so bad, also because the US tried to minimize its identification with Operation Condor. However, they were far from good (Van Wert 1982; Craig 1978: 125, 129).

With Operation Condor in 1975, the Mexican government quickly managed to establish control over poppy growing regions, despite persistent problems such as rough terrain, trafficker resistance, corruption, and bureaucratic rivalries. Mexico offered better social and political conditions for achieving a substantial reduction of drug production than Burma, Afghanistan, or Colombia. The same holds true for Turkey. The governments of both countries were able to reduce drug supplies since few drugs were consumed domestically, since revenues from the drug trade were not as important for the national economy as was the case in other countries, and since they had a relatively firm grip over the national territory. Once the US had coerced both countries to reduce drug supplies and, in the case of Mexico, provided the means to implement drug control measures, the Turkish and Mexican governments acted decisively in reducing illicit drug supplies, if only for a short period in the case of Mexico.

Contingent conditions

Contingencies apply to one case only and thus defy generalizations except of the most banal type ("contingencies are part of any social phenomenon"). Several contingent factors contributed to the Turkish opium ban, the elimination of the French Connection, a rise in drug production in Southeast Asia, increased drug smuggling from the region to the US, the eventual diversion of smuggling routes from the US to Europe and Australia, and the establishment of Mexican control over the US heroin market.

It is doubtful, for example, whether without a change of government Turkey would have banned opium production. Similarly, if the French government had not changed, the French Connection might have survived. And without the victory of the Chiu chau over the rival Green Gang criminals, Southeast Asia might have lacked the skills necessary for producing and exporting large amounts of No. 4 heroin.

Moreover, and perhaps most importantly, the Vietnam War proved decisive for the transformation of Southeast Asia into a hub of drug production and trafficking. Since the Truman administration's decision to back the French colonial empire in Indochina, until the moment when the last helicopter took off from the US embassy in Saigon in 1975, the presence of US agents and soldiers in Indochina had a crucial impact on the regional and global drug trade. US support for groups and governments involved in drug trafficking was conducive to the expansion of the illicit industry, as shown above. Furthermore, if it had not been for the presence of hundreds of thousands of GIs in Southeast Asia, the region might not have evolved from a regional opium producer into a global heroin producer and exporter. Washington's military engagement thus provided a catalyst for the development of a thriving heroin market.

Later, when the conflict was "vietnamized" and American troops withdrawn, traffickers exported increasing amounts of heroin to the US, although this trend already had begun before. These new trafficking patterns coincided with the Turkish poppy ban and the elimination of the French Connection, and entrepreneurs based in Southeast Asia were able to benefit from the resulting rise in heroin prices. Increasing exports of Southeast Asian heroin to the US was a firs step in the globalization of drug problems. This process received another boost by increasing US law enforcement pressure on Southeast Asia and the diversion of trafficking routes to other world regions

Many other conditions enabled displacement. Widespread poverty in rural Southeast Asia and Mexico made poppy cultivation attractive to peasants. Norms against heroin consumption, production, and trafficking may have been strong in some places, but those against opium were not, at least not in Southeast Asia, where people had been smoking opium for centuries. Further, the climate in Southeast Asia and Mexico was suitable for poppy cultivation. Finally, migration was conducive to drug industry displacement. In the early 1970s, all major US cities had Southeast Asian and Chinese communities. These had grown in the 1960s, not least due to the introduction of a more liberal US immigration law in 1965. Almost all members of the Chinese communities were hard working and law-abiding, but a few were Triad members. These Triads benefited from their communities, which provided, if not a safe haven, then at least some protection against police infiltration. To be sure, close ties among their members did not prevent the Triads from cooperating with other ethnic communities such as the Italian community to distribute heroin in US cities (Bresler 1980: 39, 73, 182).

All these contingent conditions did not "cause" the displacement of drug production and trafficking to Southeast Asia and Mexico in a strict, positivist sense. Rather, they made the displacement possible. Some external factors functioned as a catalyst, such as the US military presence in, and later withdrawal from, Vietnam. Others, such as poverty and corruption, can be considered background conditions enabling displacement.

Black boxes and alternative explanations

Understanding and explaining the displacement of the drug industry from the Mediterranean to Southeast Asia and Mexico is complicated by empirical black boxes pertaining both to the structure of the industry and to state policies. Moreover, one could think of alternative explanations for displacement. This part discusses black boxes and the limits they pose to causal inference and then refers to alternative explanations. A lack of data makes it impossible to disconfirm these explanations. Nevertheless, alternative explanations for industry displacement are less plausible than the explanation proposed here.

Due to the illegality of the drug trade, there is no reliable data on traffickin routes and traffickers. It is unclear, for example, how much of the heroin entering the US from Mexico was actually produced in Mexico. According to a Triad member in Canada interviewed in the 1970s, considerable amounts of Southeast Asian heroin came into the US via Mexico: "Asian heroin out of the Golden Triangle never stopped coming into the United States. What they did was, for a time, they shipped it into Mexico where they treated it by chemical process to make it look and 'taste' like 'Mexican Brown' – and then they brought it up into the States" (quoted in Bresler 1980: 209). Estimating the share of Asian heroin coming through Mexico is difficult not least because so little is known about Asian trafficking networks. There is some information about Chiu chau operations in Hong Kong and elsewhere, but overall, the linkages between traffickers laboratories, and governments are nebulous (Stares 1996: 26).

Little is also known about who was behind Mexico's drug boom. Fenton Bresler (1980: 13) writes that Mexican traffickers became entrenched in the US in 1971, but does not expand on this assertion. Peter Lupsha (1981) refers to the huge sums of money Mexican criminal groups such as the Herrera organization made in the drug trade at the time when Mexico already dominated the US drug market. He does not, however, discuss whether these groups were already active at the time of the Nixon initiative. Peter Lupsha and Kip Schlegel (1980: 5–6) write that by 1972, the Herrera group was probably well-established. However, they do not further elaborate on the group's role during the early 1970s, but focus on the late 1970s, when it had become a target of the US and Mexican governments. James Van Wert (1982) evaluates the success of the Mexican poppy eradication program. Since he looks at the period between 1976 and 1980, there is little information about the evolution of Mexican drug trafficking

Michel Lamberti and Catherine Lamour (1973: 255) offer a more detailed analysis. They write that not all traffickers were of Mexican origin, but that US citizens organized and financed illicit poppy cultivation in Mexico by buying fields under false names, lending money to peasants to buy seeds, and purchasing the harvest. Moreover, they paid members of the Mexican army and police to keep quiet. Peter Reuter, discussing the impact of the elimination of the Mediterranean heroin pipeline on Mexico, takes the paucity of data into account and wisely keeps a balance between agnosticism and causal assertions: "While we lack sufficient data to estimate how large an expansion took place in the relevant period, it appears that thousands of peasant farmers in Mexico [...] increased their acreage under drug cultivation within a few months in response to new income opportunities. This is rather sobering testimony to the adaptability and energy of these farmers, perhaps as encouraged by drug entrepreneurs" (Reuter 1985: 92).

Similarly, little is known about trafficking groups operating elsewhere. Despite the fact that numerous officials, researchers, and journalists have looked at the Mediterranean heroin pipeline, for example, many aspects remain obscure. As shown above, the French Connection procured opium not only from Turkey, but probably also from Southeast Asia, but nobody knows how much. There is also a lack of knowledge about the chain linking Turkish poppy farmers and New York heroin consumers, which is not surprising, given that this chain may have had up to 18 elements (Lamberti and Lamour 1973: 39).

Thus, analyzing even only one trafficking network poses problems. Yet in order to understand and explain industry displacement, analysts must look at several networks at the same time, as well as at several anti-drug policies, all of which are implemented in a secretive manner. This obviously yields a very complex and somewhat fuzzy empirical picture.

The scarcity of empirical data makes it difficult to assess the impact of US drug policies on the drug industry. More precisely, scholars disagree over whether drug imports from Asia to the US increased significantly in the wake of the French Connection's elimination and the Turkish poppy ban, or whether the increase was negligible. Moreover, authors cite different reasons for increasing Southeast Asian drug supplies. Alfred McCoy writes that the amount of Southeast Asian heroin smuggled into the US increased significantly in the early 1970s, and that this increase was stimulated by the withdrawal of US troops from the region. Fenton Bresler (1980), in contrast, explains the rise of Asian heroin imports to Western countries by referring, among others, to an increase in the number of Asian immigrants. Kevin Riley (1996: 256) looks at the period in a slightly different way, arguing that following the Turkish poppy ban, Asian supplies were unsteady because of the Vietnam War and the withdrawal of US troops. According to his analysis, Asian trafficking networks also found it diffi cult to smuggle drugs to the US because the Asian immigrant population was not well established in the US and because it was confronted with hostile public attitudes.

There are several alternative explanations for drug industry displacement. Black boxes and alternative explanations are interrelated: the former result in the proliferation of the latter. As some black boxes cannot be illuminated, the true extent of, and the underlying reasons for, drug industry displacement will remain controversial. Nevertheless, alternative explanations offer a less plausible account of developments in the early 1970s than the initial causal mechanism.

According to one alternative explanation, the Mexican drug industry would have expanded even without US pressure on Turkey and the French Connection, and the sequence of events was merely coincidental and not the result of underlying causal forces. This explanation cannot be excluded beyond doubt, as long as the underlying reasons of the Mexican drug boom are unclear (rising US heroin prices resulting from decreasing Mediterranean supplies, migration, etc.). However, it is likely that Mexico would not have been able to significantl increase drug exports if Turkey had not banned poppy production and if the French Connection had not been eliminated. After all, Mediterranean heroin was of a high quality and smuggled into the US by a sophisticated network that would have continued operating, and managed to retain major market shares, even when faced with competition from Mexico.

Prohibition is another explanation for displacement. In the 1960s, the UN, under US auspices, pushed for a curtailment of the production and sale of heroin, cocaine, synthetic drugs, and cannabis products. In the early 1970s, new legal provisions strengthened the global prohibition regime. Washington forced other countries to implement the ban, albeit selectively, as shown above. Prohibition stimulated the illicit drug business and constantly attracted new producing regions and entrepreneurs. Thus, US-led prohibition created dynamics on drug markets at the time when the Nixon administration put pressure on France and Turkey. However, it is unlikely that in the absence of the initiative, the restructuring of the drug economy would have occurred in the way it did. Although many more countries would probably have begun producing and exporting drugs since prohibition offered significant income opportunities for peasants and traffickers alike, Turkey as an opium producer and the French Connection as a trafficking network were too well entrenched to be quickly replaced by competing drug producing countries and trafficking networks

According to another explanation, the Nixon initiative was less of a contributing factor for displacement than the increase in international trade, finan cial transactions, and the movement of people.[13] During the 1970s, new transport and communication technologies enabled, and resulted from, more economic interdependence, and governments found it increasingly difficult to manage the international political economy. These changes were not only beneficial to market participants trading in licit goods, but also to drug smugglers. Thus, one could say that even in the absence of US pressure on Turkey and the French

Connection, the importance of Turkey and the French Connection as a US heroin supplier would have decreased anyway.

However, this explanation is plausible only at first sight. Even though the drug industry would have been in flux even without the Nixon initiative, displacement would have occurred slower and along different geographical lines than actually happened. Although other trafficking groups might have begun to operate alongside the French Connection, the Connection would probably have maintained its grip on the US heroin market. This is because an efficient and effective trafficking network cannot be established overnight. Moreover, in the absence of the US-sponsored Turkish poppy ban, Turkey would probably have remained an important opium source. After all, the Turkish opium industry, as well as the trafficking network needed to transport opium to laboratories, process it into morphine and heroin, and transport it to the US, were well established. Even though more international economic interaction would probably have increased Southeast Asian and Mexican drug supplies anyway, displacement would probably have been slower if Turkey had continued producing poppy. Southeast Asia and Mexico were ideally placed to fill the gap left by the Mediterranean heroin pipeline, but in the absence of this gap, it is likely that they would have remained suppliers of secondary rank for some time.

Another alternative explanation must be considered. Henrik Krüger argues that officials of the Nixon administration or shadowy figures backing the administration destroyed the French Connection to allow the Connection's competitors to fill the gap. Krüger is circumspect in advancing his ideas. Admitting that evidence is scarce in the realm of intelligence and crime, he proposes several possible causal pathways. Although his analysis is not rigorously scientific, as indicated by the tabloid newspaper style that marks his book, some arguments are plausible, including the argument that some individuals benefited from the dismantlement of the French Connection. If there were any truth to this conspiracy theory (not all conspiracies are fictitious), the displacement of the drug industry would not have been a side effect of US foreign drug policy, but rather the intended main outcome of a political plan.

Discussing Krüger's hypotheses is a research project in its own right, and no attempt shall be made here to disentangle the web of names, places, and organizations mentioned in his book. However, Krüger probably overestimates the planning capacities (not to mention the criminal energy) of US policy-makers. Even though some individuals may have benefited from the French Connection's demise, and even though some of these may have been close to the Nixon administration, it is unlikely that an international network of traffickers, intelligence agents, politicians, and others would have been able to implement a complex strategy over a period of several years. Although the drug industry can be restructured by design, it is unlikely that political engineering was behind the numerous political, military, economic, and social developments that led to the displacement of the drug industry in the early 1970s.

Conclusion

This chapter set out to understand and explain the displacement of the illicit drug industry in the early 1970s. During this period, illicit poppy cultivation, opium and heroin production, and drug trafficking decreased in the Mediterranean and increased in Southeast Asia and Mexico. The US government wanted to force Turkey to stop poppy cultivation, since much of the crop was reportedly diverted for illicit heroin production destined for the US market. Moreover, the US put increasing pressure on the French government to curtail the activities of the Corsican French Connection. Although the Connection was active in many countries, its center was in Marseille, where it transformed Turkish opium into heroin and from where it smuggled the drug to the US.

The chapter showed that during and after World War II, the US supported criminal elements in Italy and France, whom Washington saw as useful assets in the war effort and the containment of Communism. Not least due to these short-sighted foreign policy decisions, the US was soon confronted with a sophisticated and well-entrenched heroin smuggling network. With the disappearance of the specter of Communism in Western Europe, Corsican criminals became a liability. In an unprecedented law enforcement campaign, security forces from several countries put the once formidable French Connection out of business. Meanwhile, the US also put pressure on Turkey. Dependent on US financia and military support, the Turkish government reduced the number of poppy-cultivating provinces and finally, in 1971, instituted a comprehensive poppy ban. Both the elimination of the French Connection and the Turkish poppy ban were major foreign policy victories for the Nixon administration.

Between 1971 and 1973, the Mediterranean heroin pipeline was destroyed. Simultaneously, the drug industry grew elsewhere. Although Southeast Asian supplies were seen as being on the verge of dominating the US market during that time, the importance of the region as a US heroin supplier quickly declined. Meanwhile, Mexico constantly increased its share of the US heroin market, establishing a near-monopoly from 1975 to 1977. Southeast Asia, a relatively small US supplier in 1974 and 1975, constituted about a third of the US heroin market between 1976 and 1979.

The available data thus indicates that in the case of Mexico, displacement was significant, and that it occurred simultaneously with and after the Nixon initiative against the Mediterranean pipeline. Southeast Asia, on the contrary, had already headed the list of world opium sources at the end of the 1950s, and the Nixon initiative against the Mediterranean heroin pipeline did not coincide with a sudden increase in Southeast Asian opium and heroin production and heroin export.

To better understand and explain displacement, the discussion then turned to the initial causal mechanism. US policy-making was characterized by a high degree of selectivity. The US put pressure on Turkey and France, but made only small efforts to reduce drug production and trafficking in Southeast Asia and Mexico. In Southeast Asia, US drug policies were sacrificed to the fight against Communism, which forged alliances of convenience between poppy-cultivating groups, drug entrepreneurs, and US agents. Only after the drug industry had shifted away from its traditional transatlantic route, bringing increasing drug loads from Southeast Asia and Mexico to the US, did the Nixon administration respond. Under pressure from the US public and Congress, the administration increased its drug control efforts in Southeast Asia, thus blocking traffickers access to the US market. As a consequence, traffickers turned their attention to Western Europe and Australia. And in Mexico, a joint US–Mexican eradication program significantly reduced drug supplies during the second half of the 1970s

Traffickers proved highly innovative in their attempts to survive economically and physically. *La Cosa Nostra*, the Chiu chao, Southeast Asian government officials involved in illicit activities, and the French Connection grabbed every opportunity to retain or increase their drug market shares, sometimes foreseeing the disruption of the Mediterranean supply chain. The French Connection was unable to survive strong US law enforcement pressure despite an anticipation of an eventual closure of the Mediterranean heroin pipeline and attempts to expand activities in Southeast Asia. There were enough competitors, however, to fill the gap. These competitors benefited from Southeast Asian governmental collusion in the trade, US support to groups involved in the traffic, and the US adventure in Vietnam. Moreover, drug entrepreneurs reinforced the position of Mexico as a convenient place for US-bound trafficking

Weak law enforcement is an additional factor for explaining the displacement of the drug industry from the Mediterranean to Southeast Asia and Mexico. Drug production and trafficking can be curbed when governments control the national territory, when they have the means and the will to take action against traffickers and farmers, when drug control is not hampered by inter-agency disputes, when drug revenues do not constitute a large share of the national economy, when public disapproval of drugs is deeply anchored in a society, and when corruption is not pandemic. These conditions were partly given in Turkey and France, but not in Southeast Asian countries and Mexico, at least not at the time of Nixon's Mediterranean initiative. Moreover, an inaccessible terrain, rural poverty, and other conditions prevailing in Southeast Asian countries and Mexico were conducive to drug industry displacement as well.

Lastly, contingent conditions matter. Turkey stopped opium production and France stopped heroin exports, not least due to a change of government in both countries, and Hong Kong's drug market benefited from Mao's victory in the Chinese civil war, which led to the resettlement of criminals from Shanghai to Hong Kong. In addition, many background conditions, ranging from weak anti-drug norms to poverty and migration, enabled the displacement of the drug economy to Southeast Asia and Mexico. Yet the most important contingency was the US military engagement in Southeast Asia. In the 1950s, CIA activities helped transform the region into the world's foremost producer of opium. In the 1960s, the large-scale US military involvement in Vietnam transformed the opium economy into a heroin economy. In the early 1970s, the withdrawal of US troops from Vietnam was paralleled by a rise of heroin exports from Southeast Asia to the US mainland.

Thus, US pressure on Turkey and the French Connection was not the only reason for the boom of the Southeast Asian drug industry. Insofar as the boom was a result of US policies, it was the presence of US troops in Vietnam, and their withdrawal, that served as a catalyst for Southeast Asia's evolution from a prime opium producer into a major heroin supplier. Hence, international drug markets were already in a turbulent state before the closure of the Mediterranean heroin pipeline.

While contingent conditions make theorizing difficult, empirical black boxes and alternative explanations further complicate matters. It is unclear how much of the heroin coming from Mexico into the US was actually produced in Mexico, who transported the heroin into the US, and who had transformed Mexico into a hub of drug production and trafficking in the first place. Similarly, little is known about Asian trafficking networks, and even the relatively well-documented Turkey–Marseille–US heroin pipeline remains mysterious. It is uncertain, for example, whether much of the opium processed into heroin in Marseille actually came from Southeast Asia rather than from Turkey.

In addition, there are several alternative explanations for the displacement of the drug industry. One could argue that it was merely a coincidence that the Mexican drug boom occurred after the Nixon initiative against Turkish poppy and the French Connection, and that Mexico would have conquered the US heroin market anyway. However, the Mediterranean heroin pipeline, even though under pressure from Southeast Asia, was well-established, and probably would have continued to function if it had not been for US pressure on Turkey and the French Connection. In the absence of the Nixon initiative, Mexican-based traffickers would have found it much more difficult to dominate the US market.

Assessing the impact of US foreign drug policy on international drug markets is also complicated by the fact that in the 1960s and 1970s, many countries introduced prohibition laws and began implementing them, which put the drug economy into a state of flux. To be sure, prohibition would have led to the displacement of drug production, trafficking, and consumption, as well as increasing drug-related problems even in the absence of the Nixon initiative. However, it is likely that displacement would have occurred along different spatial and temporal paths if it had not been for US pressure on Turkey and the French Connection.

Similarly, one could argue that an increase in international economic transaction and the free movement of people in the 1970s would have led to a dispersion of drug production and trafficking even if the US had not engaged in major drug supply reduction efforts. There can be no doubt that greater economic interdependence was beneficial for drug entrepreneurs and contributed to the spreading of drugs and drug-related problems to countries formerly unaffected by these phenomena. However, if it had not been for the Nixon initiative, the French Connection would have probably continued to retain major market shares, and Turkey would probably have continued to function as a major illicit drug supplier. Displacement would have occurred, but along different temporal and spatial lines, and not as visibly and fast as was the case.

The last alternative explanation referred to above pertains to the domestic motives behind the Nixon initiative. As Henrik Krüger argues, the displacement of the drug industry was no foreign policy accident, but designed by an international conglomerate of criminals, intelligence agents, government officials and politicians. While it is possible that vested interests played a role in the destruction of the Mediterranean heroin pipeline, one should not overestimate the ability of a network to implement such a huge and complex scheme clandestinely over several years. It is unlikely that the shift of the drug industry to Southeast Asia and Mexico was purely the result of a conscious plan. Deliberately changing the structure of the global drug industry is arguably too great a task even for a sophisticated conspiracy network. Drug markets are highly complex and dynamic, and thus respond to input in unforeseen ways.

Understanding and explaining the displacement of the illicit drug industry is thus a complex endeavor. Yet two things are obvious. First, states and individuals suffered from displacement. Second, US drug policies in the early 1970s contributed to spreading drug production, trafficking, consumption, as well as violence and corruption, around the globe. Paul Stares (1996: 28) writes that "during the period from 1974 to 1988 there was an explosive worldwide growth in the production and trafficking of virtually all types of illicit drugs." Alfred McCoy attributes this effect first and foremost to US drug policies. His writings were often cited in this chapter. He shall have the last word as well.

> Despite its initial success, Nixon's drug war thus produced a paradoxical strengthening of the global narcotics traffic. By the late 1970s the simplex of the Turkey–Marseille–New York heroin pipeline had been replaced by a complex of international smuggling routes that tied the disparate zones of First World consumption to Third World narcotics production. With production and consumption now dispersed around the globe, the international narcotics traffic was far more resistant to suppression than before
>
> (McCoy 1991: 396)

3 Targeting smugglers flying over the Andes

The 1990s

Introduction

In the 1970s and early 1980s, the US was mainly concerned about heroin and marijuana. But in the mid-1980s, the focus shifted to cocaine. The US government declared a "war on drugs" at home and in Latin America, where cocaine came from. One could argue that speaking of a war on drugs makes as much sense as speaking of a war on drink driving or on AIDS. However, the metaphor is not completely unsuitable because the US armed forces have become involved in a low-level conflict since the mid-1980s that has escalated over the years and has cost many lives on all sides.

This chapter focuses on one aspect of US supply reduction efforts that has not been widely studied to date: the Air Bridge Denial Program (ABDP). One of the program's aims was to prevent traffickers from transporting coca paste from Peru and Bolivia to Colombia on small aircraft for refinement into cocaine. To disrupt this air bridge, the US cooperated with Andean states in the detection of airstrips and airplanes, the arrest of traffickers, and the interdiction of suspicious planes. Until 1995, the ABDP was only implemented sporadically. The program was then improved and possibly led to the seizure and shoot-downs of dozens of planes. However, while pressure on traffickers grew, coca cultivation increased in Colombia and decreased in Peru and Bolivia, and traffickers found new smuggling routes and methods. Aerial interdiction was suspended in 2001 after the Peruvian air force accidentally shot down a small aircraft carrying a US missionary family. By that time, Colombia was the world's uncontested producer of coca.

The fact that Colombian coca cultivation increased and that, more generally, the structure of the South American coca/cocaine industry became more complex during the implementation of the ABDP raises the question of whether there is a causal link between the ABDP and the displacement of the drug industry.

US perceptions and politics

In his bid for the US presidency, Ronald Reagan benefited from a widespread public concern about drugs. Many conservative Americans saw drug problems as symptomatic of a decline in family, community, and religious values, and they hoped that Reagan would re-establish moral order. In September 1981, Reagan emphasized his administration's determination to reduce drug problems as part of an overall strategy against a "crime epidemic" (quoted in Carpenter 2003: 19). In June 1982, his rhetoric became more militant. Standing in the Rose Garden of the White House, Reagan said: "We're taking down the surrender fla that has flown over so many drug efforts. We're running up the battle flag. We can fight the drug problem, and we can win" (quoted in Bertram *et al.* 1996: 112).

To increase coercion, the White House implemented several measures. Reagan ordered the CIA and other federal agencies to participate in drug control, amended the *Posse Comitatus Act* to enable the military to assist civilian agencies in drug control, pushed drug bills through Congress, and skillfully employed the media in a public relations campaign against drugs. Nancy Reagan toured the country and advised people to "Just Say No" to drugs. In the early stages of the campaign, policy-makers and the US public saw marijuana as the most worrisome drug. One of the conservative pressure groups supporting Reagan was a parent's movement concerned about marijuana consumption. Indeed, in the early 1980s, an estimated 20 million people in the US smoked marijuana. Yet there were also three to five million cocaine users (Carpenter 2003: 19–20). In his public relations campaign, Reagan tried to draw people's attention to cocaine. The media was not unresponsive to this campaign. Newspapers and television stations carried more and more stories about cocaine smuggling operations.

Increased cocaine trafficking was due, among other factors, to the entry of new traffickers into the market. Until the late 1970s, most cocaine trafficker were daring individuals who transported small quantities of drugs from Latin America to the US. Since then, ruthless and sophisticated Colombian trafficker had risen to prominence. These transformed Latin America's cocaine industry into the region's "only successful multinational" company, as the former Peruvian president Alan García once said (quoted in Lee 1989: 195). Journalist Michael Massing (2000: 165) vividly describes the situation in the early 1980s:

> [T]he Colombian narcos had developed a [cocaine] pipeline into the United States that, in terms of capacity and sophistication, made the old French Connection look like a capillary. Extending more than 2,500 miles, from the coca-rich highlands of Peru's Upper Huallaga Valley to the dirt airstrips of Florida, the network employed thousands of growers, chemists, pilots, couriers, communication specialists, accountants, bodyguards, spies, bribe payers, and money launderers, all coordinated from the great traffickin centers of Medellín and Cali. In the face of all this, U.S. drug agents were hopelessly outmatched. The Colombians were so effective at moving cocaine into the United States, in fact, that its price began to drop. And drop, and drop. And, as it did, the market for it would grow and grow. The result would be a dramatic transformation of the American drug world.

With supplies increasing and prices falling, cocaine was no longer a drug for the elite. In the 1970s, the drug's high price meant that use was mainly confine to the affluent classes. In the early 1980s, the user-spectrum became larger and now included high school students and also disadvantaged inhabitants of the US inner cities. These were particularly drawn to crack, a smokable cocaine derivative. In November 1985, the *New York Times* ran its first alarming story about crack (Reinarman and Levine 1994: 56). The low price of crack, as well as innovative marking strategies by dealers, made it the drug of choice for a consumer population that was mainly black or Hispanic, young, and poor. Since crack made some consumers behave violently, middle-class Americans were soon haunted by the specter of a crime wave that would ultimately affect everyone.

On June 19, 1986, 22-year-old US basketball superstar Len Bias died of a cardiac arrest after taking cocaine at a party, in an incident that had significan repercussions. Suddenly, cocaine replaced marijuana as the drug that aroused most public concern in the US, and cocaine control became a central US domestic and international policy objective (Gray 1998: 107–108). Now, the authorities could no longer ignore the fact that a large number of US citizens consumed cocaine and crack. The cocaine scare certainly took US agencies by surprise. On July 15, 1986, a senior DEA official admitted in a Congressional hearing that the agency had only begun to collect statistics on the availability, price, and purity of cocaine the week before (Massing 2000: 182).

Despite insufficient knowledge about cocaine, the administration, as well as Republican and Democratic policy-makers in Congress, hoped for quick solutions. Hence, several anti-drug measures were instituted. One of these, the drug-free workplace program, included drug testing. In August 1986, the president, vice president, and 78 other White House officials urinated into bottles, and in the campaign for the Congressional elections in November 1986, candidates challenged their rivals to take drug tests (Massing 2000: 183–184). More serious than these publicity stunts was new legislation passed by Congress. The Anti-Drug Abuse Act was signed into law in October. It significantly increased spending on law enforcement and the construction of prisons. The bill also introduced mandatory minimum sentences for drug sales. In the field of drug control, US policy-makers suddenly became very active.

Policy-makers' focus on coercive, supply-oriented strategies instead of non-coercive, demand-oriented strategies had domestic and international implications. Domestically, the Reagan years were marked by a stiffening of sanctions and a deterioration of public drug treatment facilities (Courtwright 2001: 175). Internationally, the search for quick solutions to drug problems led to spectacular foreign policy initiatives. In July 1986, the administration sent around 160 army personnel, six Black Hawk helicopters, and equipment to Bolivia. In the framework of the four-month Operation Blast Furnace, US personnel cooperated with Bolivian security forces in the destruction of cocaine laboratories in the Beni and Santa Cruz regions and in the arrest of traffickers (Mendel 1992). In spring 1987, the US launched another anti-drug campaign, Operation Snowcap.

Operation Blast Furnace, Operation Snowcap, and subsequent operations, which are described in further detail below, put the Andean governments in a difficult position. Blast Furnace, for example, led to an outburst of anger in Bolivia and almost caused the downfall of the country's government, whose willingness to give in to US demands was encapsulated in President Paz Estenssoro's January 1986 remark to US Ambassador Edward Rowell: "Mr. Ambassador, you can do anything you want to do!" (quoted in Menzel 1996: 16). Concerns about US infringement on the sovereignty of US "host nations" were aggravated by the fact that US forces sometimes assumed an operational role, giving orders to the Andean forces they had helped to create, equip, and train. US officials insisted that their role was a supporting one, "but it is quite clear that they call the shots," as one observer described the situation in Bolivia (Painter 1994: 81).

US policy-makers were not so much concerned about the sovereignty of other countries but rather about the inefficiency of anti-drug operations. Despite frequent tactical successes, the strategic objective of improving US drug problems was not reached. When fields were eradicated, labs destroyed, and trafficker arrested, the drug industry recovered, within days or months. International drug strategies seemed to have no effect on the availability, price, and purity of cocaine in the US.[1]

One should not exaggerate the increase in drug problems in the 1980s. As the previous chapter showed, drug problems are to a certain degree constructed by policy-makers and the public. Hyperbole is never far when drugs are discussed, whereas rational deliberation often is. The problem of discussing drug problems rationally is compounded by the fact that many aspects of the clandestine nature of drug trafficking do not lend themselves to systematic empirical analyses and, consequently, lead to a lack of knowledge about the true dimension of drug problems. Nevertheless, the US really did experience serious drug-related problems. According to a 1988 Senate report, 60 percent of all illicit drugs produced globally were consumed in the US. Nearly six million people in the US used cocaine regularly. Between 1983 and 1987, cocaine-related hospital emergency admissions rose nearly 600 percent, with cocaine-related deaths rising from under 400 in 1983 to nearly 1,400 in 1987. Moreover, 70 percent of all violent crime in the US might have been drug-related. Between 1980 and 1988, the US street price of a kilogram of cocaine decreased from $60,000 to around $9,000. Whereas in 1982, 31 metric tons of cocaine coming into the US were seized, this number had risen to 72.3 metric tons in 1985. In addition, the report estimated that cocaine consumption led to an annual financial loss in productivity of $100 billion (Congress 1988: 8–9).

Some developments were positive as well. Most importantly, casual cocaine consumption declined during the second half of the 1980s. The death of basketball star Bias probably played a role, since it changed the way some Americans thought about drug use. Moreover, the lifestyles of many Americans were changing. On average, people smoked less, ate healthier food, and were disinclined to take illicit drugs (Massing 2000: 189). Still, the public thought that drug problems were getting worse. Every day, newspapers and TV stations showed pictures of murdered drug dealers, pregnant women supposedly consuming crack cocaine, disfigured "crack babies," and drug users dying from AIDS. The media thus played an important role in the making of the US drug crisis (Reinarman and Levine 1994).

The new US President George Bush responded to these public concerns, among others, by appointing William Bennett as Drug Czar in 1989. A former philosophy professor, Bennett defended the view that drug consumption was a burden to society and a symptom of moral decline (Connolly 1999). As director of the ONDCP, which had been created in 1988 and which was responsible for reducing demand and supply, Bennett rallied policy-makers and the US public behind his coercive stance on drugs. In the first National Drug Control Strategy (NDCS), released in September 1989, the ONDCP proposed an increase in federal drug control spending by 39 percent, to almost $8 billion (Massing 2000: 201). Bush and Bennett sensed that the US public would support coercive anti-drug initiatives since many people were concerned about a reported rise in crime, which had transformed Washington DC into the US city with the highest murder rate.

While Bennett toured the US, Bush quickly elevated drug control to a prime US foreign policy interest. The first NDCS increased spending on international drug control by 80 percent, to $449 million (Massing 2000: 201). It is important to note that official figures often understate the US financial commitment. In the early 1990s, for example, the Department of Defense (DoD) officially spent over $1 billion on drug control per year, up from less than $5 million in 1982 (Bertram *et al.* 1996: 112). However, the real costs probably were even higher since some costs were absorbed in the department's total budget (Howard 2001: 23).

Under the leadership of Secretary of Defense Dick Cheney, the Pentagon became a pivotal drug control actor, despite the opposition of many military planners who saw drug control as a police task and who feared corruption and a detrimental impact on the morale of soldiers. But the military had to give in to pressure from Congress, the White House, and the US public. Moreover, some critics of military involvement changed their views, hoping that drug control funding would help offset cuts in military budgets after the end of the East–West conflict. In 1990, General Maxwell Thurman, head of the US Southern Command, said that the drug war was "the only war we've got" (quoted in Zirnite 1997: 11). The US Navy emphasized that its nuclear-missile equipped Trident submarines could help reduce drug supplies (Zirnite 1997: 11).

In September 1989, Cheney signed a statement that declared drug traffickin and its related problems a threat to US national security and identified drug control as a high-priority mission of the DoD. This step built upon the 1986 National Security Decision Directive 221, in which Ronald Reagan had named drug trafficking as a threat to US national security.[2] On September 5, 1989, Bush showed a bag of cocaine supposedly confiscated near the White House on national TV (later it was revealed that US agents had lured a young dealer, who did not even know where the White House was, into selling it there; see Gordon 1994: 184; Reinarman and Levine 1994: 50–52). Bush promised that he would attack drug problems on all fronts and that the military would play a comprehensive role in the effort.

Bush's rhetoric again revealed the belief in coercion as a solution to drug problems. He said that "all of us agree that the gravest domestic threat facing our nation today is drugs" and proclaimed an "assault on all fronts." Against this "evil," Americans had to stand united. According to Bush, "victory over drugs is our cause, a just cause." He defined the responsibility for drug problems in broad terms: "Who's responsible? Let me tell you straight out. Everybody who uses drugs. Everybody who sells drugs. And everybody who looks the other way." He then explained his policy program: "The rules have changed: if you sell drugs, you will be caught; and when you're caught, you will be prosecuted; and once you're convicted, you will do time. Caught, prosecuted, punished." With regard to international programs, Bush emphasized that he would make US military resources available to counter-drug missions (all quotes from Bertram *et al.* 1996: 115).

Two months before his speech, only 20 percent of the US public saw drugs as the country's most pressing problem. Shortly after the speech, the number soared to 64 percent. Moreover, 82 percent supported military involvement in drug control. It is important to note that some of Bush's statements were tame in comparison to more radical views voiced in what increasingly became a climate of hysteria. Bennett, for example, did not see the beheading of drug traffickers as morally problematic. The chief of the Los Angeles Police proposed to Congress that casual drug users "ought to be taken out and shot." The White House pushed a bill through Congress that made drug trafficking a capital crime. Forty-eight senators agreed with a proposal of a former US Customs chief to shoot down planes merely suspected of carrying drugs (see Bertram *et al.* 1996: 115–116). And Bush spoke of inner city police officers as "freedom fighters (quoted in Dorn and South 1993: 72).

These views helped Bush justify Operation Just Cause, the invasion of Panama with 26,000 troops in December 1989. The invasion's aim was to capture the country's president, Manuel Noriega, who was wanted in the US on charges of drug trafficking. Brought to the US, a Florida court sentenced Noriega, a long-time CIA informant who later had become inconvenient to Washington, to an extended prison term.

Simultaneously, a drug drama of unprecedented scale unfolded in Colombia. From the mid-1980s on, the country witnessed a surge in drug-related violence. In 1984, traffickers from Medellín assassinated Justice Minister Rodrigo Lara Bonilla, a prominent figure in the fight against drugs. Over the following years, the war between government forces and traffickers escalated. Hundreds of offi cials and bystanders lost their lives. Nobody seemed to be beyond the reach of the *narcos*, as shown by an assassination attempt on the Colombian ambassador to Hungary in Budapest in 1987. The victim, who was gravely injured, had previously served as minister of justice and had been given the diplomatic post for his protection. One factor fueling the violence was the US demand to extradite traffickers to the US. Extradition was the worst scenario for traffickers since bribing one's way out of prison was possible in Colombia, but not in the US. Traffickers thus did everything to prevent the government from yielding to US pressure. Yet some traffickers did end up in the US, including the flamboyan Carlos Lehder, who in the 1970s had invented the method of transporting drugs on small aircraft to the US. Former US Attorney and Chief Prosecutor Robert Merkle said that "Lehder was to cocaine trafficking what Henry Ford was to automobiles" (quoted in Filippone 1994: 325). Once in the US, Lehder received a life sentence plus 135 years.

On August 18, 1989, the Medellín group assassinated presidential candidate Luis Galán, who had advocated strong measures against traffickers, including their extradition to the US, despite an announcement by the traffickers that they would kill ten judges for every extradited suspect. This murder galvanized Colombian public opinion into action against Medellín-based Pablo Escobar. The government mobilized significant police, military, and judicial resources, which led to the arrest of many suspects and the confiscation of their property. Escobar's declaration of war came swiftly. In the four months following Galán's death, Escobar's men carried out 250 bombing attacks, including one on a civilian aircraft in which all 107 passengers died. The government, in turn, extradited suspects to the US and succeeded in shooting dead Medellín trafficker José Rodríguez Gacha in late 1989. Offers made by the traffickers to negotiate an end of hostilities were turned down by the administration of Virgilio Barco. In 1991, after the new Gaviria administration had confiscated a record amount of cocaine, the traffickers intensified their terror campaign by kidnapping and killing journalists, judges, and other real or potential adversaries. Judges now had to wear hoods in the courtroom so that traffickers could not identify them

US support came in the form of a $65 million emergency aid package offered days after the Galán murder, as well as a large-scale anti-drug program, the $2.2 billion Andean Initiative. The aim of this initiative was to improve the law enforcement capacities of the Andean states and to reduce the drug flow into the US by 60 percent over ten years (Isacson 2005: 23; Perl 1992). But besides helping the country, the Bush administration also put unilateral pressure on Colombia. In 1990, for example, it announced its intention to send a US aircraft carrier (!) and a frigate to Colombia's coast as part of an anti-drug blockade. Bogotá protested against this violation of the country's sovereignty (Menzel 1997: 78; Crandall 2002a: 35).

The traffickers' strategy of escalation increased public pressure on the government to do what it had vowed not to do after the murder of Galán: negotiate. While the traffickers demanded that the government did not give in to US pressure to extradite suspects, the government demanded that the traffickers end the violence and surrender. An agreement was reached, and Escobar moved into a luxurious prison that he had helped to construct, where he received guests, and from which he continued to organize his deals. Anticipating his transfer to another prison, Escobar escaped in the summer of 1992. The government, ridiculed once more, staged a manhunt that lasted for more than 15 months. With the help of US intelligence and also Cali traffickers, many of which had

had lost friends and family members to Escobar's *sicarios* (assassins), a special military and police unit arrested and killed many of Escobar's lieutenants and followed his moves. Acting upon US intelligence, which had intercepted a phone call made by Escobar to his son, security forces killed Escobar on a Medellín rooftop on December 2, 1993, to the relief of Colombia and the US (Bowden 2001). By that time, Escobar's once formidable cocaine empire had already fallen apart. The rival Cali group now controlled most of the air, river, and land trafficking routes, cocaine laboratories, coca fields, and foreign cocaine markets.

Colombia was not the only country that caused concern in the US. In Peru, the Maoist *Sendero Luminoso* (Shining Path) rebel movement asserted its authority in the country's prime coca-growing region, the Massachusetts-sized Upper Huallaga Valley, in 1983 (Riley 1996: 114). Over the following years, the Shining Path ruthlessly murdered peasants who refused to plant coca or whom it suspected of collaborating with the state, "taxed" drug sales, and killed or bribed Peruvian officials. Among the many violent acts, some stand out, such as the murder of 19 members of a US-funded coca eradication team in November 1984. Moreover, the rebels cooperated with Colombian traffickers who bought coca paste and flew it to Colombia for processing into cocaine. For the protection of airstrips against the Peruvian security forces, the traffickers paid the Shining Path handsomely. As in Colombia, the rebel–trafficker alliance in Peru was more tactical than strategic, and it was occasionally interrupted by violence. Nevertheless, it heightened a sense of insecurity among US policy-makers and increased the popularity of the narco-guerilla paradigm. This paradigm had been invented by the US ambassador to Colombia, Lewis Tambs, in the 1980s. It implied that rebels received significant funding from drug trafficking (Youngers 2001: 12–14; Tickner 2003: 79–80).

While the US demanded that the Peruvian government attack the drug trade and the guerilla simultaneously, Peruvian policy-makers and particularly the military saw that campaigns against coca growers broadened the support base of the Shining Path (Palmer 1992; McClintock 1988). To the dismay of Washington, drug control was therefore half-hearted or not undertaken at all, with the military imposing tight limits on the activities of coca eradication and police forces in the coca growing zones, and even standing by when *Senderistas* launched lethal attacks on the police. Referring to the 250,000 cocaine growers in the country, President Alberto Fujimori said in February 1992: "[N]o government may fight against an entire population" (quoted in Walker 1996: 245). The coercive momentum only increased after the capture of Shining Path leader Abimael Guzmán in September of that year.

Bolivia witnessed astonishing changes as well. In the mid-1980s, the tropical Chapare region experienced a boom in coca cultivation, not least due to an influx of laid-off miners coming down from the Andean plateau. These were a willing labor force, and their work was vital for Bolivian-based cocaine producers and transporters who had the capacity to meet the rising US and also European demand for cocaine. As in Peru, new coca producers supplied Colombian traffickers with huge quantities of coca and coca paste and thus played a crucial role in increasing South America's coca production between 1982 and 1987 more than twofold (Andreas and Youngers 1989: 553). Anti-drug operations contributed to the creation of powerful peasant unions that organized roadblocks and prevented security forces from eradicating their fields. The unions also mobilized Bolivian public opinion against the US and particularly US ambassador Robert Gelbard, whom many activists and researchers saw as acting "like a modern proconsul" (Walker 1993/94: 48).

To defend coca, farmers stressed the importance of coca for Bolivian indigenous culture. Coca had been planted in Bolivia for many centuries and was used for spiritual and medical purposes. Moreover, the country's economy depended on coca. At the end of the 1980s, around a quarter of the economically active Bolivian population were employed in the coca and cocaine economy, and the coca economy created a value equal to all other economic activities in the country (MacDonald 1988: chapter 4; Painter 1994). These factors helped those opposed to coca eradication to portray US pressure on Bolivia as an example of flagrant imperialism. Some also argued that the US used drug problems as a pretext to consolidate its economic, political, and military hegemony in Latin America (Arrieta *et al.* 1993).

Mexico was another trouble spot. As discussed in the previous chapter, US and Mexican authorities together succeeded in reducing poppy cultivation in the 1970s. By the early 1980s, however, Mexican poppy cultivation was again increasing. To make matters worse, the Mexican marijuana industry promised great profits, and Mexico became a prominent transit country for US-bound South American cocaine. New, ruthless trafficking groups emerged who colluded with elements within the Mexican security forces, and possibly even senior policy-makers. US–Mexican confrontations over the drug issue reached a climax in 1985, when traffickers kidnapped DEA agent Enrique Camarena and tortured him to death. US efforts to bring the perpetrators to justice revealed the extent of corruption in Mexico. Mutual recriminations between the two countries over the following years reached another crisis point in 1990, when the DEA sponsored the kidnapping of Mexican doctor Humberto Alvarez Machain, who was suspected of having been involved in the Camarena affair. Brought to the US and tried in a Los Angeles court, Alvarez was acquitted in 1993. The affair hardened both the Mexican view that the US was imperialist, and the US view that drug lords dominated Mexican politics. Alvarez' lawyer, speaking to the press, expressed the Mexican view as follows: "If Mexico came into [the United States] and kidnapped a U.S. citizen, I can guarantee you two divisions of American troops would be occupying Mexico City today" (quoted in Chepesiuk 1999a: 78).

Drug problems in Colombia, Peru, Bolivia, and Mexico illustrate a general trend. From the mid-1980s, drug problems seem to have increased in the Western Hemisphere, leading to a greater US commitment to address the problem. US policy-makers were concerned about the possible involvement of Nicaragua's leftist *Sandinista* government in drug-trafficking activities. They also accused the Cuban government of drug smuggling. Many people shared the view expressed by Senator Paula Hawkins in a 1985 Senate hearing that Cuban and Nicaraguan leaders wanted to "destroy American youth, cripple American society, by flooding our country with drugs" (quoted in Lee 1989: 179). In the Caribbean and elsewhere, the drug economy was seen as destabilizing US allies and as providing US enemies with large sums of money. And, as mentioned above, drug-related problems in the US put pressure on US policy-makers to reduce drug supplies. Concerns about drugs certainly did not prevent US policy-makers from applying pressure selectively.[3] Noriega, who had been a paid CIA informant as early as 1971 (Gilboa 1995/96: 541; Bagley 1988: 170), was safe as long as he was seen as serving Washington's interests. The Reagan administration also supported the Nicaraguan *Contras* despite clear evidence of their involvement in drug trafficking (Scott and Marshall 1991; McCoy 2003: 487–500).

By constructing a perception of drugs as a national security issue and by starting a "war on drugs," US policy-makers adopted coercive, oversimplifie strategies against complex problems. In short, drug problems were personalized, externalized, and linked to other problems (Friesendorf 2001: 71–74). They were personalized since "cartel bosses" and peasants were blamed for drug problems, instead of taking into account societal disintegration, rural poverty, or other factors in the complex equation of drug demand and supply (Daase 1991: 77). Drug problems were externalized because drug supply was seen as the driving force behind the industry, a perception that obscured the demand factor. Lastly, drug problems were linked to other security issues as US policy-makers saw drug control as essential for containing Communism. This construction of drug problems is essential for understanding Washington's emphasis on coercive, international, anti-supply strategies.

Given the fact that drugs were seen as a threat to US national security, it is surprising that the US spent relatively small sums of money on drug control in the 1980s. Between 1980 and 1987, the budget for international drug control increased threefold (Carpenter 2003: 21), but much more money would have been needed to match the resources of the multi-billion dollar cocaine industry. Generally, US promises to reduce drug supplies were not matched with suffi cient funding (Morales 1989: 150–153). Toward the end of the decade, however, US funding increased significantly. In fact, the "war on drugs" now achieved a self-sustaining momentum. By the late 1980s, at least 58 federal agencies and 74 congressional committees had begun to participate in drug control (Andreas and Youngers 1989: 531). Drug control had thus developed its own institutional dynamic, which contributed to the continuity and even escalation of US drug policy under President Clinton, despite the fact that Clinton had initially wanted to reduce coercion on the national and international level.

> The new administration wanted to deescalate the Reagan and Bush drug wars – to soften the rhetoric, to downsize and streamline the drug war bureaucracy, and to advance a policy that placed greater emphasis on treat-

> ment and prevention. But the drug war legacy Clinton inherited severely limited his prospects for winning even this modest reform without a fight The public had grown accustomed to hearing a get-tough line on drugs and crime; and although the economy had replaced drugs and crime at the top of America's worries, the public was in no mood to be generous toward drug users and dealers. Moral conservatives, mobilized during the Reagan/Bush years, remained organized and vigilant. The sweeping network of drug war laws and institutions, created by former presidents and Congresses, was solidly in place.
>
> (Bertram *et al.* 1996: 117)

The next section focuses on the ABDP. It first examines the question whether the ABDP coincided with displacement. In a second step, it looks at the plausibility of the causal mechanism.

The Air Bridge Denial Program

The ABDP can be divided into an early and a main phase, with the early phase lasting from the late 1980s until 1995 and the main phase lasting from 1995 to 2001. The first question is whether air interdiction was accompanied or followed by the displacement of coca production, coca paste production, and drug smuggling from Peru and Bolivia to Colombia (for maps of South America, Colombia, Bolivia, and Peru see Annex I). Second, the chapter analyses the causal link between the ABDP and new developments of the South American coca/cocaine industry such as an increase in the number of countries producing significan amounts of cocaine, and a dispersion of trafficking routes to countries other than Peru, Bolivia, and Colombia.

The early phase

To produce cocaine, drug entrepreneurs need cocaine base paste (*pasta básica de cocaina*). Coca paste is made from mashed coca leaves and chemical products and is mainly produced at or near the coca growing sites. This reduces costs, since significant amounts of leaves are needed for producing coca paste (300–500 kilograms of high-alkaloid coca leaves equal around 2.5 kilograms of *pasta básica*). Until the mid-1990s, most of the world's coca grew in Bolivia and Peru, whereas most of the cocaine refinement occurred in Colombia. Colombian traffickers came to Bolivia and Peru to buy coca paste from peasants or middlemen and brought it back to Colombia for processing into cocaine and eventual export, primarily to the US. Thus, a division of labor evolved whereby Bolivia and Peru specialized in the production of coca leaves and coca paste and Colombia in the production and export of cocaine. Although some cocaine was produced in Peru and Bolivia, and some coca was cultivated in Colombia (Filippone 1994: 329), the drug business was largely structured along these lines.

Some of the Peruvian and Bolivian coca paste was brought to Colombia on rivers by boat and by truck or carried across land routes. But the most common means of transport was by small aircraft. Traffickers had thus established a drug-trafficking air bridge. The main goal of the ABDP was to destroy this air bridge and thereby reduce US cocaine problems. Moreover, the program aimed at preventing smugglers from transporting cocaine from Colombia to the transit zones near the US borders. This chapter focuses on the program's first element, i.e. the attempt to block drug smuggling from Bolivia and Peru to Colombia. This is done for the sake of analytical parsimony. It does not imply that transit zone interdiction was unimportant. Indeed, given the size of drug smuggling in the transit zone, this strategy component was pivotal to US international drug control efforts. In 1992, it was estimated that some 1,300 to 3,000 suspected smuggling aircraft flew out of Colombia to bring drugs closer to US consumers (Menzel 1997: 113).

The ABDP was based on several assumptions. By preventing traffickers from transporting coca paste from Bolivia and Peru to Colombia, coca farmers in the first two countries would see their customers disappear. This would lead to the disappearance of Bolivian and Peruvian local trafficking structures and a drop in coca prices. On the Colombian side, Colombian cocaine manufacturers would have less raw material for producing cocaine. As a consequence, less cocaine would be produced, and this reduction of supply would translate into a shortage of cocaine on the US market, a rise in cocaine prices, and a decrease in purity, all of which would lead to a reduction of US cocaine consumption. As mentioned in the first chapter, this logic is flawed, not least because most value is added to drugs in drug consuming countries and not in producing and transit countries.

Many actors were involved in the implementation of the ABDP. In Latin America, military, police, and intelligence forces participated in the effort, with Colombian, Peruvian, and Bolivian forces playing the principal role. On the US side, various institutions contributed their resources. The General Accounting Office reported in 1998 that "more than 20 federal or federally funded organizations, spread across five cabinet level departments and two cabinet level organizations, have a principal role in collecting and/or producing counterdrug intelligence" (quoted in Roncken 1999: 26). Agencies involved in the ABDP included the CIA, the DEA, the FBI, the Coast Guard, and institutions operating under the direction of the DoD such as the Joint Interagency Task Force South, the Defense Information Agency, the Office of Naval Intelligence, the National Mapping and Imagery Agency, and the National Security Agency (General Accounting Office (GAO 1998a: 7))

The leading role naturally fell to the DoD. The Joint Air Operations Center (JAOC) of the DoD's Southern Command (SOUTHCOM), first based at Howard Air Force Base in Panama and, from 1999, in Key West, Florida, directed and coordinated the efforts of the US Army, Navy, and Air Force. The JAOC was created in 1992 after the Peruvian air force shot down a US military aircraft over Peru (see below). It played a crucial role in the implementation of the ABDP by monitoring the gigantic airspace over South America and the Central American transit zone. Although this was an enormous challenge, sophisticated technology enabled the US to track the movement of planes flyin between the Bolivian city of Santa Cruz and Florida (Fabricio 1997).

The complex task of implementing the ABDP in many countries, the need to gather complementary intelligence, and attempts by Andean governments to protect their countries' sovereignty, forced US officials to cooperate closely with Andean states. Thus, the JAOC hosted Latin American military liaison officer and let them participate in US drug surveillance flights. Further, when these flights crossed national frontiers, a military officer of the country whose airspace was used sat in the airplane (Roncken 1999: 26). And when the decision was taken to shoot down suspected traffickers, the lethal action was carried out by the armed forces of the respective Latin American country.

To cover the large areas of the Western Hemisphere, the JAOC received data and analyses from several sources. These include intelligence airplanes of the C-130, P-3 Orion, and E-3 Sentry Airborne Warning and Control System (AWACS) types, which extended the coverage of ground radar stations and provided a real-time intelligence link to the air forces of Andean states. These forces then forced down suspicious aircraft flying over the respective national airspace (Mendel and Munger 1997: 118). Moreover, F-16 fighter planes helped to visually identify suspicious aircraft. Additionally, C-130 transport planes and C-27 Spartan refueling planes supported the detection and monitoring effort.

US officials already saw a need to improve the interdiction of traffickin flights during the 1986 Operation Blast Furnace (Howard 2001: 30, fn 41). This operation reportedly achieved a 70 percent decline in coca prices in the production zone (by reducing the number of traffickers buying coca, which in turn reduced peasant income and thus incentives to plant coca). Six months after the end of the operation, however, coca prices reached nearly 90 percent of the pre-Blast Furnace level (Reuter 1994: 217). US officials working in Bolivia at the time of Operation Blast Furnace argued that air interdiction was vital for achieving a sustainable low level of coca prices, since interdiction would cut the link between coca paste purchaser and coca farmers (Roncken 1999: 36). The idea of interdicting aircraft was taken up in 1987 by US Customs Commissioner William Van Raab, who went further and suggested that the US Air Force should be given permission to shoot down suspicious smuggling aircraft that fail to respond to warning signals (McClintock and Vallas 2003: 120).

In the framework of Operation Snowcap, which began in spring 1987 and lasted well into the 1990s, the US developed an integrated militarized approach to reducing drug supplies. Snowcap was implemented in 12 countries, with a focus on Bolivia and Peru. As part of this operation, US Special Forces (Green Berets) provided training to the security forces of the Andean states (Anthony *et al.* 2000: III/31; Chepesiuk 1999b: 177), and helicopters and aircraft supported ground troop action against cocaine laboratories, coca fields, traffickers, and farmers. During the first two years of Snowcap, the US government claimed that 26 aircraft had been seized (Menzel 1996: 44). The US also sponsored the creation of special anti-drugs forces. Already in 1983, Bolivia and Peru had created the police force *Unidades Móviles de Patrullaje Rural* (UMOPAR). Later, Bolivia created the Red Devils (operating in the air), Blue Devils (operating on rivers), and Green Devils (operating on land).

In Peru, seven or eight trafficking groups were active in 1987–1988, with Colombians playing the dominant role. Coca farmers in the Upper Huallaga Valley sold coca paste to buyers who then sold the product to large traffickin groups. These either converted the paste into cocaine in Peru or, more commonly, took it to Colombia for processing. At that time, two to five traffickin aircraft per day landed on clandestine airstrips – often for no longer than ten minutes – picked up between 800 and 2,500 pounds of coca paste, and took off for Colombia. For each flight, traffickers paid the Shining Path between $3,000 and $8,000. Security forces received an equal amount (Menzel 1996: 130–134). Since 1989, the presence of Colombian traffickers from both Cali and Medellín increased, particularly in the Peruvian coca cultivation zones (Menzel 1996: 144–145). They prevented all but a few Peruvians from reaching the higher echelons of the drug business.

The Andean Initiative, announced by George Bush in 1989 and implemented from 1990 onward, channeled significant US funding to Latin American security forces and led to increased air interdiction efforts. In July 1990, the US began to share real-time intelligence about flight activities with Colombia and Peru (Evans 2001a: Overview). In addition, the US trained and equipped Andean military and police forces and gathered intelligence through so-called Tactical Analysis Teams (TATs) consisting of DEA and DoD personnel. Ground-based radar stations complemented intelligence gathered by ground forces and reconnaissance planes, and thus made aerial interdiction more effective. Peru, for example, installed ground radar in the Iquitos area in 1990. And in Colombia, US forces began installing radar facilities in October 1992. Stationed in Leticia, the radar covered an area of 240 miles (Roncken 1999: 27–29). This station was installed and operated by 30 US military officers, five Colombian air force personnel, several radar specialists and a Colombian combat pilot flying a OV-10 Bronco who was given permission to attack suspicious planes coming from the south. Apparently, this radar station spotted a daily average of two planes carrying possibly up to two tons of coca paste. From September 1992, a similar radar station was installed in an Indian reservation. The installation and operation of these radar stations was accompanied by a series of lawsuits motivated by concerns of Colombian citizens that the stations undermined Colombia's sovereignty and contributed to deforestation and pollution.

In 1991, the CIA and SOUTHCOM installed additional radar facilities and continued to do so during the following years with the installation of ground radar in Yurimaguas in 1992 and Pucallpa in 1995 (McClintock and Vallas 2003: 120). These stations helped to detect flight patterns in the tri-border area with Colombia and Brazil. The Peruvian air force supported the effort by deploying Tucanos, Machis, A-37, and Camberra military aircraft. Until 1994, the Peruvian anti-drug effort was centered at the military base at Santa Lucía in the Upper Huallaga Valley, the country's prime coca region and a stronghold of the Shining Path. In 1995, the equipment was moved to Pucallpa in the Ucayali basin.

Obtaining information about air interdiction in Ecuador is particularly diffi cult. "In the Ecuadorian case, confusion and denial reigns among official anti-drug agencies as to the operations or even existence of the radar installations" (Roncken 1999: 27). According to researchers working for Acción Andina and the Transnational Institute, a ground-based radar of the TPS-70 type was installed in the northwest of Quito and became operational in 1993 (Roncken 1999). Other radar facilities were possibly installed as well, including one near the Colombian border that was run by 30–40 US military personnel. The fact that apparently only US officials operated these radar stations again raised questions about the ability of Andean states to guard their sovereignty.

Bolivia also saw the installation of US ground radar, although much obscurity reigns here as well. In 1990, when the Pentagon announced that it would install radar facilities in the Andean countries, the Bolivian government did not give the permission because of concerns about the country's sovereignty and security. It is possible that facilities were nevertheless installed in the Beni and Santa Cruz departments in 1992. Moreover, in that year the Bolivian military said that radars would be installed in Santa Cruz, Trinidad, and La Paz with the help of the Italian government. In mid-1990s, there were signs that the radar was about to become operational. The role played by US forces in the operation of the radar stations is unclear. Three years later, Bolivian-based US personnel claimed that the US was not involved in the operation of any ground-based radar in Bolivia.

Brazil has traditionally distanced itself from US policies that could compromise its sovereignty. This stance had an impact on Brazil's participation in the ABDP. Brazil approved a shoot-down policy only in 1998 after years of debate and did not implement the policy until 2004. Nevertheless, Brazil participated in drug interdiction. From 1995, the government began to set up an impressive intelligence network, named *Sistema de Vigilância da Amazônia* (SIVAM) to protect the Amazon region from illegal deforestation, gold mining, and drug trafficking, and to mobilize police and military resources (Mora 1996: 136–137; Transnational Institute 2003a: 14). This computerized system, which was inaugurated in 2002, integrates ground-based radar stations, monitoring aircraft, aerostat balloons, and satellites. It covers the entire Amazon Basin. The fact that SIVAM was installed by a US company led to concerns that intelligence could be passed on to the US military. To make sure that this would not happen, only Brazilians were allowed to participate in the operation of the system.

During the early 1990s, the US continued to sponsor several operations whose aim was to destroy the trafficking air bridge. The most important were operations Snowcap, Safe Haven, Ghost Zone, and Support Justice. The exact relationship between these operations is unclear. Many operations were divided into different phases, and different sources provide different chronologies. The present book does not discuss the chronology of these operations in detail. What matters here are the actions taken by the US and Andean states against aerial drug trafficking

In Bolivia, Operation Safe Haven was supported by helicopters and C-130 aircraft. It may have dealt major blows to traffickers, as in June 1991, when Bolivian and US forces raided Santa Ana de Yacuma, a town that was reportedly controlled by three key Bolivian traffickers operating in tandem with Colombian drug entrepreneurs from Cali and Medellín. The raid led to the arrest of 54 suspects, the destruction of 15 cocaine laboratories, and the seizure of 42 aircraft. These aircraft were estimated to be half of all trafficking aircraft operating in Bolivia (Menzel 1996: 57–58). However, it must be noted that this operation and other operations were only temporary setbacks for traffickers

In Peru, the country's air force destroyed airstrips and intercepted suspicious planes. During Operation Support Justice III, which lasted from fall 1991 to spring 1992, Peru intercepted an estimated 55 unscheduled aircraft, forcing most of these planes to land. Six of the 55 planes may have been trafficking planes on their way to Colombia. In their interception mission, the Peruvian air force was supported by US ground radars, AWACs, and P-3 aircraft. The interception strategy was risky, as became clear on July 9, 1991 when the Peruvian air force shot down a civilian aircraft, killing 17 people on board. The Peruvian police was later reported to have stolen the belongings of the dead from the plane wreck (Menzel 1996: 165–166).

In late 1989 and during the first half of 1990, coca prices decreased sharply (Painter 1994: 86). In Bolivia, a drop in prices was followed by a first-time drop in coca cultivation. Observers also saw a reduction in the number of traffickin flights. Whereas before it had been estimated that six smuggling aircraft fle between Bolivia and Colombia every day, the number was now down to six per week. In Peru, trafficking declined from five to six per day to five to six per week (Menzel 1996: 52–53, 156–157). While one could attribute these price changes to the ABDP, other factors such as actions taken by the Colombian government against Medellín traffickers are important as well, as explained further below.

By mid-1992, air smuggling operations continued as before, with an average of 20 trafficking planes flying drug loads from Peru and Colombia every day (Menzel 1996: 75, 165, 170). US planners were also concerned about the fact that Bolivian coca prices recovered in late 1990 and that coca cultivation, after a brief slump, flourished again. The relative stability of the cocaine industry was also indicated by the price, purity, and availability of cocaine on US streets. During 1990, prices increased and purity decreased. But by late 1991, prices and purity had reached former levels (Menzel 1997: 89–90).

During Operation Ghost Zone, which began in March 1992, US and Bolivian forces interdicted trafficking flights to and out of the Chapare and tried to stop precursor chemicals needed for the production of cocaine from being flown into the Chapare (Mendel 1992: 78–79). Ghost Zone formed part of the DEA's "kingpin" strategy whereby the US would apply pressure on major trafficker (on the origins of this strategy, see Nieves 1998). Ghost Zone inconvenienced traffickers but did not stop the incursion of Colombians into Bolivia's coca zones. While the operation was in full swing, Colombian traffickers, benefitin from the partial destruction of Bolivian trafficking networks, made sure that the region supplied sufficient amounts of coca paste and also cocaine. The Colombians paid in cash, thus guaranteeing the dependency of the Bolivian coca industry on Colombian buyers (Menzel 1996: 70–71).

On April 5, 1992, Peru's President Fujimori assumed quasi-dictatorial powers by suspending Peru's constitution, as well as the legislative and judiciary. The US and other countries strongly criticized this *autogolpe* and used sanctions to back up their demands for a return to democracy. Then, on April 24, 1992, Peruvian fighter jets fired at a US Air Force Hercules C-130 surveillance aircraft flying in international airspace. The aircraft was returning to Panama after a counter-drug mission over the Upper Huallaga Valley. One crewman was killed and several injured. The Peruvian pilots were awarded medals and the Peruvian Ministry of Defense sent a $20,000 bill for treating the wounded US airmen, who had landed their damaged plane in Peru, to the US embassy in Lima. In response to the incident, and to put pressure on Fujimori to return to democracy, the US suspended its aerial surveillance operations, the delivery of anti-drug aid, and the training of Peruvian forces for a period of several months. These measures obviously reduced the effectiveness of the air interdiction effort (Youngers 1995: 6; McClintock and Vallas 2003: 118–119; Menzel 1996: 177–178).

Fujimori was surprised by the harsh international response to his coup, a step he saw as the only way to reduce governmental inefficiency and corruption, as well as the threat posed by rebels. Maintaining the momentum, Fujimori dismissed hundreds of allegedly corrupt members of the judiciary, government bureaucracy, and security forces, declared a state of emergency in the Upper Huallaga Valley, and ordered the Peruvian air force to control the region's airports. Moreover, he restructured the army and policy command systems to improve their performance against the Shining Path and the traffickers. In September 1992, US and Peruvian officials agreed on measures to avoid accidental shoot-downs of planes and began another interdiction operation in January 1993 (Operation Support Justice IV).

Meanwhile, the Colombian government undertook air interdiction measures as well. During Operation Support Justice III, which began in autumn 1991 and continued until spring 1992, the Colombian air force used signals provided by ground radar stations near the Colombian–Peruvian border, as well as intelligence from US surveillance aircraft, to interdict suspicious planes. During a one-year period, over 6,000 aircraft were reported, 1,700 of which were seen as suspicious and 42 of which were captured, although only six to ten were reportedly intercepted in the air by the Colombian air force. Interdiction was hampered by legal provisions preventing Colombian security forces from shooting down suspicious aircraft. Sewall Menzel, who served as a US military advisor in South America in the 1980s, describes the consequences of the unclear legal situation: "[D]espite the application of hundreds of millions of dollars in ground based radars, static balloons and airborne radar and support systems to identify, monitor and intercept narcotrafficking aircraft, there was no comprehensive consensus on shooting down or forcing down identified trafficking aircraft" (Menzel 1997: 102).

In November 1992, the US and Colombia began to implement Operation Support Justice IV (Anthony *et al.* 2000: III/29). But 16 months later, US–Colombian intelligence sharing ran into serious problems. On March 2, 1994, Colombian President Gaviria said that security forces would begin shooting down aircraft that had no flight plan, did not respond to radio signals, and refused to land. The Colombian government had informed the US as early as 1990 that it wanted to shoot down smuggling planes, although this would have changed provisions of Colombia's participation in the international aviation Chicago Agreement, which specifically forbids the use of force against civilian aircraft except for self-defense. US officials, fearing that Andean governments would accidentally shoot down civilian aircraft and that US officials would be held responsible, had voiced their concerns. Colombia had nevertheless changed the legal provision, but had not implemented the new policy.

Colombia announced the new policy in March 1994. On May 1, 1994, the Clinton administration stated that the sharing of real-time aerial intelligence data would be suspended. This led to Congressional criticism. One Congressman said that the decision was "the most significant retreat since George Washington retreated from New York during our revolution" (quoted in Crandall 2002a: 38). Another Congressman expressed his disappointment of the US aerial interdiction effort in the Andes as follows:

> Every six months for the last four years I have had to call successive Secretaries of Defense and ask that their intentions to close down these radars be reversed. First it was the Persian Gulf War. The radars are needed in the Middle East. By all means, take them away. Then it took months to get them back. And then six months later, they were needed somewhere else. And then six months later they wanted to close them down again. If indeed the United States Military has reached the point that they want to help and they are committed to fight against narco-trafficking, I will tell you there is precious little evidence of it. I suspect at the moment that such damage has been done to our relationship with Colombia and Peru on narco-trafficking that if the funds are available to you, you're going to have a hard time getting the same degree of cooperation [...]. They did [institute an air intercept/shootdown policy] at the request of members of this Congress, and now to have it shut off humiliates them and I think is a setback that's going to be very difficult to reverse
>
> (Robert Torricelli, D-NJ, quoted in Roncken 1999: 34)

The US decision to suspend the sharing of intelligence about aerial drug smuggling came at a time when the US reviewed its global air operations. Pending a clarification of the legal situation, intelligence-sharing remained suspended. Officials at the Pentagon and Justice Department were concerned that

US staff would be held responsible if US intelligence-sharing led to the shoot-down of aircraft and to the killing of civilians on board. These concerns arose not just from the situation in Latin America, but also from the death of civilians in a military operation in Iraq (McClintock and Vallas 2003: 121).

Many State Department officials, staff in the US embassies in Lima and Bogotá, and members of the US Congress were adamantly opposed to the suspension of intelligence-sharing. They predicted acrimonious reactions from Andean governments and negative repercussions for the US drug control effort (Crandall 2002a: 39). And indeed, the suspension of US intelligence-sharing in 1994 worsened relations between the US and the Andean states. Colombia, for example, reacted angrily to Washington's unilateral decision. Moreover, the drug control effort seemed hampered. Apparently, only four aircraft were seized in Peru in 1994, compared to the 13 claimed in the previous year (McClintock and Vallas 2003: 115 and 121). In Colombia, traffickers now flew more often, carried smaller loads, flew during daytime, and stayed longer on the ground. Hence, they felt more secure (Anthony *et al.* 2000: III/31).

It was only in December 1994 that the situation was clarified. In that month, President Clinton signed legislation that exempted US officials from liability for civilian deaths in interdiction operations against suspected smuggling aircraft, as long as the officials involved had respected specified rules of engagement. This legal clarification paved the way for the renewed interdiction effort from 1995 onward.[4]

Data problems make it difficult to evaluate the ABDP's impact on the drug industry, as shown further below. Yet this challenge notwithstanding, there is no evidence that the program's main aim – a reduction of cocaine supplies and an alleviation of US drug problems – was reached. During the early phase of the ABDP, US cocaine prices were relatively low, cocaine purity increased, and cocaine was widely available (Basov *et al.* 2001: 149; Tokatlián 2003: 24). Although casual cocaine consumption decreased from the mid-1980s, changing social attitudes toward drug consumption and domestic changes in the US, rather than US drug supply programs in the Andes, probably account for the decrease (Roncken 1999: 12).

While the ABDP did not coincide with a reduction of US drug problems, it did coincide with a restructuring of the South American drug industry. More precisely, the ABDP's early phase coincided with decreasing coca cultivation in Bolivia and Peru and increasing cultivation in Colombia (see Annex II, Chart 1 and Table 3). For Colombia, the estimates read as follows: 37,100 hectares cultivated in 1992, 39,700 (1993), 44,700 (1994), and 50,900 (1995). Parallel to this increase in Colombia, Peruvian coca cultivation declined, although the year 1995 saw a brief increase. The hectare estimates for the early 1990s are: 129,100 (1992), 108,800 (1993), 108,600 (1994), and 115,300 (1995). Colombian traffickers thus now no longer specialized exclusively in drug production and trafficking, but also produced coca in Colombia. The production of raw materials reduced traffickers' risks and costs and thus made the Colombian drug industry more efficient

Table 3 Andrean coca cultivation, 1988–2005

	Colombia	*Peru*	*Bolivia*	*Total*
1988	34,000	115,530	48,925	198,455
1989	42,400	121,685	52,900	216,985
1990	40,100	121,300	50,300	211,700
1991	37,500	120,800	47,900	206,200
1992	37,100	129,100	45,500	211,700
1993	39,700	108,800	47,200	195,700
1994	44,700	108,600	48,100	201,400
1995	50,900	115,300	48,600	214,800
1996	57,200	94,400	48,100	199,700
1997	79,500	68,800	45,800	194,100
1998	101,800	51,000	38,000	190,800
1999	122,500	38,700	21,800	183,000
2000	136,200	34,200	14,600	185,000
2001	169,800	34,000	19,900	223,700
2002	144,450	34,700	21,600	200,750
2003	113,850	29,250	23,200	166,300
2004	114,100	27,500	24,600	166,200
2005	144,000	38,000	26,500	208,500

The main phase

As shown above, legal concerns hampered the ABDP during its early phase. The US government was concerned about an accidental shoot-down of a civilian aircraft and liability claims against US personnel. These concerns notwithstanding, the Clinton administration was under pressure from Congress and from some government officials to resume aerial interdiction. In 1995, the administration resolved the legal problem by effectively granting immunity to US personnel involved in the shoot-down of aircraft over the airspace of Andean states. This clarification enabled a resumption of intelligence-sharing between the US and the Andean states and the launching of large-scale operations against suspected smuggler planes. The fact that with the new legislation, which had been sponsored by Senator John Kerry (D-MA), the US "became accessory to a policy in violation of international law and the principle of due process" (Evans 2001b) carried less weight than the hope of interrupting aerial smuggling.

The Clinton administration was now committed to military drug control, not least due to pressure from Congress, which was dominated by the Republicans following the 1994 mid-term elections. The Republicans had strongly criticized Clinton's decision, taken shortly after he had become president, to reduce the ONDCP staff and the budget for drug interdiction especially in the transit zone, following reports saying that international anti-drug programs had failed to curb supplies. Unable to surmount Congressional and agency resistance, and unwilling to lose domestic political points over the drug issue, Clinton presided over a reinvigoration of international efforts, and particularly interdiction operations in South American source countries.

In addition to political changes in the US, developments in Peru also helped to reinvigorate the air interdiction effort. Fujimori's victory in the 1995 elections strengthened his domestic and international legitimacy and made it easier for Washington to cooperate with his administration. The US saw Fujimori's efforts against cocaine as positive and embarked on a course of rapprochement with him and his close aide Vladimiro Montesinos. The close cooperation between the CIA and Montesinos was important for bringing the ABDP back on track (Rojas 2005; McClintock and Vallas 2003: 120–123).

In 1995, the US resumed information-sharing with Andean security forces. Moreover, it installed or made operative ground-based radar stations in Pucallpa (Peru), Tabatinga (Colombia), and possibly elsewhere. Most importantly, the year 1995 saw the implementation of Operation Green Clover. This was directed by SOUTHCOM and formally launched in October. During the operation, 3,000 US military personnel cooperated with their counterparts from Peru, Colombia, Ecuador, Panama, Costa Rica, and Venezuela. In Peru, CIA contractors, flyin in surveillance aircraft owned by the US military, provided information about suspicious flights to the Peruvian air force, which then intercepted the planes. As the interdiction program evolved, more US actors were drawn in, including the DEA, Customs, the National Security Agency, and the CIA (Zirnite 1998: 170–171). This proliferation of actors was not confined to Peru, but a general characteristic of interdiction in South America.

In January 1996, Clinton appointed four-star General Barry McCaffrey as director of the ONDCP. Before taking up this post, McCaffrey, whom many in the US considered a Gulf War hero, had been commander-in-chief of SOUTHCOM in Panama and the central figure behind Operation Green Clover. Clinton's decision was a move against critics accusing him of giving foreign drug control a low priority. Expectations that McCaffrey would reinvigorate the anti-drug effort were proven correct.

US anti-drug aid to Peru increased from $15 million (1995), $19 million (1996), $26 million (1997), $32 million (1998), and $75 million (1999) to $80 million in 2000. In Colombia, things were more difficult than in Peru for Washington. US relations with Colombia were complicated by the US decision to decertify Colombia in 1996 and 1997 after allegations had surfaced that the Samper administration had received funding from Cali traffickers in Samper's 1994 election campaign (see Chapter 4). Nevertheless, Colombia did receive significant funding

In April 1996, the DoD announced the beginning of Operation Laser Strike, the successor program of Operation Green Clover. Nine countries participated in the operation, which combined ground-based radar and detection and monitoring aircraft of the C-130 Hercules, P-3 Orion, and E-3 Sentry AWACS types.[5] US officials saw Laser Strike as a significant improvement over previous operations, not least because aerial interdiction was more effectively coupled with riverine and ground interdiction. Moreover, many countries participated in the effort.[6]

In autumn 1996, McCaffrey said that multilateral air interdiction was operating smoothly:

> Throughout the region, in the past year we have greatly increased our support to host nation interdiction efforts. On any particular day there are about 20 U.S. Coast Guard, Customs, and DOD aircraft involved in source country counter-drug operations. Approximately 300 additional military personnel are deployed in South America supporting Operation Laser Strike. These military personnel operate ground based radar sites in remote Andean locations, fly detection and monitoring aircraft, and provide operational and intelligence support to our allies participating in this regional operation. Our AWACS, P3s, SIGINT (Signals Intelligence), PHOTINT (Photographic Intelligence), and FLIR (Forward Looking Infrared Radar) aircraft all operate in complete prior coordination with regional governments and military authorities.
>
> (Quoted in Roncken 1999: 35–36)

Officials also said that operations Green Clover and Laser Strike had significantly increased the risks for traffickers; that many trafficking aircraft had been forced to the ground or had been shot down; and that pressure on traffickers had reduced the price of coca paste by reducing the number of potential buyers. In a Congressional hearing in September 1996, senior ONDCP official William Bonzin said:

> The results of this multinational, cooperative effort have been stunning. The so-called "air bridge" between Peru and Colombia saw a greater than 50 per cent reduction of flights as aircraft were intercepted and, in some cases, shot down. Approximately 50 narco-trafficking aircraft operating along the Peru/Colombia air bridge have been forced down and seized, or shot down. The cost of shipment has increased fivefold as pilots demand more money as their personal risk increased dramatically. Movement was reduced so drastically that there was a glut of coca base on the market and the price of the product being shipped [from Peru to Colombia] fell by 50 per cent overall and by as much as 80 per cent in some areas.
>
> (Quoted in Roncken 1999: 42)

However, official claims of success must be read cautiously for several reasons. First, it is unclear how many planes were actually intercepted in South America, as discussed further below. Second, air interdiction did not reduce drug problems in the US. During the second half of the 1990s, US cocaine consumption remained stable, and so did US cocaine prices, cocaine purity, and cocaine availability (National Narcotics Intelligence Consumers Committee 1998). As research has shown, price increases in supply zones have little impact on US cocaine prices since most of the value is added to drugs within the US (Rydell and Everingham 1994; Riley 1996). This helps to explain why changes in Latin American coca prices had no impact on the US cocaine market (see also Annex II, Chart 2). The third reason why official claims of success are dubious is the fact that the South American drug industry was undergoing a major restructuring process at the time.

This restructuring process had several facets and indicators. One of these indicators was the fact that coca prices changed. In 1995, coca prices in the Peruvian Upper Huallaga Valley declined. Between January and September 1995, prices fell from $3 to $0.40 per kilogram, and coca base prices from $850 to $100 per kilogram (Jelsma 2002: 9; Roncken 1999: 9). Subsequent price levels are controversial. Some authors write that by early 1996, coca prices were recovering, while others state that prices remained low throughout 1997 and that they did not even cover the costs of production (Roncken 1999: 9; McClintock and Vallas 2003: 126). According to one estimate, a kilogram of coca cost $1.19 in 1995, $0.65 in 1996, and then climbed again to $0.78 (1997), $1.22 (1998), $1.75 (1999), $2.03 (2000), and $2.31 (2001) (Dietrich 2002: 26). Nevertheless, although there is uncertainty when and how much prices changed exactly, it is likely that Peruvian coca prices were low in 1995 and 1996.

Another development that indicated a fundamental restructuring of the South American drug market was a drop in Peruvian coca cultivation and a concomitant increase in Colombian cultivation. Lower Peruvian production levels, which were both a cause and a consequence of low Peruvian coca prices, had already been recorded in the early 1990s, and they were even more remarkable in the second half of the decade. In 1995, 115,300 hectares of coca were planted in Peru. Cultivation then decreased to 94,400 (1996), 68,800 (1997), and to 51,000 hectares (1998) (see Table 3 and Annex II, Chart 1). This represented a decrease of 18 percent (1995), 27 percent (1996), 27 percent (1997), and 26 percent (1998), respectively (Roncken 1999: 9–10). Over the following years, coca cultivation went down further, to 38,700 hectares (1999), 34,200 (2000), and 34,000 (2001). The reduction of Peruvian coca cultivation and coca prices delighted US officials. McCaffrey, for example, described the developments in Peru as "revolutionary," "without historical precedent," and "absolutely astounding" (quoted in McClintock and Vallas 2003: 115).

A further trend showed that such views were somewhat myopic: increasing Colombian cultivation offset the gains made in Peru. For 1995, Colombian cultivation was estimated at 50,900 hectares. As illustrated in Chart 1, the following years saw significant increases: 57,200 hectares (1996), 79,500 (1997), 101,800 (1998), 122,500 (1999), 136,200 (2000), and an amazing 169,800 hectares in the year 2001 (for higher estimates, see Vargas 2002: 22). Hence, during the main phase of the ABDP, coca cultivation moved from Peru to Colombia. This displacement had begun in the early 1990s and gained momentum in the second half of the decade. In the early twenty-first century, Colombia was the world's preeminent coca producer. Ironically, increasing cultivation in Colombia compensated almost exactly the decline in Peru and Bolivia, as shown in Chart 1: From the late 1980s to the early twenty-first century, total coca cultivation was relatively stable at around 200,000 hectares per year.

The profound restructuring process of the Andean drug industry was also reflected in the "verticalization" of the Peruvian and Bolivian drug markets. Traditionally suppliers of coca leaf for the Colombian cocaine market, Peru and Bolivia began to produce and export significant amounts of cocaine from the mid-1990s. This decoupling of Peru and Bolivia from Colombia helps to explain the recovery of coca prices following the 1995 coca price crash in Peru: non-Colombian buyers filled some gaps left by the Colombians. In early 1996, Peruvians began marketing coca products to Bolivian buyers (Menzel 1996: 96; Roncken 1999: 9 and 54). In Bolivia, cocaine accounted for 61 percent of coca products seized in 1995, up from 9 percent in 1994 (Roncken 1999: 54). This verticalization process effectively limited "the impact of the air bridge denial operations since [it] decreased the importance of the Peru–Colombia and Bolivia–Colombia air link" (Roncken 1999: 54).

A last element of the restructuring process must be mentioned: changes of drug trafficking routes and methods. As shown below, the ABDP increased the risks of smuggling. Nevertheless, some smugglers continued flying drugs from Peru and Bolivia to Colombia. In early 1998, for example, residents of the Peruvian Putumayo basin reported a continuation of drug smuggling flights to Colombia. In the same year, a senior Peruvian police officer said that at least three functioning clandestine airports existed in the lower Huallaga Valley, and that seaplanes landed on the nearby Aypena River (Roncken 1999: 49–52). However, some traffickers avoided aerial smuggling altogether. According to an official US report, in 1997 traffickers continued the pattern observed since 1995 and avoided air trafficking, relying mainly on river and land transport (National Narcotics Intelligence Consumers Committee 1998: 4, 25). Significant drug loads were transported through the jungle, and some traffickers also moved drugs along the Pan-American Highway and by ship on the Pacific Ocean

Although land and water transport was an alternative to aerial smuggling, it was less convenient since traffickers lost time and risked falling prey to interdiction and banditry (Anthony *et al.* 2000: 11; CIA 1998). To avoid the risks associated with the traditional Peru/Bolivia–Colombia air link on the one hand, and land and water transport on the other hand, many traffickers dispersed air routes. In Ecuador, traffickers rerouted flights from the Amazonian region to the coast. Some smugglers also avoided Ecuador and flew to other countries (CIA 1998). From Peru and Bolivia, traffickers imported coca paste and cocaine into Brazil. From there, the drugs were exported to Colombia, the US and to Europe, and they also supplied a rising Brazilian demand. In 1996, the DEA reported that the ABDP in Colombia and Peru had led traffickers to carry coca base via land and rivers to aircraft waiting at clandestine airstrips in the tri-border area of Brazil, Peru, and Colombia (Roncken 1999: 51). Other countries such as Venezuela were used as transshipment countries and for laundering money and purchasing precursor chemicals.

In October 1998, the US Congress again increased drug control funding, this time under the Western Hemisphere Drug Elimination Act. In May 1999, the closure of Howard Air Force Base in Panama, which resulted from a 1977 agreement stipulating a return of the Canal Zone to Panama, forced US strategists to change their tactics. SOUTHCOM facilities were transferred to Florida and Puerto Rico. Moreover, the US began to establish Forward Operating Locations (FOLs) in Ecuador, Aruba, and Curaçao. FOLs had airports for various types of aircraft, intelligence equipment, radar facilities, and large antennae. Planners saw FOLs as cheaper than Howard Air Force Base and as covering a larger geographic area. The FOLs were apparently not only used for counter-drug missions, but for various other military activities as well. Critics argued that these activities included counter-insurgency operations that violated legal restrictions imposed on US forces. After a US drug reconnaissance plane crashed in Colombia in July 1999, a knowledgeable source said: "We're not supposed to be monitoring guerillas, but that's what they were doing" (quoted in Transnational Institute 2003a: 9).

Peru now caused less concern among US officials than before. By 1997/1998, the Peruvian–Colombian air bridge seemed to be in a shambles. US officials saw it as insignificant enough to halt AWACS and P-3 Orion surveillance flight over Peru in May 1998 and to use the equipment to track aerial smuggling in Colombia. Ceding to protests from the US embassy in Lima, which feared that reduced US anti-drug efforts would lead to an increase in aerial smuggling, the Clinton administration, in August 1998, said that P-3 flights over Peru would resume again (Krauss 1999). To be sure, Peruvian coca prices were again high from 1998 onward, following the historically low prices of 1995 and 1996. Moreover, rising prices led to some increase in Peruvian coca cultivation. However, much less coca was cultivated than in the early 1990s.

Meanwhile in Bolivia, the former military dictator and President Hugo Banzer committed himself to an aggressive eradication campaign. From 1998, the government implemented Plan Dignity, whose aim was to eliminate all illicit coca cultivation within five years. Despite fierce resistance from coca farmers that led to numerous deaths, Bolivia reduced coca cultivation significantly. Between 1998 and 2001, coca cultivation was halved and cocaine production possibly reduced by a third (European NGO Council on Drugs and Development 2001: 2).

US drug policy in Latin America now clearly focused on Colombia. The country led the global list of coca producers and was also a hub of drug production and trafficking. In addition, US economic interests were at stake. According to US General Charles Wilhelm, new oil explorations increased Colombia's "strategic importance" (quoted in Dunning and Wirpsa 2004: 93). Moreover, left-wing rebels, and most importantly the FARC and *Ejército de Liberación Nacional* (ELN) controlled large parts of the country and received revenues from the drug trade. As a consequence of these and other motivations, the US significantly increased support for the Colombian government, as discussed in more detail in Chapter 4.

The chronology of this chapter ends on April 20, 2001. On that day, the Peruvian air force shot down a small civilian aircraft over Peruvian air space carrying a US Baptist missionary family. The wife and her infant died in the crash. The Peruvian personnel had been supported by intelligence gathered by a private company flying a Cessna Citation V airplane. The company, Aviation

Development Corporation, had been hired by the CIA. Following the shoot-down, a heated debate erupted in the US over the outsourcing of US intelligence activities, leading a veteran of counter-drug missions in Latin America to complain that "[t]here wasn't one person aboard that [CIA-commissioned] plane sworn to uphold the Constitution of the United States. They were all . . . businessmen!" (quoted in Tamayo 2001a). As a consequence of the shoot-down, the US government suspended the ABDP.

Until this point, the aim of the discussion was to determine whether the ABDP was accompanied by the displacement of the coca and cocaine industry from Peru and Bolivia to Colombia and, more generally, by a restructuring of the South American drug industry. The answer to this question is positive. However, was the ABDP the main cause of the displacement? Which other factors played a role?

Explaining displacement

This section examines the initial causal mechanism and its constituting elements: the selectivity of US drug policy, the flexibility of the drug industry, weak law enforcement capacities of drug producing and trafficking states, and contingent conditions. It also discusses empirical black boxes and alternative explanations.

US selective pressure

US foreign policy selectivity has often been conducive to the displacement of the drug industry. This also holds true with regard to the ABDP. US forces failed to coordinate their activities properly, to implement anti-drug operations in a way that prevented the displacement of the drug industry, and to counterbalance coercion with more sustainable non-coercive anti-drug policies. However, the displacement of coca cultivation from Peru and Bolivia to Colombia occurred despite significant US-sponsored eradication efforts in Colombia. One should therefore not rush to the conclusion that the US did not make any efforts to prevent displacement from occurring.

As shown above, US legal concerns impeded the implementation of the ABDP during the program's early phase. Declassified documents issued by the National Security Archive reveal the difficulties of US agencies to respond to Colombia's and Peru's adoption of a shoot-down policy against suspicious aircraft. Some agencies demanded that the campaign be continued and others that it be stopped (Evans 2001a). US agencies also failed to agree on the choice of military hardware and its use. In 1989/1990, the DEA wanted to use helicopters at the Santa Lucía base in Peru for operations against drug laboratories, but the Narcotics Assistance Unit lobbied for using the helicopters for coca eradication (Menzel 1996: 147). In the early 1990s, the US military wanted to use E2C AWACS reconnaissance planes, but the CIA preferred Schweitzer planes, the US Customs its P-3 aircraft, and the National Guard contributed F-16 jets (Menzel 1997: 125).

The usefulness of technology was not always the main factor behind their use. In 1993, the GAO wrote that "[s]ensors designed to detect large supersonic aircraft and nuclear-powered submarines are less proficient against low-flying planes and small wooden boats" (cited in Zirnite 1998: 169).

Different technologies and standard operating procedures, as well as inadequate technology, made the implementation of the ABDP a real challenge. Scholars have described the difficulty of the many US agencies and departments involved in the counter-drug effort to coordinate their activities as "bureaucratic balkanization" and "ad-hoc-racy" (see McClintock and Vallas 2003: 139). When Bill Clinton assumed the presidency, the situation was bad indeed.

> While President Clinton [early on during his first administration] was reviewing his administration's narcotics-control policy [. . .], officials at different ranks and at different bureaucracies were making their own policies. The CIA, Department of Defense (DOD), DEA, and State Department were at odds over policy in the Andean nations. Complained one SOUTHCOM analyst: "With the Department of Defense barely on speaking terms with its number one customer – DEA – [in many areas of Latin America it] is the equivalent of two battalions going into combat, with one having the bullets and the other having the guns."
>
> (McClintock and Vallas 2003: 120)

Coordination problems between US agencies contributed to the application of local law enforcement pressure, instead of countrywide or region-wide pressure. In the 1980s, the selective application of pressure sometimes allowed trafficker to avoid arrest and property seizure by moving into another country. During Operation Blast Furnace, for example, up to 800 persons escaped from Bolivia, some of them on small trafficking aircraft, an evasion strategy that US planners had not foreseen (Menzel 1996: 18). This was despite the fact that the Bolivian country team had presented a detailed plan that included road and riverine checkpoints, air interdiction, and development aid. Washington only implemented part of this plan, which led to the displacement of drug trafficking structures (Menzel 1996: 20–21). Generally, Washington relied on

> a series of operations and programs, sometimes operating in tandem and sometimes not. Highlighting this fact was General Fred Woerner's annual SOUTHCOM conference on Latin American issues in early 1988. When queried at the conference if the Department of State had an anti-drug strategy for the Andean region, Ann Wroblesky, the Department of State's Assistant Secretary of State for International Narcotics Matters stated openly to those in attendance that: "We have no strategy; we just operate!"
>
> (Menzel 1996: 33)

The lack of a regional US strategy led to inefficiencies and was conducive to the displacement of the drug industry. The DEA team in Bolivia complained that it did not receive information from US teams in Peru, Colombia, and other countries, even though this information was vital to US drug control in Bolivia (Menzel 1996: 72–73). Similarly, the anti-drug effort in Peru was not part of a regional strategy, but was often decoupled from activities in other countries (Riley 1996; Menzel 1996: 215). Even within Peru, the US approach was relatively selective and un-coordinated. Until the mid-1990s, the US focused on supply reduction in the Upper Huallaga Valley and neglected dynamics taking place in other coca growing areas in the departments of Cuzco, Ayacucho, Pasco, and Puno (Menzel 1996: 185).

During the main phase of the ABDP, these problems persisted, revealing a lack of institutional memory. Personnel of the Southern Command did not have adequate knowledge about earlier air interdiction operations, the problems that were encountered, and the way these problems had been dealt with. US personnel said that this was a result of the continual turnover of personnel and the legal obligation to destroy documents (Zirnite 1998: 30; GAO 1997: 15–16). Implementation problems were not confined to Bolivia and Peru. In 1998, the GAO (1998b) reported that the failure to deliver spare parts for aircraft and helicopters was hampering the US anti-drug effort in Colombia.

However, it is important to note that the ABDP was not decoupled from other anti-drug measures. During the implementation of the ABDP, Andean governments, in close collaboration with the US government, eradicated coca fields arrested peasants and traffickers, destroyed cocaine laboratories, and seized the property of traffickers. Although these operations were sometimes chaotic, not properly integrated into a regional strategy, and interrupted by political tension and legal concerns, they were undertaken simultaneously with the ABDP.

This becomes obvious when looking at Colombia. As shown above, coca cultivation in Colombia began to increase in the early 1990s and climbed to dramatic heights in the second half of the decade. This displacement coincided with the ABDP. However, it also coincided with efforts by the Colombian government to destroy coca crops through a large-scale aerial fumigation program. This program began in 1995, after several trials in the Colombia Amazon the year before and after the government's decision, on February 11, 1994, to eliminate illicit coca plants within two years (Coffin 1998; Vargas 2002: 23, 25). Whereas in 1994 only 1,420 hectares of Colombian coca had been eradicated, in 1995 the figure stood at 25,402 hectares, and then at 23,025 (1996), 41,797 (1997), and 49,527 (1998). Between 33.3 and 52.8 percent of Colombia's total planted area was eradicated. Despite this campaign, the Colombia land area used for coca cultivation was two and a half times larger in 1998 than in 1992 (Vargas 2002: 22–23).

Since displacement increased simultaneously with eradication, it would be wrong to argue that displacement resulted from Washington's focusing on the ABDP to the detriment of eradication. After all, Washington sponsored the Colombian eradication program financially and logistically, even if to little effect. Colombian researcher Ricardo Vargas (2002: 14) shows that the eradication effort was a resounding failure.

> Between 1992 and 1998, $19,051,676 was spent fumigating coca crops with glyphosate, yielding operational costs in the order of $22,354,164. This means that there was a total expenditure of $41,405,840 without counting the investment in aircraft, anti-narcotic bases and interdiction infrastructure [. . .]. According to the U.S. Departments of State and Defense, nearly $625 million in equipment (helicopters and fixed-wing aircraft, weapons, ammunition, training and logistical support) were supplied to the Colombian National Police and the Colombian Armed Forces between the fiscal years of 1990 and 1998. The end result of this investment was staggering; during that period, the initial coca-growing areas actually tripled in size. This suggests that the nearly $41 million in overhead costs and $625 million in military aid, corresponding to almost an entire decade of funding, were a total waste, given their stated objective.

While US drug control in the Andes did not only focus on air interdiction, US policy was selective in that preference was given to coercive strategies for reducing drug supplies. In a rather myopic fashion, Washington looked at the complex issue of drug production as a military and law enforcement problem, thus neglecting myriad political, economic, and social issues. The US did spend significant sums of money on crop substitution and other strategies designed to draw Andean farmers away from coca cultivation, but the distribution of economic aid was normally tied to strict conditions that did not take into account the dire economic reality in coca producing regions. Moreover, non-coercive strategy elements were closely coupled with military and law enforcement operations, a strategy that antagonized farmers who often saw development aid workers as potentially threatening their survival (Vellinga 1998; Tullis 1995: 163).

The flexibility of the drug industry

Traffickers are often able to evade US-sponsored law enforcement through adaptive and innovative behavior. Traffickers responded to the ABDP by displacing their trafficking routes and by using modern equipment superior to the one of Andean security forces. Moreover, they adapted to air interdiction by increasing cocaine production in Peru and Bolivia. In addition, Colombian trafficker increased coca cultivation within Colombia to avoid the risk of losing their planes or lives while transporting coca paste from Bolivia and Peru to Colombia. Hence, responses to the ABDP increased the displacement of the drug industry in South America and contributed to the verticalization of the Peruvian, Bolivian, and Colombian drug industries.

Trafficking groups used sophisticated techniques to avoid interception. In the early 1990s, for example, the Peruvian air force lacked the equipment necessary for flying and fighting at night, and their planes were relatively slow. Trafficker thus often flew at night, switched to twin-engine planes that were faster than Peruvian fighter planes, and flew very low to avoid radar detection (Anthony *et al.* 2000: III/27; Roncken 1999: 52; Menzel 1997: 125). Traffickers also reduced the number of flights by increasing the size of drug shipments, flew zigzag patterns, flew in the shadow of legitimate commercial aircraft, and took off in groups of several aircraft that then used distinct flight routes to confuse interdiction teams (Howard 2001: 31; Riley 1996: 191). Moreover, they avoided detection by US ground radar installed in Peru and Bolivia by flying into Brazil and Ecuador where radar coverage was less dense. In their attempts to avoid detection, traffickers benefited from past experiences. Operation Blast Furnace, for example, taught the traffickers some valuable lessons (Menzel 1996: 100; Riley 1996: 194–195). And since they had enough money, they purchased technology that was not only superior to the technology used by Andean security forces but even to that of the US military. Researcher Robert Filippone (1994: 341) underlines the importance of technology:

> [The traffickers] have state-of-the-art equipment, including satellite radios, digital decryption devices, and voice privacy mechanisms, that makes it difficult for even the U.S. armed forces to penetrate. [U.S.] General Gorman made this clear when he said, "I have seen equipment used on the aircraft that fly between the United States and Colombia, and I can assure you that it is more sophisticated and more facile than the equipment that I had on my aircraft of the U.S. Air Force in the U.S. Southern Command". He went on to say that the government's communication system is regularly intercepted by the traffickers and that traffickers can track the movements of armed forces units better than the respective commanders.

Often, however, traffickers did not need high-tech equipment. Motorboats, canoes, trucks, cars, and other standard means of transport were often superior to the high-tech interdiction equipment used by states, since drug loads could easily be concealed and since the vastness of the Andean region made it impossible to survey the movement of every boat and car. One should not underestimate the total size of drug loads carried by backpackers across borders on jungle paths.

The innovation capacity of peasants and drug entrepreneurs is also evident when looking at the verticalization of the Peruvian and Bolivian cocaine market described above. Colombians showed Peruvians how to make coca paste and how to operate small cocaine base preparation laboratories, which produced *agua rica* (liquefied cocaine base). This helped the traffickers to reduce costs, as well as to disperse the cocaine industry and thereby to reduce the damage of drug and laboratory seizures (Menzel 1996: 167). Of course, the ABDP was only one reason for this verticalization strategy. Law enforcement operations on the ground were probably the more crucial factor. However, US-sponsored air interdiction was one of the factors that forced traffickers to reduce risks by increasing the number of potential law enforcement targets.

Traffickers also showed that they were able to respond to law enforcement pressure by increasing coca cultivation in Colombia, a growth that was particularly visible from 1995 onward. They forced Colombian farmers to plant coca and/or provided financial incentives to farmers. The increase in Colombian cultivation reduced traffickers' dependence on Bolivian and Peruvian coca, which translated into a reduced interdiction risk. However, some Colombian traffickin groups, and particularly the smaller ones, did not deliberately choose whether to continue their operations in Peru and Bolivia or whether to stay in their home country. Due to a lack of means to engage in bilateral smuggling, they had to operate from Colombia. Cultivation thus increased in the 1990s and reached staggering levels at the end of the decade.

Weak law enforcement

In addition to US foreign policy selectivity and the ability of drug entrepreneurs to adapt to law enforcement pressure, analysts should also examine the capacities of drug-producing and transit states to implement laws against drugs. Particularly corruption and a lack of governmental control over the national territory undermined the effectiveness of the ABDP and contributed to the displacement of coca cultivation from Bolivia and Peru to Colombia, the verticalization of the Bolivian and Peruvian drug industries, and the displacement of trafficking routes

Corruption is a perennial obstacle to drug control. In Bolivia during the 1980s, traffickers reportedly offered *Unidades Móviles de Patrullaje Rural (*UMOPAR) officers and town officials between $15,000 and $25,000 for keeping quiet for 72 hours to allow small aircraft to land, pick up drug loads, and take off again (Menzel 1996: 45). Some officials, due to a small salary and a monthly US supplement ranging from $50 to $100, found it difficult to turn down such offers. In Colombia, officials often warned traffickers of drug raids in advance. The criminal justice system also suffered as traffickers paid judges, witnesses, and others who participated in what frequently resembled mock trials (Lee and Thoumi 1999: 69). During Operation Support Justice in 1992, corruption probably lowered interdiction rates as Colombian air controllers, working at the 497 authorized airports, informed smugglers about interdiction operations (Menzel 1997: 113). In Peru, aerial interdiction was plagued by corruption as well. There are even indications that the country's second most powerful man, Vladimiro Montesinos, had sided not only with US forces but also with traffick ers through the 1990s (Rojas 2005). In Venezuela, corruption, counter-coup measures, and other factors helped traffickers to exploit the national territory and airspace for their operations, as described by Sewall Menzel (1997: 119):

> While the US sought to incorporate the Venezuelan government more and more into its anti-drug policy effort in order to stem the trafficking taking place in that country, effective narcotics control measures were significantl impeded. Control measures announced by President Carlos Andres Perez in 1991 never came to fruition. The continuous scandals over corruption rocked the government's leaders and resulted in a number of military coup attempts which diverted the national focus away from the anti-drug effort to

> attempting to restore internal domestic order. As a result, up to 2,500 Air Force pilots and aircraft technicians found themselves in prison as part of the government's counter-coup backlash. In short, the Air Force's counter-drug reconnaissance activities were significantly reduced as an entire OV-10 squadron was grounded. In addition, SOUTHCOM saw several of its radars working inside Venezuela malfunction for periods lasting up to several weeks which lessened further the interdiction capability of the Venezuelan authorities [. . .] General officers in the Venezuelan military were also found to have been involved in trafficking operations, indicating the extent of the corruption now taking place within that country.

A lack of governmental control over the national territory additionally undermined the ABDP and contributed to displacement. Despite intense US pressure on Andean states to reduce drug supplies, traffickers found relatively safe havens in these countries and were able to use their territory and airspace to smuggle drugs into all directions. Peru, for example, had an estimated 396 airports in the early 1990s. Of these, the government's civil aeronautics agency controlled 58, with another nine airports controlled by the Peruvian air force. Thus, the Peruvian government had no control over 80 percent of the country's airports, essentially leaving them open to traffickers (Menzel 1996: 167). Weak territorial control resulted not least from the presence of the Shining Path. Colombian traffickers benefited from the insurgency, since the rebels induced peasants to grow coca and since they protected rural areas from incursions of Peruvian security forces.

From 1992/1993, security forces put strong pressure on the Shining Path, and Colombian traffickers found it more difficult to operate in Peru. In the second half of the 1990s, the Shining Path was pushed back even further. However, rebels still made their presence felt. To reduce drug smuggling on rivers, the US wanted to cooperate with the Peruvian military in a riverine interdiction program. This was not easy, as a State Department official acknowledged on February 3, 1997 in the *New York Times*: "[Y]ou still have to deal with the insurgency at night. What you are talking about is imposing control over areas that the central Government has never controlled" (quoted in Independent Task Force 1997: 42).

Weak territorial control was also a problem in Colombia. The inability of the Colombian government to prevent left-wing guerillas and right-wing paramilitaries from ruling many rural regions was a prime reason for the displacement of coca cultivation from Peru to Colombia. For both rebels and paramilitaries, revenues from the drug trade were crucial. As a consequence, they increased coca cultivation in their respective areas of control. In addition to their activities in the cocaine business, armed groups profited from the production of opium (Labrousse 2000: 97). Increases in coca cultivation were particularly visible in areas controlled by the guerilla. These were also the most dangerous areas for fumigation planes, which the guerilla often opened fire on

However, it would be wrong to label the FARC a drug cartel. State Department allegations that the FARC was involved in international cocaine traffickin notwithstanding, the rebels were mainly taxing coca fields, as the DEA confirmed (Tickner 2003: 80). Paramilitary groups were probably deeper involved in the drug business due to their often close relationships with traffickers. Some of the new trafficking groups that rose to prominence during the destruction of the Medellín and Cali groups were formed with the help of paramilitary outfits As shown below, the greater prominence of these groups was conducive to the displacement of coca cultivation to Colombia.

Contingent conditions

The ABDP, as well as US policy selectivity, industry flexibility, and weak law enforcement capacities of South American governments, are insufficient for explaining displacement. Contingent conditions that are not related to US anti-drug efforts, or only indirectly related to these, must be taken into account as well. A combination of military, social, and economic developments in the Andes helps to explain the decreasing importance of the drug air bridge and the concomitant decoupling of the Peruvian and Bolivian drug industries from the Colombian drug industry.

Developments in one country affect another country. In the present context, developments in Colombia had a direct impact on Peru. Above it was shown, for example, that in the late 1980s and early 1990s, trafficking flights between Peru, Bolivia, and Colombia experienced a brief slump. This slump was not so much a result of the ABDP. Rather, it reflected developments in Colombia. The Colombian government put significant law enforcement pressure on the Medellín traffickers after their assassination of presidential candidate Galán in August 1989. At the time of the murder, Escobar and his allies controlled most of the aircraft that were carrying coca paste and cocaine across South America. The mobilization of significant state resources forced the traffickers to keep a low profil for a couple of months. Medellín traffickers then resumed the transport of coca paste from Bolivia and Peru to Colombia for processing, yet possibly on a lower scale than before.

With law enforcement pressure concentrating on Medellín traffickers, the rival Cali group became more powerful. From summer 1992, when Escobar decided to leave his prison, until his violent death on December 2, 1993, the Medellín "cartel" disintegrated. Cali traffickers played a prominent role in the manhunt for Escobar, providing a vigilante force called Los PEPES (*Perseguidos por Pablo Escobar*, or People Persecuted by Pablo Escobar), which decimated the Medellín group. This was done together with Colombian security forces, which benefited from US law enforcement, military, and intelligence aid (Bowden 2001). Whereas the Medellín traffickers had killed officials, Cali traffickers preferred to pay them. This obviously stifled Colombian law enforcement efforts against the Cali group. Corruption also benefited the group, since it reduced public pressure on the government to end trafficking. After all, corruption campaigns are less visible than bombing campaigns.

Given this power transition, air trafficking again resumed, Bolivian and Peruvian coca prices recovered, and cocaine purity increased. The Cali group now dominated international cocaine smuggling. The group was probably the leading air bridge user and also increased Colombian coca production by offering coercive or financial incentives to peasants to grow coca. The financial benefit of a verticalization of the Colombian cocaine industry was probably recognized by the shrewd Cali traffickers. But smaller trafficking groups sprang up as well. These did not have the means to import coca paste from Peru and thus increased coca cultivation in Colombia. This process was accelerated by the arrest of leading Cali traffickers in 1995. Vargas (1999) writes that since "the demise of the Medellín and Cali cartels, drug trafficking has undergone a process of decentralization. The many unknown trafficking groups provide the financial incentive to spread illicit crops." Hence, the verticalization of the Colombian cocaine industry resulted not only from strategic choices made by Cali traffickers, but also from the rise of smaller trafficking groups.

The rise of smaller trafficking groups and an increase in coca cultivation formed part of a general worsening of security problems in Colombia. Myriad reasons transformed Colombia into the world's most important coca-cultivating, cocaine-producing, and cocaine-exporting country. These reasons include widespread corruption, the rise of non-state armed groups, a lack of governmental control over the national territory, and other factors discussed above. Moreover, weak anti-drug norms, a delegitimized state, and poverty played a role as well. The reasons behind Colombia's preeminent role as a drug-producing and trafficking country are discussed in Chapter 4. At this point, it is only important to note that the ABDP was not the only reason for the increase in Colombian coca cultivation.

There were complex developments in Peru as well. In 1987, it was reported that the fungus *Fusarium oxysporum* had a destructive effect on coca (Riley 1996: 49). In 1991, the fungus appeared on Peruvian coca fields and soon destroyed as much as 30 percent of the Upper Huallaga Valley's coca (Riley 1996: 107–108), although total cultivation levels were not greatly reduced since coca increased along the Ucayali River, the Lower and Middle Huallaga Valleys, the Ene Perené, the Apurimac River Valley, and other regions (Youngers 1995: 3–4). Until 1991, the Upper Huallaga Valley produced half of Peru's coca, but by 1994, cultivation only made up 27 percent (Kay 1999: 109). The displacement of coca cultivation within Peru was related to the migration of many farmers, although some had already begun to migrate before the onset of the fungi plague. It may well be that these changes made it more difficult for traffickers to transport coca paste from Peru to Colombia, since the change in flight routes from the Upper Huallaga Valley to other parts of the country increased risks and costs. Moreover, the fungus probably functioned as an incentive for traffickers to reduce their dependence on Peruvian coca and increase Colombian cultivation instead.

Insurgency and counter-insurgency in Peru changed the drug industry as well. The Peruvian government and military saw that coca eradication increased resentment against the government and the popularity of the Shining Path. Thus, Army General Alberto Arciniega, who was appointed commander of the Peruvian military forces in the Huallaga region in August 1989, ordered a suspension of forced eradication. Many Peruvian officials shared his view that the eradication program antagonized farmers and made the Shining Path more popular (Kay 1999: 105–106; Menzel 1996: 145). Arciniega was replaced in December 1989, but his successors stuck to his course, and so did the newly elected President Alberto Fujimori. Following the example of the former García administration, Fujimori rejected a $35.9 million US military aid package in September 1990. The package was accepted only in May 1991. Moreover, between early 1989 and 1995, only coca seedbeds were eradicated. Mature coca plants were left untouched in order to mitigate the anger of coca farmers (McClintock and Vallas 2003: 115). Fujimori argued that drug control should focus on economic development instead of coercion to improve Peru's dire social, narcotics, and insurgency situation. Drug flows were not the main concern in a country where the Shining Path insurgency had led to the death of tens of thousands of people, where 80 percent of the population was unemployed or underemployed, and where the inflation rate had reached 3,500 percent (Menzel 1996: 158–159)[7]

On September 12, 1992, Peruvian security forces arrested Shining Path's charismatic leader Abimael Guzmán in a Lima suburb. That year and the following year, numerous rebel cadres and fighters were arrested. Slowly, the anti-drug campaign gathered pace, and the Peruvian government increasingly tried to deprive the Shining Path of its revenues by attacking traffickers and eradicating coca. Between 1996 and 2001, around 40,000 hectares of coca were destroyed (Dietrich 2002: 26). Peruvian farmers still saw eradication as a threat, but most were also relieved to see the rebels retreat. Security operations, particularly in the Upper Huallaga Valley, as well as violent encounters between traffickers and rebels probably led some traffickers to reduce their dependency on Peruvian coca paste and instead increase cultivation in Colombia. The partial withdrawal of Colombian traffickers from Peru, in turn, may have enabled Peru-based traffick ers to fill the gap and verticalize the Peruvian cocaine industry. In addition, the withdrawal of Colombians may have helped Bolivia-based traffickers to procure more coca paste from Peru and thus to increase Bolivian cocaine production.

To explain the decrease in Peruvian coca cultivation, one must also look at socio-economic changes in Peru. During the 1990s, alternative development helped to improve the rural infrastructure and provided farmers with income. In addition, annual Gross Domestic Product (GDP) increases of more than 7 percent between 1994 and 1997 were accompanied by a reduction in the number of people migrating from the Andean high plateau to warmer regions where coca grows (Dietrich 2002; Kay 1999: 114–115). A relative improvement of the economic situation also resulted from a rise in coffee prices. In 1993, a kilogram of coffee cost around $1.5. In 1997, the price had risen to over $3. Coffee is one of the most viable alternatives to coca, which is why high prices probably helped to reduce coca cultivation (Dietrich 2002: 27). To be sure, coca remained a lucrative crop. However, fewer Peruvian farmers may have been faced with the choice between coca cultivation and starvation in the second half of the 1990s than in the first half

Many other factors and processes changed the South American drug industry. For example, a border conflict between Ecuador and Peru, which erupted in fighting in January 1995 and ended with a peace treaty in October 1998, probably influenced the behavior of traffickers. The conflict led to the deployment of significant military assets to the jungle region along the border of the two countries and thereby increased traffickers' risks (McClintock and Vallas 2003: 78–84).[8] Besides human agency, traffickers also had to take into account natural phenomena. It is possible that *El Niño* rains made some airstrips inoperable and thus reduced air smuggling (National Narcotics Intelligence Consumers Committee 1998: 25).

Analysts are thus faced with a fuzzy empirical picture, which means that oversimplified assertions concerning the impact of the ABDP are unwarranted. US policy-makers who attribute the decline of Peruvian coca cultivation to air interdiction operations provide a monocausal, and obviously politically motivated, account of a complex process.[9] But the overall picture is even more complicated.

Black boxes and alternative explanations

Assessing the links between the ABDP and displacement is further complicated by empirical black boxes. One of the (scientifically *and* politically) most troubling black boxes is the lack of knowledge about the number of traffickin planes forced down, shot down, or seized in the course of the ABDP. The obscurity of this pivotal question was noted already in 1994. During a Congressional hearing, it was unclear how many suspected trafficker planes had been shot down over Peru. With the figures ranging from 0 to 31, one participant remarked that "it would be sort of nice to have our three top experts be prepared to answer such an unbelievably elementary question" (quoted in Roncken 1999: 7). Similarly, it was unclear how many aircraft had been intercepted. The Peruvian military was reported to have claimed that 124 trafficking aircraft were intercepted or shot down from 1991 to mid-1993 (Menzel 1996: 184). Cynthia McClintock and Fabián Vallas (2003: 115), however, write that only ten aircraft were seized in 1991, seven in 1992, and 13 in 1993.

Interdiction figures remained controversial during the main phase of the ABDP. In January 1996, SOUTHCOM reported that Operation Green Clover had led to the shooting down of 27 smuggling aircraft. Three months later, US Secretary of Defense, William Perry said that only 12 aircraft had been interdicted or shot down (Zirnite 1998: 170–171). Looking at other sources, the number of planes seized in 1995 ranged from 20 to 39 (Independent Task Force 1997: 48; Roncken 1999: 48; McClintock and Vallas 2003: 115). From then, the number of interdicted planes seems to have declined, albeit unevenly, from seven (1996), 11 (1997), and zero (1998 and 1999) to two (2000) (McClintock and Vallas 2003: 115). However, these are only the figures for Peru, and seizures particularly in Colombia may have been higher. US General Charles Wilhelm, for example, said in a Senate hearing on July 14, 1999 that states participating in the ABDP had "shot down, forced down, seized or destroyed 26 narcotrafficking aircraft [in 1998], bringing the total to 123 narcotrafficking aircraft taken out of action since 1995" (quoted in Lessmann 2000: 348, fn 31). According to Bruce Bagley (2001: 5), the Colombian Air Force began to intercept suspicious aircraft by force in 1998 and intercepted 36 planes in 1998/1999. Six of these planes were shot down, and the others were destroyed after having been forced to land.

In addition, it is impossible to say how many smuggling flights the ABDP helped to prevent. Traffickers analyze risks and change their behavior continuously, but do not publicly document their adaptive behavior. Figures indicating a reduction of trafficking flights are unreliable, since they imply that the total number of flights is known. In October 1997, for example, McCaffrey said that Operation Green Clover had led to a 47 percent decrease in drug flight (Roncken 1999: 48). But since he did not know the total number of drug flights this figure is yet another "mystical number," with which official statements are replete (Reuter 1984). As a matter of fact, many success stories can be read as failures. An increase in the number of interdicted planes, for example, can result from increased trafficking flows. In this case, air interdiction would have failed to deter drug flights

The number of hectares used for coca cultivation is another uncertainty. As further discussed in Chapter 4, farmers often hide coca among licit crops, and the surveillance of coca-producing areas is technically difficult due to frequent cloud coverage and other obstacles. Moreover, simply listing the number of hectares under cultivation is only of limited use, since that figure does not say anything about yield (the amount of coca that can be produced on one hectare and the potency of the leaves). As a matter of fact, although the South American coca cultivation area was relatively stable during the period analyzed in this chapter, the potential production of cocaine increased significantly due to an increase in yield. This increase in yield became particularly visible from 1998 to 2001 and partly resulted from innovative agronomical methods (Transnational Institute 2003b: 3–4).

Causal reasoning is further limited by insufficient knowledge about the actors involved in the drug business. The discussion above emphasized the role of Peruvians and Bolivians as coca farmers, paste producers, and middlemen, and the role of Colombians as traffickers. However, this gain in analytical clarity comes at the price of neglecting empirical fuzziness. In 1993, for example, Mexican traffickers entered Peruvian coca markets. This sometimes led to conflict with Colombians, although there were instances of cooperation as well (Hoffmann 1995: 587, fn 3). The presence of Mexicans continued to be felt in late 1997, when the Peruvian police "disbanded a fledgling drug 'cartel' operating out of the coastal cities of Callao, Pisco, and Nazca. A senior police officia told reporters for a local newspaper that the cartel was being formed with the help of Mexicans, who wanted to find a cheaper source for cocaine" (CIA 1998)

To make matters more complex, Peruvians were not only involved in coca farming, but also in trafficking. In 1994, Demetrio Limoniel Chavez, nicknamed *Vaticano*, was captured in Cali and extradited to Peru. In Peru, he had supplied his colleagues in Cali with cocaine base and cocaine. By the time of his arrest, he had come close to forming a cartel-like structure, exporting an annual estimated 50 metric tons of cocaine to the US (Riley 1996: 183).[10] Similarly, some Bolivians also reached the higher echelons of the drug business. In an anti-drug operation in 1990 in Santa Cruz, one of Bolivia's estimated 35 major narcotraffickers, Carmelo "Meco" Dominguez, was arrested. Bolivian forces also arrested almost all of the leading members of his trafficking groups and seized valuable data and assets, including nine aircraft (Menzel 1996: 54).

Another black box pertains to coca prices. Explaining coca price changes is one of the trickiest issues facing drug policy researchers. Kevin Riley (1996: 123) writes that "coca prices often fluctuate, but that no authoritative explanation for these fluctuations exist." James Painter (1994: 91) underlines the obscurity of the issue as well. He writes that it is "almost impossible to ascertain the exact balance of factors in determining coca prices: whether the buyers do operate a cartel (given their numbers), whether they can maintain low prices, and what is the relationship between Colombian and Bolivian buyers." Moreover, during interviews with the author conducted in 2003, US drug control officials at the US Embassies in Peru and Bolivia confirmed that they did not know the mechanisms behind fluctuating coca prices, as prices depended on numerous factors.[11] The difficulty of explaining coca prices compounds the diffi culty of explaining displacement. To arrive at more fine-grained explanations of displacement, fluctuations in coca prices must be explained. After all, high coca prices can induce peasants to plant coca, and low prices can lead them to abandon their coca fields

Furthermore, it is unclear whether the ABDP reduced the availability of coca paste in Colombia. Some observers say that Colombia never experienced a shortage of coca paste, while others argue to the contrary. A DEA report from June 1996 states: "Although the air bridge interdiction initiative is considered to be a counter-drug success, this year long campaign does not appear to have caused any measurable shortage of cocaine paste for processing in Colombia" (cited in Roncken 1999: 10). Colombian drug policy expert Ricardo Vargas (1997: 64), however, notes an increase in coca paste prices in Colombia. From late 1995 until July 1996, he writes, buyers had to pay $1,200 for one kilogram of coca paste, a 100 percent increase when compared to previous prices.

The last black box that deserves mentioning pertains to drug demand.[12] Particularly during the later 1980s and early 1990s, the demand for cocaine was rising in countries other than the US, particularly in Europe and Japan. Since traffickers could fetch higher prices for cocaine in these countries than in the US, they diverted some supply routes. Moreover, this demand-induced incentive brought new traffickers to the fore, with local Brazilian traffickers forging alliances with Bolivian and Colombian coca producers and cocaine traffickers Hence, the verticalization trend particularly of the Bolivian cocaine industry cannot be explained without reference to changing patterns of drug demand. However, it is not clear how and to what extent this factor has influenced the restructuring of the Andean drug industry.

The difficulty of assessing the impact of the ABDP on the South American drug industry sometimes leads analysts to eschew a systematic treatment of the issue, and to shift the explanatory focus instead. In the first chapter of a Pentagon-commissioned report on the ABDP, analysts write that in 1994, Colombian traffickers began to increase coca cultivation in Colombia, and that this "may have been in response to new felt price rises from pilot fees for flying coca base from Peru during Support Justice IV or an anticipation of the vulnerability of the air-bridge to more concerted interdiction."[13] (Anthony *et al.* 2000: I/14). In the third chapter, things suddenly appear to be simpler. "Very likely, Colombian traffickers recognized the vulnerability of the air-bridge to Peru and began investing in new cultivation as early as 1994" (Anthony *et al.* 2000: III/35). Another example illustrates the point. It is difficult to estimate whether the arrest of leading Cali traffickers in 1995 or the ABDP led to low coca prices in Peru and Bolivia. In his 1996 book on drug policies in Peru and Bolivia, Sewall Menzel (1996: 199) writes that the ABDP "caused" a drop in coca leaf and coca paste prices. In his 1997 volume on drug policies in Colombia, however, he writes that the "arrest of leading Cali narco-kingpins, in conjunction with successful radar guided intercept operations of trafficker aircraft coming out of Peru, did cause the price of coca leaf to plummet [. . .] in Peru and Bolivia" (Menzel 1997: 169).

These black boxes and uncertainties pose serious analytical challenges, and they lead to a proliferation of explanations for displacement. One could even argue that the ABDP did not contribute to displacement at all. According to this explanation, US-sponsored air interdiction was not necessary for an increase in Colombian coca cultivation, the dispersion of trafficking routes, or the verticalization of the Bolivian and Peruvian drug industries. Along this line of thought, other factors and processes were sufficient for displacement. These include an increase in the number of Colombian small trafficking groups, rebels, and paramilitaries, an increase in Colombian poverty and Peruvian prosperity, the disintegration of the Shining Path and the coca-destroying fungus, and other factors and processes.

However, this view underrates the contribution of the ABDP to displacement. After all, traffickers took the ABDP into account. Deterrence can be feeble as smugglers alter their routes and smuggling methods, find new business partners, or simply wait until equipment is withdrawn. This was confirmed by imprisoned traffickers interviewed in the framework of a ONDCP-sponsored investigation into the risk assessment of traffickers (Transnational Institute 2003a: 22). Nevertheless, the ABDP influenced traffickers' decisions. In Colombia in the late 1980s, for example, "the Gonzalo Rodriguez Gacha organization is believed to have grown its own coca inside Colombia as a means of protecting itself from interruptions in the Peruvian and Bolivian supply" (Filippone 1994: 329). Traffickers take deterrence particularly seriously when it is backed up by lethal force. In 1995, the enforcement of the shoot-down policy in Peru posed a problem to traffickers. Then, in late November, security forces interrupted potentially lethal interdiction for more than a month. "Traffickers quickly took advantage of this opportunity because what had been 5 or 6 flights per month jumped to 22 flights in December of 1995 and fluctuated between 7 and 10 flights per month for the next 8 months" (Anthony *et al.* 2000: IV/44). Pilot fees also illustrate changing risk perceptions. In 1994, pilots demanded about $30,000 to fly one drug-smuggling aircraft across the Peruvian–Colombian border. In 1997, when the risk of interdiction was substantially higher, the fee stood at around $180,000 (McClintock and Vallas 2003: 126).

In the 1990s, the Pentagon commissioned the US Institute for Defense Analyses (IDA) to analyze the effects of the ABDP. IDA reports on interdiction must be read cautiously, since they received devastating reviews. Reviewers argued that IDA staff overestimated the effects of interdiction, since they had "started with a conclusion and tried to fit a model that would support it rather than starting from the data." Moreover, reviewers suspected the authors of being "neither well versed in the drug policy literature nor in the standard social sciences, particularly economics" (quoted in Roncken 1999: 83). While it is important to keep these review results in mind, an IDA report published in 2000, nevertheless, illustrates the point that a relatively high risk of being shot down by interdiction forces can lead to the abandonment of air smuggling:

> Between 1989 and 1995, three only moderately successful operations had seldom interdicted more than 2.5 per cent of the known trafficke flights [. . .] [From 1995], the Peruvians achieved a remarkable degree of success. From March through November, air interdiction rates averaging 13 per cent deterred another 64 per cent of trafficker flights [. . .] From a pilot's perspective, an interdiction rate of 12 per cent backed by lethal force would be daunting. If a pilot expects to smuggle six times in his career – the average number for inmates in federal prisons – surviving six flights with an 88 per cent chance of success on each yields only a 46 per cent chance of surviving all six attempts. Less than 50:50 chances of survival cannot be very attractive to pilots.
>
> (Anthony *et al.* 2000: ES/1, ES/3, IV/44)

To be sure, the figures listed in the report are dubious. They reflect the futile attempt to quantify an essentially unquantifiable phenomenon. But even if interdiction rates were lower than 13 percent, the ABDP still provided some form of deterrence. Moreover, the decrease in trafficking flights was probably the main cause for the decline in Peruvian coca prices in 1995. The spread of the coca-destroying fungus mentioned above, by comparison, seems to have played a less important role. If the fungus had had a greater impact, one should have been able to observe an increase in Peruvian coca prices since supply would have become scarcer. Similarly, alternative development, the exhaustion of coca fields, and coca eradication are unlikely to have been the main causes of the

Peruvian coca price crash, since they all limited supply and would therefore have increased prices. Hence, lower coca prices resulted mainly from the ABDP (Clawson and Lee 1998: 224–233; CIA 1998: fn 1). In the absence of air interdiction, the decline in Peruvian coca cultivation and prices would probably have been less dramatic.

Moreover, the ABDP contributed to the dispersion of trafficking routes and an increase in Colombian coca cultivation, as indicated by traffickers' changing risk assessments. And since the withdrawal of Colombians from Peru was conducive to the verticalization of the Peruvian and Bolivian cocaine industries, the ABDP also contributed to this verticalization, albeit indirectly. Hence, it can be concluded that the ABDP was not the only reason for displacement, but an important one.

Conclusion

This case study has disregarded some aspects related to aerial interdiction. These include human rights violations through the diversion of US anti-drug aid to ruthless anti-insurgency campaigns by Andean states; environmental destruction through the construction of air bases and radar stations; and a weakening of state legitimacy through the imposition of coercive drug policies that antagonized rural populations (Evans 2001b; Youngers 2001; Tickner 2003; Vargas 2002; Jelsma 2001). Cynthia McClintock and Fabián Vallas (2003: 123) remind us that whatever the impact of the ABDP on the Peruvian drug economy, air interdiction "raised many questions about the overall war."

The ABDP came at a particularly high cost for Peruvians. As shown above, air interdiction led traffickers to divert smuggling routes. New routes often went through Peruvian coastal cities, where traffickers sold cocaine base at low prices, causing a surge in drug consumption and drug-related problems. In the early twenty-first century, Peruvians regarded drugs, after the economic situation, as the country's most pressing problem (El Comercio 2003). Moreover, US officials forged a close alliance with the repressive Fujimori–Montesinos administration. Many US policy-makers saw the regime as a loyal ally in the anti-drug effort, and whenever criticism surfaced in the US, Fujimori and Montesinos skillfully played the card of the air interdiction and eradication program. Yet at the same time as he was cooperating with US forces, Montesinos may have been participating in illicit activities. Drug policy researcher Isaías Rojas (2005: 222) writes that Montesinos "manipulated Peru's military, police, and intelligence apparatuses to set up and run a parallel criminal network that allowed him to engage in and benefit from the very crimes he was supposed to be preventing." Fujimori's and Montesinos' fall from power came only in 2000 following a scandal over rigged elections.

With regard to the question of whether the ABDP coincided with displacement, this chapter has shown that this was the case. During the early phase of the ABDP, coca cultivation decreased in Peru and increased in Colombia. During the main phase, this process was even more remarkable. In the late

1990s, Colombia produced most of the world's coca. Moreover, coca prices crashed in Peru in 1995, i.e. in the same year that the US resumed air interdiction. In addition, traffickers diversified their smuggling routes and used new smuggling methods, particularly during the ABDP's main phase. Furthermore, in the 1990s, a trend toward verticalization, i.e. a drug production cycle ranging from coca cultivation to cocaine exports, could be noted, not only in Colombia, but in Peru and Bolivia as well. All these changes meant that the South American drug industry was much more complex in the late 1990s than it had been in the early 1990s.

Explaining displacement is difficult. Still, the initial causal mechanism helped to bring order into a very complex episode. It was shown that US foreign drug policy was sometimes marked by a selective application of pressure. US agencies frequently failed to coordinate their activities, to develop a regional approach to drug-trafficking, to prevent traffickers from escaping across borders, and to exert simultaneous pressure on different trafficking groups. Moreover, Washington favored coercion over more sustainable, non-coercive strategies against drugs, and thus perpetuated the conditions of poverty, violence, and insecurity that had given rise to illicit crop cultivation and drug production in the first place. However, US policies were not selective in one important respect: while the US implemented the ABDP, it simultaneously sponsored large-scale aerial fumigation in Colombia. Hence, more coca grew in Colombia despite US attempts to reduce coca supplies.

The second element of the causal mechanism pertains to the innate flexibilit of the drug industry. Faced with potentially lethal air interdiction, pilots displayed considerable skills in their attempts to evade radar surveillance and interdiction planes, not least because they used sophisticated technology that was often superior to that available to Andean security forces. Moreover, the ABDP seems to have led to a reduction of air trafficking and to more smuggling on rivers and along land routes, for which basic means of transport were sufficient In addition, traffickers based in Peru and Bolivia made more money by producing more cocaine in these two countries, while Colombian traffickers responded to the ABDP, the coca-destroying fungus in Peru, and the dismantling of the Shining Path, by increasing Colombian cultivation. However, this increase was not only the result of a conscious choice by traffickers but also reflected the fact that smaller Colombian groups had come to the fore who could not buy coca paste in Peru.

In addition, corruption and a lack of territorial control enabled the shift of coca production to Colombia. In Peru, the Shining Path helped to establish the drug industry in the country. In Colombia, the growing strength of armed non-state actors and smaller trafficking groups provided a fertile ground for displacement at a time when the Peruvian government had partly dismantled the Shining Path and thus improved territorial control.

This leads to contingent conditions. The displacement of coca to Colombia, the verticalization of the Bolivian and Peruvian drug industries, and the dispersion of trafficking routes resulted to a certain extent from factors that were unrelated, or only indirectly related, to the ABDP. In Peru, operations against the Shining Path and a coca-destroying fungus made it more difficult for Colombian traffickers to operate in the country. An aggressive eradication campaign by the Fujimori administration also reduced Peruvian coca cultivation. In Colombia, the destruction of the Medellín group benefited the Cali group, which may have decided to expand coca cultivation in Colombia to make the Colombian drug industry more efficient. The arrest of leading Cali traffickers in 1995 benefite smaller trafficking groups that had a similar interest in having more home-grown coca and consequently expanded cultivation, a process that had already begun in the early 1990s. In addition, and related to the rise of various non-state armed groups, the 1990s were a period of political, economic, and social upheaval in Colombia. Other factors that contributed to the displacement of the drug industry include the spread of a coca-destroying fungus in Peru in the early 1990s; a relative economic recovery in Peru; the border war between Ecuador and Peru; and *El Niño* rains. In combination, these contingent conditions underline that the ABDP was not the only element driving displacement. A complex empirical picture challenges mono-causal accounts.

To make matters more complicated, the number of trafficking airplanes shot down, forced down, seized, or deterred is unclear. The real size of the area on which coca was cultivated might be different from official figures, and even if figures were accurate, they would still conceal potential cocaine production due to differences in yield. Moreover, it is unclear whether the ABDP led to a shortage of coca paste in Colombia. Furthermore, although in the 1980s and early 1990s Colombia specialized in cocaine production and trafficking, and Peru and Bolivia in coca cultivation, the structure of the drug business, and particularly the actors involved, was more complex. There is also a lack of knowledge about the underlying reasons for changes in coca prices. Lastly, it is unclear whether, and to what extent, the verticalization particularly of the Bolivian drug industry was a result of a rising demand for cocaine in countries other than the US.

Due to these empirical black boxes, the debate about the impact of the ABDP will remain controversial. While policy-makers oversimplify matters by saying that the ABDP was the only reason for the Peruvian price crash and the decrease in Peruvian coca cultivation, it would be equally exaggerated to say that the ABDP did not play any role at all. After all, there are many indications that traffickers took the ABDP into account when planning and executing their operations. In the absence of US-sponsored air interdiction, coca cultivation might still have increased in Colombia, the Peruvian and Bolivian drug industries might still have become more vertical, and traffickers might still have diversifie their trafficking routes and methods. However, these developments would have been slower and smaller in scale. Hence, this chapter proposes a compromise: dynamics on South American drug markets during the 1990s resulted from many factors. One of these was the Air Bridge Denial Program.

4 Targeting the Colombian drug industry

The early twenty-first centur

Introduction

Over recent years, the US has attempted to reduce the import of Colombian drugs through Plan Colombia and the Andean Regional Initiative. Whereas the US and Colombian governments presented these multi-billion dollar programs as necessary for stabilizing a war-torn country, critics around the world argued that US military aid led to human rights abuses and environmental destruction, weakened the Colombian state and society, and strengthened paramilitaries. This chapter largely disregards these important issues. Instead, it explains the displacement of the South American drug industry in the early twenty-first century

US perceptions and politics

During the second half of the 1990s, US policy-makers became increasingly concerned about Colombia. Large rebel and paramilitary groups roamed the cities and countryside, the illicit drug industry was thriving, and the Colombian government was unable to exert control. These problems directly affected US perceived security interests, prompting US policy-makers to redefine the US role in Colombia. Drugs were the most obvious reason for an increase in US aid. Every year, the US federal government and the state governments spent many billions of dollars to combat the narcotics trade, but drug consumption continued unabated.

While US drug problems continued to make headlines in the US, the Clinton administration changed its rhetorical stance toward drugs. Already in 1994, Robert S. Gelbard, US Assistant Secretary of State for International Narcotics and Law Enforcement, had said that the "main line of defense" against drugs was in the US, and that the world's largest drug market should do more to reduce drug demand (cited in Chepesiuk 1999a: 92). In its 1999 National Drug Control Strategy, the ONDCP emphasized that the US should focus on drug demand reduction. And ONDCP director, Barry McCaffrey, considered the drug war metaphor inappropriate, preferring instead to speak of drug control as a continuing challenge (ONDCP 1999: Section 1).

Nevertheless, the course of US drug control under Clinton essentially remained the same, with coercion at home and abroad receiving priority over non-coercive strategies. As shown in Chapter 3, this inability to change policy resulted from several factors, including a lack of public support for non-coercive measures, political pressure from moral conservatives, and an entrenched drug war bureaucracy (Bertram *et al.* 1996: 117). Moreover, the martial rhetoric did not disappear. Both administration officials and members of Congress continued to use bellicose language when talking about drugs. In 1998, for example, DEA Administrator Thomas Constantine applauded the "heroes in the war on drugs" and talked about a "global battle against international drug trafficking" (quoted in DEA 1998: 3 and 8). Such militancy helped the DEA to secure higher budgets and allowed the Clinton administration to steer a repressive course. As before, US drug policies continued along familiar lines, or even escalated, because offi cials did not want to be accused by the political opposition of being "soft" on drugs. In 1998, the US federal drug control budget was $15.8 billion. Over the following years, it increased to $17.7 billion (1999), $18.5 billion (2000), and $19.2 billion (2001). Only one-third of the funds were invested in non-coercive strategies against drug demand. Two-thirds were spent on coercion at home and abroad, despite calls from reform groups to change the allocation of funds and spend two-thirds on prevention, treatment, and research (ONDCP 2000; Network of Reform Groups 1999).

US drug problems were intimately related to Colombia. In the late 1990s, Colombian cocaine production accounted for 80 percent of global production, and almost all the cocaine found on US streets originated from that country. Moreover, in the early 1990s, Colombian traffickers had diversified and begun to produce large amounts of heroin (Claudio 1992). Compared to Burma and Afghanistan, which together produced an estimated 90 percent of the world's opium, Colombia was a small opium and heroin producer. But for the US heroin market, Colombia played a crucial role. In the late 1990s, 70 percent of the heroin consumed on the East Coast of the US came from Colombia (ONDCP 1999: Section IV).

In 1996 and 1997, the US denied certification to Colombia, accusing President Ernesto Samper of having received money from Cali traffickers during his presidential campaign. Washington even revoked Samper's visa in July 1996, a step that had been taken against a foreign head of state only once before. Yet, despite acrimonious US–Colombian relations during this period, US anti-drug aid continued to flow. The aerial fumigation of coca fields reached record levels, and the US cooperated closely with the Colombian National Police (CNP) while effectively circumventing Samper. Between 1995 and 2000, the influence of the chief of the Colombian police in Washington equaled, or even surpassed, the influence of the Colombian ambassador (Crandall 2002a: 4, 40)

Despite US aid, the situation in Colombia deteriorated. Corruption was rife, and the arrest of leading Cali traffickers had made little difference. In 1999, Transparency International ranked Colombia as one of the world's most corrupt countries (Bagley 2001: 6). This made life difficult for Colombians and for US agents who needed reliable Colombian counterparts in their operations against traffickers. Another disturbing trend was the fact that Colombia's non-state armed groups expanded their activities. US policy-makers were particularly worried about left-wing rebels. Fighting left-wing insurgency has always been a central tenet of US policy in Latin America because insurgents are seen as threatening US economic interests and US citizens based in Latin American countries.

Many US policy-makers therefore had reservations about attempts by the Colombian government in the 1990s to negotiate with the insurgents. Nevertheless, the Colombian government at times tried to stabilize the country by negotiating with the guerilla. The administration of César Gaviria (1990–1994), for example, struck peace deals with the smaller guerilla groups. Yet while smaller groups were demobilized and incorporated into the political system, the two main rebel groups, the FARC and the ELN, expanded their activities to advance their agenda of land reform, political decentralization, income redistribution, and a curtailing of paramilitary power.

The FARC was nominally Marxist and grew from an estimated 3,000 troops in 1985 to around 15,000 combatants in 1999, making it the largest insurgent force in Latin America (Shifter 1999: 15; Carpenter 2003: 61). With a presence in most Colombian departments, the FARC engaged the Colombian state in jungle warfare, and even conducted conventional military operations. The ELN only counted around 5,000 troops in 1999 (Shifter 1999: 15). Inspired by the Cuban revolutionaries, the ELN was mainly confined to Colombia's northeast, a region of strategic importance because most of the oil pipelines run through it. The ELN frequently bombed these pipelines, which led to a daily average finan cial loss of $3 million in the late 1990s, as well as a drop in national oil production. Theses losses were painful for the Colombian state, since oil exports had replaced coffee exports as the leading source of foreign revenue (Crandall 2002a: 75). The attacks affected the US as well, since US companies had stakes in many pipelines. These companies not only lost oil revenues, but also had to invest in private security firms that protected the pipelines from rebels, who portrayed the companies as part of a US plot to subject Latin America to hegemonic rule.

Gaviria's successor Samper was willing to negotiate with rebels as well. The initial response of the ELN and another guerilla group was positive. The FARC, however, began a large military operation in May 1995 that hardened the view held by many within the Samper administration and the Colombian military that there was no point in negotiating with insurgents. When Samper proposed to withdraw the military from a region where peace negotiations were to take place, the military vetoed the idea, thus revealing Samper's domestic political weakness. The FARC was similarly reluctant to negotiate with a president whom it saw as lacking the ability to implement a peace deal. The US decision to ostracize the Samper administration and decertify Colombia twice further undermined Samper's credibility and diminished his negotiating position.

To receive US aid, the Colombian military alerted the US to alleged links between the FARC and drug traffickers (Tickner 2003: 79–80). However, the

Clinton administration was reluctant to support the Colombian military for several reasons. Guerilla activities were less visible in the mid-1990s than toward the end of the decade. There were fewer indications that the FARC received significant revenues from the drug trade. US officials regarded the Colombian military's performance in drug supply reduction efforts as poor. And the US decision to deny certification to Colombia in 1996 and 1997 impeded enhanced military cooperation between the two countries.

Moreover, the appalling human rights record of the Colombian military was an obstacle to an increase in US aid. In the so-called Trujillo massacres, for example, government security forces, in cooperation with drug traffickers, had carried out more than 100 assassinations between 1988 and 1991. Human rights violations continued over the following years, and sometimes the US was indirectly implicated. In 1992 and 1993, for example, Colombian military units responsible for human rights violations benefited from US counter-narcotics funding (Tickner 2003: 82). To assure the correct use of US aid, US Senator Patrick Leahy (D-Vermont) sponsored a constitutional amendment. This Leahy Amendment, which came into force in September 1996, stipulated that the US must suspend counter-narcotics funding to military units accused of human rights violations unless the US Secretary of State can confirm that the perpetrators have been brought to justice. Although the bill prevented cooperation with some notorious Colombian human rights violators, it was no panacea, partly because US Special Forces, whose involvement in foreign drug control deepened over the 1990s, were exempt from these restrictions (Farah 1998; Priest 1998).

In August 1997, the Colombian military accepted the terms for US aid as laid out in the Leahy Amendment, despite reservations about the imposition of unilaterally defined conditions. This step facilitated an increase in US support to the Colombian armed forces, not least because it helped US proponents of increased US aid to bolster their claims that the time was right for such an increase. But US policy-makers also began to consider an increase in US aid because the Colombian war, which had been going on for decades more or less intensively, shifted into higher gear. In October 1997, for example, the US media widely covered guerilla activities during the municipal elections in Colombia (Youngers 2001: 20).

Moreover, it became increasingly evident that drugs and the insurgency were linked. The FARC, in particular, seemed to profit from the drug trade by encouraging peasants to cultivate coca, taxing coca fields, and protecting drug laboratories as well as landing strips and other trafficking infrastructure. In 1999, the Colombian government believed that the FARC had earned as much as $400 million per year from the drug trade. To this, the government added the estimated $500 million derived from kidnapping, extortion, and various other crimes, as well as legal business investments. Total FARC earnings were thus estimated at $900 million in the late 1990s (Bagley 2001: 7). Although this figure was probably inflated, few observers doubted that the FARC leadership was able to fund a large number of combatants.

The FARC's involvement in the illicit drug industry led US policy-makers, who were reconsidering the US role in Colombia, to rediscover the "narco-guerilla" paradigm invented by the US ambassador to Colombia, Lewis Tambs, in the 1980s. In the late 1990s, the term implied that the Colombian guerilla were involved in all stages of the drug industry, that the state could not cope with this challenge, and that the US had to help Colombia to drive the guerilla out of drug-production regions. As early as 1996, senior State Department offi cial Robert Gelbard had said that the FARC was Colombia's third-largest drug cartel (Tickner 2003: 79). US policy-makers greatly oversimplified the guerilla–drug connection when describing the FARC as a "narco-guerilla." First, traffickers and rebels have distinct and often conflicting goals. Second, it was doubtful whether the guerilla actively participated in the higher stages of the illicit drug business. The DEA itself stated that there were few indications that the FARC was engaged in cocaine trafficking (Tate 1999: 2; Tickner 2003: 80). With regard to the ELN, their involvement in the drug business was even less obvious, since that group specialized in kidnapping and extortion. However, these subtleties did not prevent US officials from linking the insurgency and the drug trade in order to show that the Colombian state found itself in a desperate situation and that it needed US help.

Colombia was thus faced with several interrelated problems: large-scale drug production and trafficking, widespread corruption, and an increase in guerilla activities. Moreover, the human rights situation grew worse and worse, with increasing numbers of Colombians killed or displaced by different factions. During the late 1990s, violence led to the death of an estimated 30,000 people in Colombia every year (The Economist 1998).

The US was directly affected by the Colombian conflict. Drug problems were a burden to the US economy, US businesses lost investment opportunities or investments, and US citizens based in Colombia were threatened. In addition, the conflict risked destabilizing Colombia's neighbors, some of which were of strategic interest to the US. In Panama, for example, the US transferred authority over the canal to the Panamanian government in December 1999. The possibility of the Colombian conflict spilling over into the Canal Zone caused great concern in Washington (Shifter 2000: 53). Moreover, the US felt migration pressure from Colombia. Between 1996 and 2001, over one million Colombians (out of a total population of around 40 million) left the country (Carpenter 2003: 61). Migration was motivated by high levels of violence and a bad economy. Historically, Colombia has had one of the healthiest economies in Latin America, despite prolonged violence. In the second half of the 1990s, however, unemployment, inflation, public debts, capital flight, and migration increased sharpl

To improve the situation, the US needed a more cordial relationship with the Colombian government. This was made possible by a change in Colombia's government. In August 1998, Andrés Pastrana replaced Samper as President, to the relief of Washington. Now, as many times before, Bogotá had to perform a difficult balancing act. On the one hand, the Colombian government had to prove to the US that it was making progress against drug traffickers and rebels. On the other hand, it had to negotiate with the rebels to make them lay down their weapons. In July 1998, president-elect Pastrana met with FARC leader Manuel Marulanda in a FARC-controlled area. Following this rather daring visit, the government and FARC began to negotiate the creation of a demilitarized zone. This *zona de despeje* (also known as *zona de distensión* or, more polemically, "FARC-landia") was about the size of Switzerland, had an estimated 100,000 inhabitants, and comprised several municipalities in the south–central departments of Meta and Caquetá (see Annex I, the map of Colombia). The agreement came into effect on November 7, 1998 when the Pastrana administration gave the FARC a guarantee that all military units would be withdrawn from the region for an initial period of 90 days. It also agreed not to gather intelligence in the zone and to allow the FARC to establish a quasi-government in the zone. Thus, the Colombian government effectively ceded control over a sizable part of the national territory, although, one might argue that it gave up something that it did not possess anyway. By giving the FARC a sanctuary, the government wanted to reduce pressure on the rebels and thus induce them to negotiate some form of power-sharing (Bagley 2001: 8; Carpenter 2003: 69).

From the official US perspective, the peace process was a Colombian affair. In reality, however, the US was deeply involved in the Colombian conflict. US material and intelligence support was crucial for the aerial fumigation campaign and for operations against non-state actors. These operations entailed significan risks for the personnel involved. In two incidents in 1997 and 1998, three US pilots working for private military companies contracted by the Pentagon died when their crop-dusting aircraft crashed during eradication missions. On July 23, 1999, five US military personnel and two Colombian military personnel died when a US Army helicopter loaded with high-tech equipment used for the interception of trafficker communication crashed in southern Colombia (Ruiz 2001: 147–150). There was no evidence that the FARC was responsible for these crashes. However, the guerilla had sufficient firepower, and many Colombian and US officials argued that drug control necessitated a reduction of guerilla activities. In late December 1998, a US official said: "Colombia poses a greater immediate threat to us than Bosnia did, yet it receives almost no attention. So policy is set by default" (quoted in Shifter 2000: 52).

On February 25, 1999, the FARC kidnapped three US indigenous rights activists. Two weeks later, their bodies were found. It was unclear which FARC members were responsible, and the FARC leadership promised that it would punish the perpetrators (Crandall 2002a: 161). Yet this promise could not prevent an outburst of anger in the US against the FARC. The murders "effectively constrained an American role in any peace effort, since the incident made further meetings between State Department officials and FARC representatives (which had taken place in December 1998) politically impossible" (Shifter 2000: 52). Other spectacular acts such as the ELN hijacking of an Avianca aircraft flying between a provincial city and Bogotá on April 12, 1999 and an ELN kidnapping of 143 churchgoers in Cali six weeks later additionally hardened feelings against the guerilla.

A new US role in Colombia implied an increase in military aid. Since 1989, the CNP had been the main beneficiary of US anti-drug aid, which came in the form of hardware and training. The US rationale was that the CNP should focus on domestic law enforcement, while the Colombian military should protect the country's borders and focus on international operations such as the ABDP. This strategy not only laid out a seemingly neat division of labor between the police and military, but, as discussed above, also reflected US concerns about human rights violations by the Colombian military.

But in October 1998, the US changed course. Congress resumed military assistance to Colombia, which had been suspended since 1996. In a bilateral agreement signed in December 1998, the two countries institutionalized meetings between military officials and defined the terms of an increase in US aid. In fiscal year 1999, the US allocated $289 million to Colombia. This sum was three times the 1998 amount, and it made Colombia the third-largest recipient of US aid after Israel and Egypt (see Annex II, Chart 3). Most of the funding went to the CNP, which was now able to purchase, among other items, six Black Hawk helicopters. But the Colombian military received assistance as well, amounting to $40 million. This funding was used to establish an elite, mobile anti-drug battalion composed of 950 Colombian Army personnel whom the US would train and equip. The battalion's task was to support National Police operations by pushing guerillas out of coca-growing regions and protecting eradication and police teams against attacks from armed opponents. The US also shared more intelligence with the Colombian military (Ramírez *et al.* 2005: 107; Shifter 2000: 51).

In the late 1990s, roughly 250–300 US military trainers and advisors – largely Special Operations Forces – and more than 100 US law enforcement and intelligence agents were operating in Colombia. Moreover, private contractors participated in the drug control effort. Even though military outsourcing is problematic because private companies lack democratic accountability, their use for dangerous missions became increasingly popular among US policy-makers during the 1990s. Former US ambassador to Colombia Myles Frechette explained the reasons for this in blunt terms: "Congress and the American people don't want any servicemen killed overseas. So it makes sense that if contractors want to risk their lives, they get the job" (quoted in Tamayo 2001a).[1]

In addition to implementing US policies, private companies also influence policy-making. In September 1999, Lockheed Martin, a manufacturer of military hardware used in Colombia, commissioned a poll. The results showed that many US citizens were unsatisfied with the Clinton administration's drug policies and thought that the Republicans would do better. During this period, before the US presidential elections in 2000, Lockheed Martin and several helicopter manufacturers were lobbying for an increase in US anti-drug efforts in Colombia (Isikoff and Vistica 2000). Similarly, oil corporations lobbied for more US involvement in Colombia (Scott 2003: chapters 4 and 6). Often, they were preaching to the converted. In 1998, the head of the US Southern Command, General Charles Wilhelm, said that new oil discoveries had increased Colombia's "strategic importance." Two years later, two senior US policy-makers wrote that Colombia's oil reserves would "remain untapped unless stability is restored." These words were echoed by a US Senator: "A decade ago the United States went to war with a powerful enemy partly to stabilize a major oil-producing region . . . The oil picture in Latin America is strikingly similar to that of the Middle East, except that Colombia provides us with more oil today than Kuwait did then" (all quotes taken from: Dunning and Wirpsa 2004: 93).

While Washington changed its policy toward Colombia, many US observers were uneasy about an increase in military aid. They feared that the Colombian military would use the money against rebels instead of traffickers, and that the US would become involved in a Vietnam-like quagmire (Rohter 1999; Darling 1999). Critics also drew parallels with the wars fought in Central America during the Reagan era. Indeed, in terms of funding and personnel, the US engagement in Colombia in 1999 was similar to the US engagement in El Salvador in the 1980s (Tate 1999: 3). In Colombia, many even anticipated an outright US military invasion (Johnson 1999). These fears and analogies should not be discarded easily. After all, US personnel trained and equipped Colombian military units and shared military intelligence with Colombia. The information passed on to Colombia pertained not only to the activities of traffickers, but also to those of insurgents (Tate 1999: 4).

Fears about a blending of counter-drug and counter-insurgency missions were closely related to concerns about human rights abuses. US officials argued that the US would not cooperate with perpetrators of human rights violations, that US training included courses on human rights, and that US funding for the Colombian security forces and judiciary would make the Colombian state more accountable and transparent. Critics, however, said that the Colombian military would continue to violate human rights. Moreover, they said that US military aid would aggravate human rights violations by strengthening right-wing paramilitary forces. These were organized under the umbrella institution *Autodefensas Unidas de Colombia* (AUC). Having grown in strength during the 1990s, the number of AUC fighters was estimated at around 7,000 at the end of the decade (Bagley 2001: 8). The AUC was led by the ruthless Carlos Castaño and supported by large landowners, some Colombian government officials, and Colombian citizens who sought protection from rebels. Moreover, the AUC cooperated with drug traffickers and derived large sums of money from their involvement in the illicit drug industry. In March 2000, Castaño publicly said what many people had known for some time: drugs represented the AUC's largest source of income (Tickner 2003: 80). In addition, the AUC had close relations with members of the Colombian military, who provided the paramilitaries at times with intelligence and logistical support against the rebels. In mid-1999, the military apparently even saved Castaño from FARC forces that had surrounded the headquarters of the paramilitary leader (Bagley 2001: 9).

The close ties between paramilitaries and the Colombian military meant that an increase in US military aid risked strengthening paramilitaries and thus aggravating human rights violations. In 1999, the Colombian government reported 402 massacres, which together cost the lives of 1,863 people. Most of the victims died at the hands of paramilitaries (Shifter 2000: 53). Many terrifie Colombians fled from the paramilitaries, who often massacred villagers whom they suspected of collaborating with the rebels. Paramilitaries thus contributed to creating one of the worst humanitarian catastrophes in the post-Cold War era. In 1999 alone, the number of Colombians driven from their homes and communities by political and drug-related violence was estimated at 225,000, with paramilitaries held responsible for almost half of all forced displacement. The guerilla, state security forces, criminal groups, and traffickers together were held responsible for the other half, with the guerillas taking the lead (Bagley 2001: 12).

Plan Colombia and the Andean Regional Initiative

This section examines Plan Colombia and its successor program, the Andean Regional Initiative. It shows that these US-sponsored anti-drug initiatives have coincided with a displacement of drug production and trafficking within Colombia and to neighboring states.

Plan Colombia

From mid-1999, US policy-makers tried to muster public support for a signific ant US involvement in the Colombian conflict. On July 13, 1999, ONDCP director, Barry McCaffrey, arguing that Colombia represented an "emergency," leaked a memo of the Department of State that proposed to increase US funding for Colombia to $1 billion. According to Russell Crandall (2002b: 162), this proposed increase in aid "served to take the wind out of the sails of Republican critics in the House of Representatives, who had been claiming for years that the Clinton White House had not been doing enough to fight the drug war in Colombia." At a press conference on July 21, President Clinton expressed his support for Pastrana's peace efforts and said that improving the situation in Colombia was in the "national security interest" of the US. On August 10, Secretary of State Madeleine Albright wrote in the *New York Times* that the US should support the peace process (Shifter 2000: 54). That same day, US Under-Secretary of State, Thomas Pickering, was dispatched to Colombia, becoming the highest-ranking US government official to visit the country in years. Upon his return to Washington, Pickering endorsed McCaffrey's view that a massive increase in US aid was needed (Crandall 2002b: 162).

Backed by these reassurances, Colombian President Andrés Pastrana launched Plan Colombia in September 1999. The plan was essentially a White House text. The Spanish version of the text was only available months after the circulation of an English-language version. The version of Plan Colombia presented by Pastrana replaced an earlier peace plan that had been drafted by his administration and that had emphasized negotiation and peacemaking with the rebels as a precondition for a comprehensive reconstruction of Colombia. As it had not sufficiently accommodated US preferences for military solutions, it was replaced by the new version (Cooper 2001; Ramírez *et al.* 2005: 107–108).

Not before early January 2000 was this new version revealed to the Colombian public by a Colombian newspaper. Neither the Colombian Parliament and its committees, nor the National Council for Peace (*Consejo Nacional de Paz*), an important Colombian institution at the time, had been invited to discuss the plan. The FARC had not been informed either (Zinecker 2002: 43). Yet, despite the strong US role in drafting the plan, Pastrana presented it as a Colombian plan, as he had to defend himself against accusations of giving in to US demands. The White House consented to this public relations move, since it could now argue that by increasing its aid to Colombia, it was merely responding to calls for help from an important US ally (Crandall 2002a: 149, 150, 163).

Plan Colombia was ambitious and was advertised as a comprehensive scheme for curing the country's many ills. It envisaged an improvement of Colombia's economy, a reduction in poverty and violence, and negotiations for a sustainable peace agreement between the different armed groups and the government. A reduction of drug supplies was another important element. In fact, it was a main component of the new approach. While the earlier version of the peace plan had emphasized the need to find a peaceful solution to the Colombian conflict in order to reduce drug supplies, the new version was based on the rationale that a reduction of drug supplies was a precondition for achieving peace. If rebels were deprived of their income, they would be weakened and would thus be more willing to accept demands from the government. Rather optimistically, the plan foresaw a reduction of coca and poppy cultivation, drug production, and drug trafficking by 50 percent over a period of six years

Achieving this objective and the other objectives mentioned above would cost $7.5 billion. Of this sum, the Colombian government would provide $4 billion and the US between $1.5 and $2 billion, with the remainder covered by European and other countries as well as multilateral institutions. It was foreseen that the US would focus on military aid and the other donors on non-coercive elements.

On January 11, 2000, the White House announced that the US would contribute about $1.6 billion to Plan Colombia. Following this proposal, Congress debated US policies toward Colombia for several months. An agreement was reached in summer 2000, and on July 13, 2000, President Clinton signed the Plan Colombia legislation. Overall, the US would supply Colombia and its neighbors with roughly $1.3 billion in aid for fiscal years 2000 and 2001. With $860 million, Colombia received the overwhelming share of this funding. Around 75 percent of the money for Colombia, or $642 million, was designated for the Colombian military and police (see Annex II, Chart 3; and Ramírez *et al.* 2005: 107–108; GAO 2004a: 8).

The most expensive items on the military procurement list for Plan Colombia were dozens of high-tech Black Hawk and Huey helicopters. These would form the backbone of two more anti-drug battalions that would complement the single existing battalion that had become operational in December 1999. These three battalions, which constituted a brigade of 2,300 men, would be deployed to the southern departments of Caquetá and Putumayo (see Annex I, the map of Colombia). In the latter department, located along the border with Ecuador, more than 100,000 residents cultivated enough coca to produce about half of Colombia's total annual cocaine output, estimated in 2000 at about 600 tons (Gutierrez 2000). Parallel to military and police operations against traffickers coca was to be destroyed through massive aerial spraying. This "push into southern Colombia" was a cornerstone of the US contribution to Plan Colombia.

Non-coercive program elements were given low priority, as Chart 3 illustrates. Investments in human rights programs, judicial reform measures, and AD were overshadowed by the increase in military aid. As a consequence, human-rights groups accused the US government of fueling the Colombian conflict by delivering more arms to a country that possessed too many already. They argued that links between Colombian military units and paramilitary forces continued to be strong and that US military aid would inevitably increase human rights violations. Moreover, NGOs described US and Colombian deliberations to develop and set free a fungus against coca plants as preparations for biological warfare (Sunshine Project 2001).

Observers criticized fumigation as well. Under Plan Colombia, fumigation was to reach unprecedented levels, and more destructive herbicides would be used to destroy as much coca as quickly as possible. The new defoliant was a mixture of glyphosate known as Round-Up, a commercial product produced and patented by the Monsanto company, and added surfactants. Critics argued that fumigation would contaminate water supplies and kill animals and plants, and that it would have a negative effect on the health of people living in or near sprayed areas. Indeed, many residents reported eye and skin afflictions and respiratory illnesses after fumigation. In addition, fumigation inevitably affected not only coca and poppy, but also legal crops, and even AD projects financed by international donors (Cederstav and Puentes 2004).

Plan Colombia also threatened rural populations by prompting reactions from non-state actors. In November 2000, the FARC, anticipating the government's push into southern Colombia and responding to paramilitary advances, set up roadblocks around the commercial center of Putumayo, thus preventing the delivery of food and medical supplies for almost six weeks. Although the Colombian military eventually airlifted supplies to the region, the security situation in the country was obviously untenable. According to Bogotá, more than 126,000 people were made homeless by the war in 2000. Human rights groups said that the number was much higher (Carpenter 2003: 61).

Criticism of Plan Colombia was particularly strong in Europe. In February 2001, the European Parliament voted 474 to 1 against European support for the project. Eventually, the EU provided some funding, but much less than envisaged by the US and Colombia. Moreover, most of the EU funding was given to NGOs and was earmarked for programs not directly related to Plan Colombia (Transnational Institute 2001). The European refusal to foot the bill for what most Europeans regarded as a counterproductive military campaign came despite a clever public-relations move contrived by Washington and Bogotá. To satisfy both Europe and the US, two versions of Plan Colombia were circulated. One version, circulated in Colombia and Europe, emphasized the need to achieve a peaceful solution to the Colombian conflict. The other version, circulated in the US, pointed at the need to reduce drug supplies in order to improve the Colombian situation (Tickner 2003: 84).

The Clinton administration was worried about the lack of international and domestic support for Plan Colombia. The most troublesome accusation was that the US was being dragged into a Vietnam-like counter-insurgency adventure. To counter this assertion, the White House argued that Plan Colombia was an anti-drug and not a counterinsurgency program. Since both Republicans and Democrats agreed on the need to reduce drug supplies, Plan Colombia enjoyed strong bipartisan support (Crandall 2002b: 163). Besides mustering domestic support, the presentation of Plan Colombia as an anti-drug program also imposed limits on US support for the Colombian peace process, which was linked to the politically perilous counter-insurgency question. Since the White House wanted to avoid becoming entangled in the peace process, it allocated a mere $3 million to it. However, drawing a clear line between drug control on the one hand and insurgency and the peace process on the other hand was unrealistic. Colombian non-state armed groups were present in, or controlled, important coca cultivation and drug production zones, and there were signs that rebels had become deeper involved in the drug trade. Thus, attempts to force the rebels out of the coca production zones would increase US involvement in the Colombian civil conflict

While the White House presented Plan Colombia as a drug-control issue only, the political situation in Colombia worsened. The peace process was repeatedly interrupted by hostilities. Due to US arms deliveries, provocations by the Colombian military, and paramilitary attacks, the conflicting parties failed to trust each other and to negotiate peace. But the FARC and ELN were also to blame. Hostile acts committed by the guerilla raised suspicions over whether the rebels really wanted peace or whether they were seeking strategic advantages over the government. Reports indicated that the FARC, which stationed around 5,000 of its troops in the *zona de despeje*, violated both the letter and the spirit of the peace agreement it had negotiated with the Colombian government. As Bruce Bagley (2001: 8) writes, the FARC was accused of

> carrying out selective assassinations, harboring kidnap victims, threatening local mayors and judges, conducting illegal searches and seizures, detaining innocent civilians, improperly re-routing public moneys, forcibly recruiting children into their ranks, training new troops and terrorist commandos, and constructing anti-aircraft batteries and other military fortifications to strengthen their defenses. They have also been accused of exploiting some 35,000 hectares of coca within the zone, of buying up coca leaf from peasant farmers in surrounding departments [. . .] and selling it directly to the drug cartels, and of utilizing the 37 landing strips at their disposal inside the demilitarized zone to fly [. .] cocaine to virtually any part of the country.

Despite this unhelpful behavior, Pastrana extended the deadline for the zonal agreement repeatedly during his tenure, not least because the Colombian military would have been unable to retake the area even if ordered to do so. The FARC was too well entrenched, organized, and financed to be defeated militarily. Thus, while officially there was peace, the war continued

It was very dangerous for the Colombian and US armed forces to fly over territories infiltrated or controlled by the rebels, who would fire at their aircraft from the ground. In January 2000 alone, the FARC fired missiles at aircraft eight times, although none of the missiles seem to have hit their targets (Shifter 2000: 52; Bagley 2001: 8). In October 2000, the FARC dealt a significant blow to the Colombian armed forces when it killed many soldiers during three days of fight ing. The Colombian military also lost one of the prestigious Black Hawk helicopters. In spring 2001, for the first time, one of the US-trained and equipped anti-drug battalions killed Colombian rebels during an anti-drug operation (Evans 2001b). These developments showed that anti-drug and anti-insurgency operations were becoming increasingly intertwined and that the US, despite official announcements to the contrary, was deeply implicated in the country's conflict

Plan Colombia caused concern not only in the US, Europe, and Colombia, but also in the countries sharing borders with Colombia. Neighboring states feared that rebels and traffickers would respond to military pressure by relocating bases, coca fields, and drug laboratories across Colombia's borders. As a consequence, Venezuela, Brazil, and Panama distanced themselves from Plan Colombia in 2000 (the following year, criticism was more muted because Latin American governments saw their participation in Plan Colombia as an opportunity to receive US funding) (Carpenter 2003: 79). To avert the feared spillover, Colombia's neighbors reinforced their military presence in the border region. For example, Brazil purchased new helicopters from France to improve its air mobility along the border with Colombia, over 1,500 kilometers long, and Peru redeployed some of its helicopter fleet to the border region (Crandall 2002b: 166). Yet despite these preventive measures, there were signs that the Colombian conflict was spilling over. In the summer of 2000, US media reported new plantings of coca and poppies in Peru (Krauss 2000). In November 2000, US State Department official Thomas Pickering acknowledged that "there is already a balloon effect" (quoted in Crandall 2002b: 160).

In December 2000, the Colombian military began its push into southern Colombia, and the large-scale fumigation campaign began with a focus on the Putumayo. In Colombia, farmers protested against fumigation. Internationally, donors were concerned about the impact of fumigation on AD projects. Indeed, fumigation in late 2000 and early 2001 damaged at least 11 AD projects financed by Colombia and the UN (Marsh 2004: 11). Nevertheless, despite national and international protests, fumigation continued. With this new phase of US drug control starting in earnest, the spillover of the drug industry became very visible. In Colombia, many farmers whose fields had been sprayed, sometimes several times, were forced to migrate to other regions.

Officially, the fumigation campaign targeted large "industrial" farms that were assumed to be owned by traffickers or rebels. In reality, however, small farms were sprayed as well (Marsh 2004: 5; Cooper 2001). Many farmers who had to leave moved to the sprawling barrios of Bogotá and other cities. But thousands of families also migrated to new rural areas where they grew coca again. The displacement of people occurred mainly in the areas affected by fumigation. In Putumayo, for example, over 55,000 people were displaced between the beginning of Plan Colombia and August 2003. Before the implementation of Plan Colombia, only 415 displacements had been registered (Marsh 2004: 28).

By May 2001, 75,000 acres of coca had been fumigated in Colombia. This campaign was effective in reducing coca cultivation in the sprayed areas. However, in the summer of 2001, aerial surveys showed that a lot of previously unnoticed coca was being cultivated on Colombia's eastern plains, where the presence of rebels was strong. Worse still, it became apparent now that more coca was cultivated in Colombia after the initial phase of the spraying campaign than before. The US ambassador to Colombia, Anne W. Patterson, was obliged to acknowledge the sobering situation regarding illicit crop cultivation in late July 2001, saying that "[i]t's quite possible we've underestimated the coca in Colombia. Everywhere we look there is more coca than we expected. There's just more out there than we thought" (quoted in Carpenter 2003: 77).

Neighboring countries were affected by Plan Colombia as well. Ecuador faced thousands of Colombian migrants. Armed groups came as well. In January 2001, Ecuadorian troops killed six men believed to be FARC members at a drug laboratory near the Colombian border. In August 2001, Ecuadorian troops discovered a FARC camp in the jungle near Colombia. In the second half of 2001, three Ecuadorian policemen were killed, presumably by intruders from Colombia. For the Ecuadorian vice president, these incidents were "a product of Plan Colombia. [T]he guerillas feel harassed and seek a place where they can act more calmly, which is worrisome" (quoted in Carpenter 2003: 82).

Moreover, Colombia's neighbors experienced an increase in illicit crop cultivation, drug production, and drug trafficking. In Ecuador, Colombian trafficker increased coca cultivation by offering money to farmers (Cooper 2001; Crandall 2002a: 160). In Brazil, new coca plantations were reported in the country's northwest in the spring of 2001 (Stanton 2001). And in Venezuela, Colombian trafficking organizations continued to expand their operations. Venezuelan security forces spotted and eradicated coca fields as large as eight hectares and, for the first time, discovered several large coca paste processing laboratories (Department of State 2002: Venezuela).[2]

Peru was affected as well. In early 2001, journalists reported new coca field (Marshall 2001). This prompted fear in the Peruvian government of a return to the 1980s and 1990s, when coca cultivation, forced eradication, and political violence had mutually reinforced each other (as described in the previous chapter). In addition, there were concerns that the Colombian conflic would lead to a rise in Peruvian poppy cultivation. Undeniably, Peruvian poppy cultivation was on the rise. In its narcotics control report for 2001, the Department of State (2002: Colombia) wrote that "Colombian narcotraffickers supply Peruvian farmers with seeds from Colombian poppies, offering technical assistance and cash loans." Peruvian sources confirmed the new dynamics. A Peruvian intelligence report warned that "Plan Colombia is forcing Colombian guerillas, drug trafficking firms, coca and marijuana growers, as well as gunrunners to Peruvian border villages" (cited in Crandall 2002a: 167). In mid-2001, the Peruvian ambassador wrote a letter to US policy-makers stating that the increase in poppy production "is a clear indication of the first effects of the spillover of Plan Colombia: Intelligence information shows that Colombian cartels are relocating their opium poppy operations in Peru" (cited in Hedges 2001). The rise in Peruvian poppy cultivation was also reflected in higher eradication figures. Whereas in 2000 only 26 hectares of opium were eradicated, in 2001 the number jumped to 135 hectares (*The Economist* 2002).

Hence, it was evident in 2000 and early 2001 that Plan Colombia was severely criticized by the international community; that a speedy implementation of the plan was unlikely; that insurgents were a difficult and dangerous negotiating partner; that Plan Colombia aggravated social and environmental problems; and that there were signs of a spill-over of the drug industry and rebel activities within Colombia and to neighboring states. As part of their effort to counter criticism of Plan Colombia, US government officials replaced the term Plan Colombia with the term Andean Regional Initiative, the new label under which US aid would be provided to Colombia from fiscal year 2002

The Andean Regional Initiative

When George W. Bush succeeded Bill Clinton as US President in early 2001, the future of US drug policy toward Colombia was unclear. On the one hand, there were signs that the new administration would focus more on drug demand reduction. The new Secretary of Defense Donald Rumsfeld, for example, said that drug problems resulted mainly from the demand for drugs (Stanton 2001). On the other hand, many in the administration supported coercive drug policies. It soon became clear that the Bush administration would not disassociate itself from the Colombia policy it had inherited from the Clinton administration. Some adjustments were made, but overall the US continued on the same militarized course. In fact, it soon became clear that the Bush administration would escalate US involvement in Colombia.

As one of the first steps toward improving the record of Plan Colombia, the Bush administration increased funding for Colombia's neighbors to help them cope with the negative externalities of Plan Colombia. In March 2001, the administration proposed to spend $731 million dollars on the Andean Regional Initiative in fiscal year 2002.[3] Of this sum, $332 million was earmarked for Colombia's neighbors, with $156 million to be given to Peru, $101 million to Bolivia, and $75 million to Brazil, Ecuador, Panama, and Venezuela. On May 16, 2001, the administration officially announced the Initiative. In late 2001, the

US Congress reduced the Initiative's budget to $567 million, thus forcing Colombia's neighbors to be content with much less money than they had hoped for (Carpenter 2003: 84; Isacson 2005: 46). Still, from the perspective of Colombia's neighbors, the Andean Regional Initiative was an improvement over Plan Colombia.

In 2001, the US lifted restrictions on the use of US funds against insurgents, thus effectively merging the wars on drugs, terror, and insurgency. In a June 2001 report, the RAND Corporation had advised Washington to no longer distinguish between drug control and counter-insurgency, arguing that Bogotá needed to control the national territory to reduce drug supplies (Carpenter 2003: 62–63). In August 2001, three members of the Irish Republican Army (IRA) were arrested in Colombia. Reports that they had operated in the FARC's *zona de despeje* heightened US anxieties about international terrorist networks. In response to criticism that it was treating paramilitaries softly, the US government, on September 10, 2001, added the AUC to the State Department's list of foreign terrorist organizations (the FARC and ELN had already been placed on the list on October 9, 1997). Concerns about terrorism in Colombia became even more urgent after the attacks of September 11, 2001 on New York and Washington. US policy-makers now saw the fight against Colombian non-state armed groups as part of the global US "war on terror." In October 2001, the State Department called the kidnapping and murder of a popular former Colombian politician an act of terrorism (Crandall 2002b: 169). In the same month, US Ambassador Patterson said that "there is no question we are now focusing more on terrorism in Colombia" (quoted in Carpenter 2003: 63–64).

One of the strongest supporters for US counter-insurgency aid was the Colombian government itself, which wanted to free itself from previous constraints on the use of US aid. Skillfully playing on US opinion, Pastrana argued that "narcoterrorists" were financing violence not only in Afghanistan, but also in Colombia (quoted in Carpenter 2003: 64). On February 20, 2002, the Colombian government labeled the FARC a terrorist organization. In March, the White House asked Congress to lift restrictions preventing the Colombian government from using US aid for counter-insurgency operations. The Republican-dominated Congress readily supported this policy change, and later in the year, a law allowing the use of lethal assistance to Colombian counter-terrorist operations came into effect. From then onwards, Colombian security forces could legally use US aid and training against non-state actors. Although this decision marked a change in official policy, US aid had been used in counter-insurgency operations before. Documents published by the National Security Archive (Evans 2002) show that the line between counter-drug and counter-insurgency operations had become increasingly blurred ever since the US government began to militarize drug control, despite legal restrictions and public assurances to the contrary.

The official decision to merge the wars on drugs, insurgency, and terrorism also led to an increase in US funding for the protection of critical infrastructures. In February 2002, Washington allocated around $100 million for protecting the

770-kilometer Caño Limón–Coveñas oil pipeline, 44 percent of which was owned by the US company Occidental Petroleum. In 2001, rebels had bombed the pipeline 170 times, which had led to the spilling of 2.9 million barrels of oil, 11 times the amount spilled in the Exxon Valdez catastrophe (Congress 2002: 20). According to US Ambassador Patterson, the pipeline was "important for the future of [Colombia], for our petroleum supplies and for the confidence of our investors" (quoted in Dunning and Wirpsa 2004: 95). The decision to train and equip Colombian army units who were tasked with protecting the pipeline showed again that the US involvement in Colombia was strongly motivated by energy interests.

In early 2002, the Colombian peace process, which had always been a fragile affair, broke down completely, and the Colombian war escalated once more. Many reasons contributed to this development, including fighting between paramilitaries and rebels, and increasing military pressure on the rebels. In January 2002, negotiations between the FARC and the Colombian government collapsed. Pastrana announced the end of his sanctuary policy, and ordered the military to prepare to retake the zone given to the rebels. A first deadline for the rebels to withdraw was extended at the last moment due to international mediation. On February 20, 2002, however, Pastrana responded to the FARC's hijacking of an airplane and the kidnapping of a Colombian senator on the plane by ordering the armed forces to move into the *despeje*. This decision, taken on the same day that Pastrana called the FARC a terrorist organization, ended a situation that had become increasingly embarrassing for the Colombian government.

US figures published in March 2002 showed that 2001 had not been a good year for the joint US–Colombian anti-drug effort. Coca cultivation increased by almost 25 percent compared to 2000. It now stood at an estimated 169,800 hectares (see Table 3 and Annex II, Chart 1). In addition to this troubling news, coca cultivation migrated within Colombia, with most of the increase occurring outside the eradication areas (Department of State 2002: Colombia). This displacement of coca cultivation was enabled, among other factors, by a record number of internally displaced people. In 2001, the number of Colombians fleeing political violence was estimated at 341,000. Colombia now had over two million internally displaced people, making it the world's fourth-largest country of internal displacement (Washington Office on Latin America 2002: 1)

In August 2002, Alvaro Uribe became the new president of Colombia. Having won the presidential election on a law and order platform, he quickly moved to reestablish governmental control over previously ungoverned parts of Colombia. His administration also lifted restrictions on areas where spraying could take place, which had been imposed earlier out of concern about peasant protests and the environment. This, as well as a huge increase in the number of people extradited to the US, made clear that Uribe was doing what the US had hoped he would do. As a consequence, Uribe became very popular among US policy-makers, who tirelessly praised his efforts.

At first glance, Uribe's hard-line policies seemed to pay off. In 2003, the number of encounters between the military and the FARC was higher than in

2002, and more municipalities had a military or police presence. According to the US government, by October 2003, the Colombian National Police had reestablished a police presence in 140 municipalities out of a total 158 that had no police presence in late 2002 (Charles 2003). Moreover, several FARC commanders were captured or killed, and the Colombian government reported fewer guerilla attacks on population centers, fewer massacres committed by non-state armed groups, and an increase in guerilla desertions (Felbab-Brown 2004: 16–17).

One should not overestimate these trends, however. Although the guerillas suffered setbacks, their retreat from some areas was probably also a tactical maneuver. They simply responded to military operations of the Uribe administration by holding out in the jungle (Canby 2004). Moreover, rebels continued to attack government forces. In 2005, the FARC staged 342 attacks on Colombian military and police targets. In the same year, 271 Colombian soldiers and police were killed in combat operations with guerillas, up from 212 in 2003 (Isacson 2006). Hence, the guerillas were far from ineffective in combat, as claimed by the Colombian and US governments. The Colombian government tried to keep the guerilla at bay by bombing rebel-controlled areas, with the support of the US. The US made its presence felt in other ways, too. In early 2006, in the largest drug trafficking indictment in US history, a $75 million bounty was placed on the heads of 50 alleged rebel leaders whom Washington saw as responsible of supplying 60 percent of the US cocaine market (Blum 2006).

At the same time, paramilitary forces underwent a transformation. During the implementation of Plan Colombia, paramilitaries had become more powerful, with their numbers increasing from an estimated 8,000 in 2000 to 12,000 in 2002 (Felbab-Brown 2004: 19). Uribe took some measures against paramilitaries, and negotiated a demobilization of paramilitary units. As of March 2006, some 23,000 paramilitary fighters had laid down their weapons (Forero 2006). During this demobilization process, the paramilitaries were treated much more gently than rebels. In response, they generally refrained from openly massacring people and thus causing public outrage, preferring to act more discreetly instead. This did not prevent the paramilitaries from continuing to commit human rights abuses. In fact, there are indications of increasing attacks against civilians. In the first quarter of 2003, about 30 such attacks were reported. In the second quarter of 2005, there were over 80 reported attacks (Isacson 2006). Moreover, the political power of the paramilitaries was increasing. As the *New York Times* (Forero 2006) reported, "commanders use bribery and intimidation to control local lawmakers and even blocks of representatives in the Congress while they reshape their militias into criminal networks that traffic in cocaine, extort businesses and loot local governments."

One of the main reasons for Washington's enthusiastic support of Uribe was a reported decline in Colombian coca cultivation in 2002 and 2003. After an increase in coca cultivation in 2001, cultivation decreased in 2002, to 144,450 hectares (see Chart 1). This was a 15 percent reduction compared to 2001, and the first decline in Colombian coca cultivation after eight years of steady increases. US officials responded jubilantly to this news. ONDCP director John Walters referred to the decrease as a "turning point" (quoted in *The Economist* 2003). According to Walters and other US government officials, the decrease showed that US support to Colombia was finally paying off. They attributed the 2002 decline in coca cultivation to record levels of aerial fumigation. In 2002, the Colombian government sprayed 122,695 hectares of coca. This represented a 45 percent increase over 2001 (Department of State 2003: Colombia).

In 2003, the downward trend in Colombian coca cultivation continued. Coca was grown on 113,850 hectares, a 33 percent reduction compared to 2001, when coca cultivation had reached a peak at 169,800 hectares. As a consequence of the Colombian decline, world coca cultivation decreased. Whereas in 2001, total coca cultivation had stood at 223,700 hectares, in 2003 it was down to 166,300 hectares. As before, the decline in Colombian coca cultivation in 2003 was accompanied by record levels of aerial fumigation, with over 132,000 hectares of coca and nearly 3,000 hectares of poppy sprayed (GAO 2004b: 5, fn 7). Record fumigation levels were made possible, among others, by the lifting of restrictions forbidding the spraying of small plantations and plantations where coca was mixed with licit crops. From 2000 through 2003, an estimated 380,000 hectares, which is 8 percent of Colombia's arable land, were fumigated (Ramírez *et al.* 2005: 112). In addition to aerial fumigation, thousands of hectares of coca and poppy were uprooted manually. Eradication continued at record levels in 2004 and 2005.

However, during these two years, Colombian coca cultivation increased – to the dismay of many US policy-makers. In 2004, the plant was grown on an estimated 114,100 hectares. In 2005, this figure jumped to 144,000 hectares, a level not seen since 2002. The Bush administration argued that this 30,000-hectare increase over 2004 levels was due to a much larger search area, and that cultivation had slightly declined in the areas surveyed in 2004 (White House 2006). Still, even if one accepts the argument that a direct year-to-year comparison was no longer possible because satellites were now monitoring a larger area, the new figures represent a defeat for US drug policy. After all, the initial aim of Plan Colombia had been to halve Colombia's drug industry by 50 percent over six years, and the 2005 figures clearly indicated that this objective had not been reached – despite a total of $4.72 billion in aid that the US gave to Colombia between 2000 and 2006 (Isacson 2006).

Regarding the displacement of the drug industry within Colombia, the US State Department acknowledged that law enforcement shifted the industry to other areas. In 2002, traffickers, under pressure in Colombia's South, moved elsewhere, for example to the West where important cocaine transshipment points were located (Department of State 2003: Colombia). Coca cultivation dropped significantly in the Putumayo and Caquetá departments, but increased in other departments. The Guaviare, for instance, registered a 163 percent increase, from 29,800 in 2001 to 78,500 hectares in 2002. In the Norte de Santander region, located in Colombia's north, cultivation even increased by several hundred percent in 2002. In Nariño, a province bordering the heavily sprayed

Putumayo, coca cultivation doubled in 2002. Farmers even began to grow coca in remote areas outside their traditional agricultural zones (Marsh 2004: 7).

The displacement of coca cultivation continued in 2003. Significant reductions were reported from Putumayo, Guaviare, and Norte de Santander, while cultivation increased particularly in Nariño and Meta. At the end of December 2003, coca was grown in 23 out of the 32 Colombian departments, compared to 21 departments in 2002 (United Nations Office on Drugs and Crime 2004a: 7 and 11). This increase becomes more staggering when one considers the fact that in 1999, only 12 departments had reported cultivation (Vargas 2004). In 2004 and 2005, displacement continued, with coca moving from heavily fumigated zones to new areas. When looking at the entire period analyzed in this chapter, the coca cultivation area had increased by 72 percent over 2000 when Plan Colombia began (Center for International Policy 2006: 3), despite escalating law enforcement. Hence, the US–Colombian fumigation and police/military machinery was unable to keep pace with this geographical spread of coca cultivation across Colombia.

Environmentalists were particularly worried about the spread of coca cultivation to Colombia's National Parks and about US and Colombian plans to lift restrictions and fumigate these parks. They are world-famous for their plants and animals and play an important role within the global ecosystem. While the US claimed that deforestation resulted from coca cultivation and that fumigation would thus stop an environmentally harmful practice, environmentalists argued that fumigation increased the negative effects of cultivation by displacing coca and poppy around the country and thus multiplying the pace of deforestation in the Amazon and Andean region. In early 2006, the Colombian Air Force strafed and bombed a national park where the FARC was allegedly growing coca and where the rebels had allegedly killed a dozen police officers. Environmentalists said that the bombing was destroying decades of conservation work (Molinski 2006).

Colombia was not the only country experiencing difficulties. As mentioned above, Colombia's neighbors were worried about the effects of Plan Colombia, and they had seen a rise in illicit activities in 2001. This trend continued over the following years. Venezuela, Brazil, and Ecuador all saw an increase in coca cultivation, cocaine production, and cocaine trafficking. Moreover, poppy cultivation and heroin trafficking increased, particularly in Venezuela, where Colombian traffickers imported large heroin loads. Yet, although these trends were worrying, it is important to note that there was no massive shift of the drug industry to those countries. The number of hectares used for coca and poppy cultivation was counted in the hundreds and not in the thousands, and cocaine and heroin production was no match to the output of Colombia (Department of State 2004, 2005).

Peru was also affected by events in Colombia. Peruvian coca prices had increased significantly since the late 1990s. For other crops to be competitive, the value of coca should not exceed $1 per kilogram. But by late 2001 and early 2002, farmers received over $4 per kilogram of coca, up from less than $2, two years earlier (Carpenter 2003: 116). Over the following years, prices remained high. The US and Peruvian governments feared that these high prices would lead to an increase in coca cultivation. This did happen to some extent, especially in 2005 (see Table 3 and Annex II, Chart 1). In 2001, with an estimated 34,000 hectares, cultivation was roughly the same as in 2000. For 2002, the State Department noted an increase to 34,700 hectares. Moreover, poppy cultivation and opium trafficking increased in 2002. In 2003 and 2004, coca cultivation declined to the lowest levels registered in Peru since 1986. But in 2005, cultivation increased significantly again, reaching an estimated 38,000 hectares, including 4,000 hectares in new areas. That was more than at any time since 1999.

In Bolivia, coca cultivation increased, too. Until 2001, US policy-makers were relatively content with the situation in the country. Through *Plano Dignidad* (Plan Dignity), launched in late 1997, the administration of former general Hugo Banzer had wanted to remove Bolivia from the list of illicit drug producing countries by 2002. Aggressive coca eradication led to a significant reduction of coca cultivation, with the most dramatic decrease recorded in the Chapare, the country's main area of illicit cultivation. But President Banzer was replaced in 2001, due to ill health, *Plano Dignidad* was put on hold, and the eradication campaign was left in a state of limbo. It thus did not come as a surprise when US figures for 2001 showed an increase in Bolivian coca cultivation to 19,900 hectares, a significant increase when compared to the 14,600 hectares cultivated in 2000. This increase resulted from coca replanting in the Chapare region and an increase of illicit cultivation in the Yungas region, the traditional center of Bolivia's licit coca crop (Department of State 2002: Bolivia).

Cultivation increased further in 2002 and now reached 21,600 hectares, despite the eradication of nearly 12,000 hectares of coca, the second highest eradication level ever recorded for the country. However, eradication was not undertaken in the Yungas. Consequently, replanting and increased cultivation in the Yungas offset eradication efforts in other parts of Bolivia. With 18,700 hectares, a level exceeding the limit of licit cultivation by 6,700 hectares, the Yungas became Bolivia's prime coca-producing region in 2002 (Ledebur 2005: 158, 178).

Developments in 2003 continued along these lines. The Chapare was no longer a major source of coca, with cultivation falling 15 percent compared to the 2002 levels. In the Yungas, however, coca cultivation increased by 26 percent. With 23,200 hectares under cultivation, coca was clearly making a comeback. In 2004 and 2005 there was a further increase in cultivation. Although these developments represented a setback for US drug control efforts, it must be noted that coca cultivation was still far below the levels recorded in the late 1980s and first half of the 1990s

By producing more coca, Bolivia helped to keep total South American coca cultivation levels relatively stable. Between 1999 and 2003, for example, cultivation shrank only a little, from 183,000 hectares to 166,300. This decrease is much less impressive than the decrease between 2001 and 2003. Understandably, the US government preferred to cite the latter percentage figure rather than the former one. Looking at a longer period, more coca was grown in South America in 2005 than in 2000, when Plan Colombia started. This increase cannot be dismissed as a result of new measurement techniques. Rather, it showed that the US had, once more, failed to reduce the supply of illicit drugs.

Perhaps even more disturbing for the US government, Plan Colombia and the Andean Regional Initiative did not alleviate US drug problems. In April 2004, the US Department of Justice reported that US cocaine and heroin prices were stable and even falling, drugs were widely available, and drug purity was high (see National Drug Intelligence Center 2004; Walsh 2004; and Annex II, Chart 2). To make matters worse, the rates of heroin use among high school students increased between 1997 and 2002. This reflected a general trend of increasing cocaine, crack cocaine, and heroin use in the US since the early to mid-1990s (Transnational Institute 2004: 3; Williams *et al.* 2006).

To foster domestic and international support for its drug policy in Colombia, the Bush administration reported a significant increase in cocaine street prices in the US and a drop in purity for the period between February and September 2005 (National Drug Intelligence Center 2006). The administration linked these alleged trends to coca eradication in South America and drug interdiction. However, experts were quick to point out that fluctuations in price and purity occur frequently on drug markets and that they can have various causes, including a rise in consumer demand (Adams 2005).

In combination, the displacement of the drug economy within Colombia, the amount of South American coca grown and cocaine produced, and continuing US drug problems contradict the claim of many US and Colombian policymakers that Plan Colombia and the Andean Regional Initiative were milestones in the fight against drugs. But similar caution is warranted against the view that drug industry dynamics solely resulted from Plan Colombia and the Andean Regional Initiative. How can one then understand and explain the displacement of the drug industry in the early twenty-first century

Explaining displacement

To explain the displacement process, this section examines the various elements constituting the initial causal mechanism: the selectivity of US foreign drug policy, the flexibility of the drug industry, the capacities of drug producing and transit states to implement laws against drugs, and contingent conditions. Empirical black boxes and alternative explanations are discussed as well.

US selective pressure

To explain the dynamics of the drug industry, it is important to note that the US implemented its drug policies selectively. By focusing Plan Colombia on Colombia's south, the US and Colombian governments pushed coca cultivation into new regions. Furthermore, US policies were selective in the sense that the emphasis was on military and police operations instead of social and economic programs that could have alleviated some of Colombia's root problems. Lastly, in its dealings with the Andean states, Washington pursued several bilateral strategies instead of a multilateral strategy.

As mentioned above, Plan Colombia really began with the push into the southern Colombian departments of Putumayo and Caquetá in December 2000. In these departments, military operations accompanied intense aerial fumigation. Already in spring 2000, a senior US narcotics official said that eradication would start in the south of Colombia, since this was the area with the largest concentration of coca fields (Rohter 2000). Hence, from 2000 to 2002, fumigation was concentrated in Putumayo, and particularly in the department's southwest (Marsh 2004: 4). Due to the local application of pressure, coca cultivation rose in other areas that were sprayed less or not at all. In 2002, Guaviare became Colombia's most important coca-growing province. This province borders Caquetá (see Annex I, Map 6), which was heavily sprayed. Ironically, the Guaviare department had been subjected to massive fumigation in the 1990s, as a consequence of which coca farmers had moved elsewhere. Fumigation works, but only in areas permanently sprayed with chemicals.

Of course, spraying only occurred in areas where coca and poppy were planted. Hence, one could argue that the displacement of coca production was inevitable as there was always some area to which production could move. However, this argument is flawed, since a presence of security forces could have prevented the establishment of new coca fields. But such a presence is precisely what was missing. US support for the Colombian security forces was significant but it was still insufficient to enable full territorial control. The US thus helped Colombian forces to apply local pressure in the south of the country, but Colombia's forces were too weak to prevent the establishment of new coca fields or drug laboratories in other regions. From this perspective, US claims of success can also be read as evidence of failure. In April 2002, for example, US Assistant Secretary of Defense for International Security Affairs, Peter Rodman, said:

> Based on the success of the first [counternarcotics Brigade], the U.S. government is supporting Colombia's request to train and equip a second CN Brigade in FY 2003 for employment elsewhere within the country. The existing CN Brigade has been successful in forcing the drug traffickers to move their operations outside of the Putumayo and Caquetá departments. A second CN Brigade will enable the Colombians to attack the other main coca growing areas to the east of the Andean Ridge or elsewhere in the country.
>
> (Quoted in Congress 2002: 28)

The US tried to enable the Colombian government to control the entire territory, but US aid often arrived late and thus led to a gradual implementation of Plan Colombia and the Andean Regional Initiative. In March 2002, in an attempt to explain the rise in Colombian coca cultivation in 2001, the White House

(2002) stated that "[a]lthough the full complement of counter-drug and development resources is still arriving in Colombia, we recognize that our efforts to date have not yet produced the results we had hoped to achieve. The security environment in Colombian drug cultivation regions has made it difficult to implement counter-drug programs."

Since US aid arrived slowly, Bogotá could apply local pressure only. It took until late 2002, for example, for the Colombian military to receive the Black Hawk and UH-1H (Huey II) helicopters procured under Plan Colombia (Congress 2002: 26). It is true that various technical, financial, and organizational problems prevented a speedy delivery of aid. But US planners knew already in 2000 that many programs would not operate until at least 2001, and that much of the US aid would not be delivered until 2002 (GAO 2000: 19). So did Colombian military officials. In spring 2000, they thought that at least six years were needed to reduce coca cultivation in areas infiltrated or controlled by armed groups, with different areas targeted at different times. First, they wanted to break the FARC's control of southern coca-growing areas for a period of two years. Then they would focus on the Guaviare region in Colombia's center for two years. Lastly, territorial control was to be wrested from paramilitary groups in the north for a similar period (Rohter 2000).

Hence, everything was set for an intervention in several stages – and for the displacement of the drug industry. The department of Nariño illustrates the impact of the anti-drug campaign's selective nature. In 1999, this department accounted for less than 6 percent of Colombia's coca cultivation, but in 2003, the department's coca represented 20 percent of the national total. According to the UN, the increase in the department's cultivation during 2002 and 2003 "might have been a consequence of the significant reduction in coca cultivation in neighboring Putumayo, following the intense spraying campaign carried out in this department in 2002. The decrease in coca cultivation in Putumayo would have driven landless labourers to move to Nariño in 2002" (United Nations Office on Drugs and Crime 2004a: 27). To be sure, the UN also notes an increase in fumigation in Nariño, from 8,200 hectares in 2001 to 18,000 hectares in 2002 to 36,900 hectares, or 28 percent of the national total, in 2003 (United Nations Office on Drugs and Crime 2004a: 15). This shows that cultivation can increase despite fumigation. Still, the US and Colombian response to developments in Nariño came late, which helps explain the increase in coca cultivation in that department.

Slowly, the US and Colombian governments extended the scope of law enforcement operations across the country. In 2002, responding to the shift of traffickers to the west of Colombia, the US embassy, together with the Colombian military, tried to enable the US-funded and trained counter-narcotics battalions to operate throughout the country. As noted above, the UH-60 Black Hawk helicopters procured under Plan Colombia finally became operational in late 2002. Thus, in 2002 and 2003, the Colombian armed forces were much stronger than in 2000 and 2001, with the number of spray aircraft and helicopters increasing from 22 to 35 from the end of fiscal year 2001 through May 2004 (GAO

2004b: 17). Concomitantly to the strengthening of military capabilities, the US invested more money into aerial eradication. US funding for the Colombian fumigation campaign·increased from around $49 million in fiscal year 2001 to over $100 million in fiscal year 2003 (GAO 2004a: 14). This upward trend continued over the following years. Despite these investments, there were still vast, remote areas with little or no government presence where coca could be grown. As the Center for International Policy (2006: 4) reported in spring 2006, these zones "are at least the size of California – yet since 2000 the U.S. spray fleet has only been able to cover an area a bit larger than Delaware."

The escalation of US involvement is also shown by the fact that the US Southern Command increasingly defined US policies toward Colombia and Latin America; that the Pentagon expanded its control over foreign military training programs formerly controlled by the State Department; that the number of Colombian trainees increased significantly under the Andean Regional Initiative amid weakening civilian oversight (Latin America Working Group Education Fund *et al.* 2005); and that in 2004, the US embassy in Bogotá had the largest number of staff of any US embassy in the world (Independent Commission 2004: 31). Moreover, in August 2003 interdiction was boosted with the resumption of the ABDP in Colombia. As described in Chapter 3, the program had been suspended in 2001 following the shoot-down of a civilian plane carrying a US missionary family. Now, new detailed interdiction procedures were devised to avoid any mistakes and liability claims in the future. Most importantly, US personnel would not participate in decisions to shoot down planes. Peru also asked the US to resume the interdiction program, arguing that its suspension had increased the number of trafficking flight

As a result of these efforts, the ability of Colombian and US forces to conduct operations across Colombia improved. In June 2004, ONDCP Director, John Walters (Walters 2004), said:

> Helicopter security and search and rescue support availability has generally been the limiting factor for coca fumigation in more isolated growing areas, but this year, spraying has also been successful in such sectors because of advanced deployment of helicopters from temporary bases supplied with fuel bladders and protected by the Colombian military.

To further reduce the selectivity of the Colombian anti-drug program, in October 2004, Congress voted in favor of a proposal by the Bush administration to double the US military forces supporting US drug policies in Colombia from 400 to 800, and the number of civilian contractors from 400 to 600.

Escalation did not greatly improve the effectiveness of US policy, however. In September 2005, for example, the (renamed) Government Accountability Office (2005) reported that the effect of the air interdiction program, which had been resumed in Colombia in August 2003, was unclear, and that the program was marred by numerous problems. Moreover, violent non-state actors continued to control many parts of the country, and, as shown above, fumigation was unable to keep pace with the displacement of the drug industry across Colombia.

US drug policy toward Colombia was also selective in that the US focused on coercion instead of social and economic programs. Of the $4.72 billion that the US gave to Colombia between 2000 and 2006, 81 percent went to Colombia's military and police forces (Isacson 2006). This coercive bias contributed to the displacement of the drug industry. Without economic alternatives, farmers whose fields were sprayed often had no choice but to resume coca cultivation in new areas or to replant their sprayed fields. As Adam Isacson (2004: 3–4) writes, "a lack of government presence, roads, clear land titles, and credit continue to make most legal crops unprofitable, while U.S. and Colombian investments in development and infrastructure haven't come close to keeping up with sharply increased fumigation." As early as 2001, the US Agency for International Development (USAID) acknowledged that development aid could not keep pace with the fumigation campaign (Kotler 2001). Hence, many farmers left their homes, and some joined the guerilla. In mid-2002, a Colombian farmer from a heavily fumigated community said: "There is no work, nothing to do since the fumigations. Some have left to find work or to look for another place to farm. A lot of the young people joined the guerilla. Of course this was going to happen. With no work, the young people looking for work and money join the guerilla" (quoted in Marsh 2004: 27).

Yet despite the displacement of populations and illicit crops, US policymakers continued to give priority to fumigation over development. In mid-2003, for example, the US tried to reduce coca cultivation in the department of Guaviare, which had a high guerilla presence, through large-scale aerial fumigation. At this time, AD projects in the department were negligible. As one US official said at the time: "Right now, the plan in Guaviare is just to spray them" (quoted in Marsh 2004: 26).

Apart from the fact that military programs received a much higher priority than AD, the effectiveness of AD also suffered from a slow distribution of aid. In 2001, for example, the US allocated $56.6 million for AD. At the end of the fiscal year, only $5.6 million had been spent (WOLA 2002: 8). A further problem was that US aid agencies often used the presence of illicit crops as their sole criterion for defining their geographical focus. Poor communities that did not grow coca or poppy, but were ready to do so given their desperate economic situation, rarely received financial support. Moreover, the distribution of aid was often made conditional upon the rapid destruction of coca and poppy. Objections by farmers that there was no market for alternative crops or that US funding was not distributed quickly enough to offset losses resulting from voluntary eradication were to no avail.

While the US focused its drug policies in Colombia on coercion, it adopted a less repressive approach toward other countries, in particularly toward Peru and Bolivia where the majority of US funds were invested into non-coercive programs. In Bolivia, AD and other "soft" programs received 67 percent of US funds between 2000 and 2004 (Independent Commission 2004: 109). Of course, the US maintained its huge influence over Bolivia, and coercive programs constituted a main pillar of the US–Bolivian relationship. In 2004, for example, the Bolivian police and military were the second-largest Latin America recipients after Colombia of US military training (Latin American Working Group Education Fund *et al.* 2005: 7). Nevertheless, AD received the largest share of US funding. The US increased funding for non-coercive programs especially in the framework of the Andean Regional Initiative, and thus partly responded to calls for the need to protect these countries from a spillover of drug production, insurgency, and other Colombian problems. In Peru, the US spent a total of $156 million in 2002, three times the amount of money invested in 2001. Although coercive programs received a significant share of US funds, with $30 million allocated for the upgrading of helicopters and the eradication of opium fields $80 million was invested in AD (The Economist 2002).

US drug policies were selective in another way. Instead of developing a multilateral strategy, the US nurtured bilateral relationships, not least because these gave the US more leverage over each Andean state. This was despite the fact that US policy-makers anticipated a spillover of Colombian problems to other countries. Already in late 2000, US Undersecretary of State, Thomas Pickering, said that the US would increase its funding for Colombia's neighbors. He explained the reasons for an increase in US funding to Colombia's neighbors by saying: "As we increase our efforts in Colombia, there will be a tendency [for traffickers] to find new areas, either in Colombia or outside Colombia, in which to move the cultivation and production of cocaine and heroin" (quoted in Carpenter 2003: 83–84). Similarly, in October 2003 a senior US narcotics officia said in Congress after the ouster of Bolivian President de Lozada: "[W]e must buttress the effort of [Andean] governments as we anticipate the 'balloon effect' – whereby anti-narcotics efforts in one country may increase narcotics production in a different country – which *will* result from our successes in dismantling the narcotics and terrorism infrastructure in Colombia" (Charles 2003 [emphasis C.F.]).

Yet despite the certainty that the campaign in Colombia would affect other countries, the US failed to coordinate its policies on a regional basis. Rhetorically, US policy-makers embraced a regional approach, but in practice, they eschewed it. As Michael Shifter argues, "[w]hat the United States calls a regional approach means us dealing with each country separately. There's still a lack of the Latin Americans working among themselves and the United States being part of that" (quoted in The Economist 2001a). There was no lack of US reassurances that a regional approach would be adopted. In late November 2000, before the beginning of the push into southern Colombia, Thomas Pickering said that US planning was informed by the understanding that a regional effort against the region's problems was needed (Carpenter 2003: 84). But more than three years later, an independent expert commission supported by the US Council on Foreign Relations published a report revealing the continuous US penchant for bilateral instead of multilateral drug diplomacy: "Regionalizing supply-side efforts – that is, formulating and implementing counterdrug policy on a regional rather than bilateral basis – would improve the effectiveness of U.S. counterdrug activities. The drug industry's ability to operate fluidly across borders is well-established; thus, working only bilaterally to fight drugs is detrimental to the scope and efficacy of U.S. policy" (Independent Commission 2004: 20).[4]

The flexibility of the drug industry

Chapters 2 and 3 show that the drug industry has an impressive ability to adapt to political pressure. This ability to adapt was also the case during the implementation of Plan Colombia and the Andean Regional Initiative. Farmers and drug entrepreneurs behaved innovatively in various ways. Farmers sometimes limited the effects of fumigation by washing coca leaves after fumigation and by treating them with chemicals to rescue the crop. Moreover, many farmers replanted fields that had been destroyed by fumigation (United Nations Offic on Drugs and Crime 2004a: 26). To prevent replanting, fields were often fumigated several times. Nevertheless, replanting posed considerable challenges to the joint US–Colombian fumigation effort. And when fumigation did lead to the abandonment of coca fields, many farmers migrated to new areas where they recommenced cultivation. As one Colombian farmer besieging the capital of the Colombian province Caquetá said in the 1990s: "If they fumigate 20 hectares here, we'll cultivate 200 hectares over there. They'll have to get rid of the whole forest" (quoted in Carpenter 2003: 164).

To make matters worse from a US perspective, farmers and trafficker increased the yield of coca leaves through an increase in plant density, the use of fertilizers, and new types of coca that grew faster and were more resistant to herbicides. During the period analyzed, the average yield of leaves per hectare rose, which meant that a decrease in coca cultivation did not translate into less cocaine production. Moreover, agronomical innovations allowed the cultivation of coca at lower elevations, for example in the Amazon Basin. Coca cultivation was thus no longer confined to the foothills of the Andes. In addition, farmers responded to the fumigation campaign by mixing coca with licit crops and by minimizing the size of coca fields, which helped them to reduce the risk of having their fields detected and sprayed. In June 2004, Adam Isacson, after visiting the department of Putumayo which US officials presented as a success story in terms of eradication, said that cultivation in the department continued, although now mainly on small and scattered plots. Locals had also told him about successes in growing coca in shade where it cannot be detected (Congress 2004: Testimony of Adam Isacson).

Similarly, to the peasants, traffickers behaved innovatively as well. On numerous occasions, traffickers successfully evaded law enforcement operations in Colombia, often through means of violence and corruption. Moreover, they induced peasants to start growing coca in various parts of the country and became more efficient in the conversion of coca leaf into cocaine through a better use of chemical precursors. Colombian drug entrepreneurs also became active in neighboring countries. Often, traffickers applied the latest, university-level, research insights, as in Peru. There, they increased coca cultivation by offering cash loans and technical advice to farmers.[5]

In 2003, a senior US official in Peru said to a US journalist: "We are seeing a large increase in the number of people clearing out old coca fields, and getting back into it." According to the official, Colombians were "paying money to the Indians" to plant coca. He and other US officials attributed the resurgence of Peruvian coca to the US-supported anti-drug campaign in Colombia. By financing the planting of new coca bushes in Peru, which need 18 to 24 months to reach peak production, Colombian traffickers may have anticipated a reduction in the availability of Colombian coca leaf (Hall 2003). Colombians also provided incentives to farmers to grow poppy. This was a smart move, as poppy is easier to grow than coca and even more lucrative. Furthermore, poppy is more difficult to detect and eradicate, partly because it can be grown at altitudes that are too high for some helicopters to reach.

Weak law enforcement

Weak law enforcement helps to understand and explain the displacement of the drug economy within Colombia, a spillover of drugs to neighboring countries, and an increase in Bolivian coca cultivation. The present analysis is more sketchy than systematic, since a thorough examination of the different aspects, causes, and consequences of weak law enforcement would be a work in its own right. Nevertheless, the analysis underlines a major challenge for US policy-makers, i.e., the frequent inability of Andean governments to implement laws against drugs.

To curb illicit activities, a state must control the entire national territory. But the Colombian government did not exercise full territorial control during the early twenty-first century since it lacked the manpower, hardware, and logistical means to cope with strong non-state armed forces. In 1999, armed non-state groups controlled roughly half of Colombia (Reuters 1999). In April 2002, a US official said that the FARC, ELN, and AUC effectively controlled over 40 percent of the Colombian territory (Congress 2002: 19). It is questionable whether the situation improved significantly over the following years. In July 2004, the GAO (2004a: 26) wrote that the Colombian government still did not control up to 40 percent of the national territory. In the same report, the GAO (2004a: 3) stated that the State Department had trained and equipped more than 16,500 Colombian police officers. "While this allowed the Colombian National Police to move into areas of the country that previously did not have a state presence, some police units cannot safely leave town limits, and some mobile squadrons have limited patrolling capability." While the rebels continued to hold onto many parts of Colombia, the territorial grip of paramilitaries and traffickers (two often indistinguishable groups) became ever stronger. In mid-2005, the Colombian government's comptroller reported that nearly 50 percent of cultivable land was believed to be in the hands of traffickers (Comptroller's Office 2005).

The significance of weak territorial control becomes obvious when taking into account the fact that the amount of land used for cultivation was tiny. In 2001, the total amount of coca grown in South America added up to 864 square miles, or 63 percent the size of Rhode Island (Congress 2002: 57, 61) – Colombia alone is as large as Texas, New Mexico and Oklahoma combined. In 2003, the UN said that the land used for coca cultivation in Colombia was 0.09 percent of the national territory (United Nations Office on Drugs and Crime 2003a: 9). Even if the state had been stronger, there would always have remained enclaves allowing cultivation to continue.

All too often, the Colombian military and police found themselves overpowered and outwitted by rebels. In 1999, the commander of the Colombian armed forces, General Fernando Tapias, deplored the poor state of equipment of the Colombian military as follows: "The head of the FARC has a [satellite] phone. I have to climb to the top of a mountain and try to get a radio signal" (quoted in Darling 1999). The relatively small size of the Colombian military was worrying as well. In late 2003, non-state armed groups in Colombia had an estimated 50,000 combatants. The Colombian armed forces regularly deployed only 40,000 troops, out of a total of 55,000 combat-ready soldiers. Over half of the Colombian armed forces, whose total strength was 125,000, worked in offices or guarded infrastructure (Independent Commission 2004: 63, fn 69). A lack of military hardware was another handicap. In spring 2000, the Colombian armed forces had only 16 helicopters, even though they would have needed at least 30 to better control the country's gigantic expanses (Wagner 2000).

Although the US tried to alleviate the problem, US support came too slow. There were several reasons for this. During the Colombian peace process, which only broke down only in early 2002, US planners had to move cautiously so as not to allow the FARC to use US military support as a pretext to call off their participation in the process. Moreover, NGOs closely watched the military build-up, forcing Washington to avoid any incident where it could be proven that US military aid led to human rights violations. Another reason for US difficulties in building up the Colombian armed forces were delays in the manufacture and delivery of helicopters, as well as a lack of coordination among US agencies involved in the Colombian anti-drug program (Crandall 2002a: 158).

In a Congressional hearing in April 2002, US government officials said that the Colombian armed forces lacked the airlift capabilities and manpower required to control the national territory, and that they did not know how much time and money was needed to enable the Colombian military to perform this task. One participant said: "At the end of the conflict in El Salvador, the military had 50 helicopters while Colombia, 50 times larger, has only roughly four times as many" (Congress 2002: 19). A lack of military hardware means that fumigation could not be undertaken too far away from military bases, since there were no refueling planes. Moreover, a lack of helicopter gunships to accompany fumigation aircraft meant that spraying operations often had to be cancelled, as rebels fired at the aircraft from the ground making fumigation too dangerous. Similarly, there were not enough search and rescue helicopters to reduce the risk of rebels kidnapping or killing the crews of crashed aircraft or helicopters (Congress 2003: H6336). Indeed, ground fire increased: "In 2001 and most of 2002, the number of ground-fire hits on spray aircraft averaged fewer than ten per month. But in late 2002 and during 2003, the number of hits increased – peaking at 73 in January 2003 and averaging more than 26 per month – and, in 2003, two spray aircraft crashed and two were forced to land because of ground fire" (GAO 2004b: Summary).

Adverse climatic and geographical conditions compounded these problems. Coca and poppy often shifted to those Colombian departments that had high mountains, access to a coast, that shared borders with other countries, and whose territory was frequently draped in clouds. These conditions made coca and poppy cultivation, drug production, and drug smuggling easier and anti-drug operations more cumbersome and also more risky for eradication teams, which not only had to cope with ground fire, but also with the possibility of accidental crashes.

Weak law enforcement also explains an increase in illicit activities in other South American countries, since it made these countries susceptible to absorbing Colombia's problems. In early 2002, the State Department described the situation in Ecuador in bleak terms, referring to a weak state, a poorly regulated financial system, unreliable border controls, and poorly equipped and trained security forces. Corruption was a further problem, as illustrated by the fact that even the Ecuadorian chief of police intelligence was implicated in drug trafficking activities (Department of State 2002: Ecuador). The State Department report on Venezuela was gloomy as well:

> Prosecutors and judges often lack computer or even telephone equipment in their offices, having to rely on typewriters and personally owned cellular telephones to do their jobs. Another drug control agency reported major staffing cutbacks. Venezuela's participation in a major region-wide chemical control operation was entirely contingent upon funding from the U.S. to cover routine operating expenses. During 2001, incumbents of several high-level law enforcement positions were replaced, some of these reportedly involving allegations of corruption.
>
> (Department of State 2002: Venezuela)

In Peru, law enforcement was weak which partly accounts for an increase in illicit activities. However, problems were less a result of greater pressure emanating from Colombia but more to do with Peruvian politics. Hence, it would be misleading to oversimplify matters by seeing the increase in illicit activities in Peru as a spillover product of law enforcement operations in Colombia. The main challenge for the Peruvian government was to eradicate coca and poppy without allowing farmers' protests to escalate to a point that would cast in doubt the future of the government. Moreover, the government still had to take into account the possibility of insurgency. After years of relative calm following successful counter-insurgency operations in the early and mid-1990s (see Chapter 3), the Shining Path rose up again. Its veterans and new members killed police, tried to gain the support of coca farmers, and allegedly struck alliances with drug traffickers (McDermott 2006; Rojas 2005: 220–222). The influence of the rebels was almost negligible compared to the power they had wielded earlier. Nevertheless, the Peruvian government knew that ruthless coca and poppy eradication carried the risk of strengthening the rebels.

Still, the Toledo administration reassured the US that eradication would continue despite the insurgents. In September 2002, it announced that forcible coca eradication would commence in those areas previously left untouched out of fear that eradication would help the Shining Path to muster support among coca farmers. This decision triggered violent unrest, including attacks on government offices. In the face of an increase in Sendero activities, a weak state presence in some areas, and coca farmer protests, the Peruvian government slowed down the eradication campaign in later 2002 and early 2003. It now emphasized voluntary and gradual eradication and signed an accord with cocaleros to this effect. Moreover, the government did not approve eradication in the Apurimac and Monzón areas and other key coca cultivation zones (Department of State 2003: Peru; Rojas 2005: 216).

Nevertheless, tensions continued for various reasons, including doubts as to whether AD projects provided a viable economic alternative for peasants, the arrest of cocalero leaders, and political violence. Attempts to reduce poppy, opium, and heroin supplies were challenging as well. Despite repeated efforts, security forces were often unable to locate poppy fields and destroy smuggling rings, not least because poppy was grown on small fields in remote and rugged terrain and was often mixed with other crops. Moreover, the Peruvian military and police lacked equipment and training, the Peruvian intelligence apparatus was in a poor state after years of abuse by the Fujimori–Montesinos regime, and turf battles prevented cooperation among the different branches of the security forces (Department of State 2003: Peru; Franco 2004: 516).

The Bolivian government found it difficult to implement laws against drugs as well. While Peruvian coca cultivation remained in check, Bolivia saw an increase in illicit coca cultivation in the early twenty-first century, as shown above. It is important to note here that developments in Colombia probably had a relatively minor influence on Bolivia. In contrast to the 1980s and early 1990s, relatively few Colombian drug entrepreneurs were active in Bolivia during the period analyzed in this chapter, and the displacement of farmers and coca field resulted mainly from a combination of economic problems and opportunities, and law enforcement operations, in Bolivia.[6]

Bolivia is a politically very unstable country, yet it is different from Peru and Colombia in that left-wing insurgency has traditionally been less of a problem to the government than in the latter two countries. However, the Bolivian government has had to face well-organized cocalero groups. These were led by the charismatic Evo Morales, an Aymara Indian whose defense of peasants' rights and coca cultivation catapulted him to the second place in the 2002 presidential elections. Morales and other protagonists defended coca against US–Bolivian law enforcement on the political stage. At the same time, farmers organized roadblocks and strikes to defend their coca fields and to protest against economic hardship and political disenfranchisement in a country largely ruled by a small, rich, and nepotistic elite. These protests often escalated into violence, not least due to heavy-handed tactics by the Bolivian security forces whom observers accused of numerous human rights violations such as unlawful detention, torture, and the shooting of unarmed peasants (Transnational Institute 2004).

Peasant protests achieved a slowing down of coca eradication, and they were conducive to the shift of coca cultivation from the Chapare to the Yungas. The Chapare had only become a major coca producer in the 1980s, when thousands of laid-off tin miners moved to the region. Most of the region's coca was reportedly used for illicit cocaine production. In the Yungas, the situation was different. This region had been a long-time supplier of coca leaves, and the Bolivian government had to act with circumspection to avoid antagonizing large parts of the population. After all, many Bolivians use coca against altitude sickness, hunger, and work-induced exhaustion. Moreover, they regard coca as part of their ancient heritage and use it for spiritual purposes. Hence, Colombian-style aerial fumigation was out of the question. Even manual eradication was politically challenging, as a senior US official in Bolivia conceded in 2003.[7] A difficul terrain was an additional obstacle for reducing the amount of illicit coca cultivation in the Yungas. Whereas the Chapare is flat, the Yungas is a hilly region hidden by high mountains, making access difficult for helicopters. Moreover, the region is linked to La Paz by perilous roads that are easy to blockade.

For these reasons, eradication efforts focused on the Chapare instead of the Yungas, which helps to explain the Yungas coca boom. In 2004, the UN reported a movement of people from Chapare and other parts of the country to the Yungas, and particularly to the municipalities of Caravani and La Asunta, which experienced the largest growth in coca cultivation in 2002 and 2003. This shift occurred at the same time as political turmoil marked the country (United Nations Office on Drugs and Crime 2004b: 11). In January 2003, cocaleros organized countrywide strikes that effectively blocked the main roads and led to the death of at least 20 people. These strikes and other protests prevented the execution of a plan devised by the US and the administration of President Gonzalo Sanchez de Lozada to eradicate coca in key areas. In August 2003, de Lozada abdicated in the face of public outrage over a proposed natural gas export deal that would have given most of the profits to US companies. Cocalero pressure also played a role. The incoming administration of Carlos Mesa backed away from eradication and tried to encourage the substitution of coca with coffee and cocoa. Mesa knew that he had to tread cautiously so as not to increase peasant support for Evo Morales.

Despite the efforts to prevent Morales from rising to the top, he won a landslide victory in the December 2005 presidential elections and was inaugurated in January 2006. His victory was a major blow to the US eradication policy. Once in office, Morales, under the slogan "coca is not cocaine," said he would halt forcible eradication and push for the legalization of coca-based tea and other products whose export would help improve the Bolivian economy.

Contingent conditions

As emphasized in this book, contingent conditions influence foreign policy outcomes. This section examines Colombian contingencies that help to comprehend Colombia's preeminent position in the illicit drug industry and the dynamics of the industry.

Numerous conditions have enabled Colombia to become a pivotal drug-producing and trafficking country. Geography is one factor. Colombia is a large country. This makes the detection of illicit crops and drug laboratories difficult Many areas are remote from urban settlements and, as shown above, are poorly controlled by the state. In addition, Colombia's large size made bribery easier. Whereas in smaller countries traffickers often need to bribe high-level officials in Colombia they frequently bribed only local authorities, thus saving money and lowering risks (Thoumi 1994: 88). Moreover, Colombia shares a border with five neighboring states. This border is around 6,000 kilometers long and poorly controlled. And Colombia's proximity to Central America and the Caribbean made it relatively easy for Colombian traffickers to establish traffick ing routes leading toward the US.

Poverty is another driving factor behind illicit activities. According to a 2004 World Bank study, over half of the Colombian population lived in poverty or extreme poverty (United Nations Office on Drugs and Crime 2004a: 33). In 2003, 1 percent of the Colombian population owned 55 percent of all arable land (Independent Commission 2004: 107). This highly unequal distribution of wealth resulted in part from the economic reform programs of the 1990s that benefited the rich, and not the poor. Moreover, the prices of coffee and other licit crops were often below the cost of production, not least because international trade mechanisms gave most profits to international export companies. Given these circumstances, many destitute Colombian peasants and poor, unemployed urban dwellers migrated to coca regions to start growing coca or to work as *raspachines* (harvesters of coca leaves).

Yet geography and poverty do not satisfactorily explain why Colombia came to dominate the cocaine economy. An answer to this puzzle that helps to understand and explain drug industry displacement within Colombia better is advanced by drug policy researcher Francisco Thoumi. He argues against the popular notion that drug problems are primarily a result of poverty, instead focusing on different norms prevailing in different societies. From this vantage point, he shows why Colombia has attracted coca and poppy cultivation, drug production, and drug trafficking. According to Thoumi (1994: 82), a "set of factors, many of which were present in other countries, but which – as a package – are unique to Colombia, gave the country its cost advantage in cocaine production and distribution."[8]

One of the main reasons for Colombia's competitive advantage was a growing de-legitimization of the governmental system. Weak state legitimacy is an endemic problem in many Latin American and Caribbean countries. Colombia is different, however, since the de-legitimization process began very early and the history of Colombia has known more extreme violence than most other countries (Thoumi 1994: 86, 89). During a civil war period known as *La Violencia*, which lasted from the late 1940s to the early 1960s and which was marked by extreme violence and cruelty, about 2–3 percent of the population was killed. The period was symptomatic of a weak state and societal disintegration. Over the following decades, the state continuously failed to protect its citizens from violence and thus lost legitimacy, while Colombian society suffered from excessive individualism and winner-takes-all attitudes epitomized by drug traffickers

The view held by many US policy-makers that drug production and traffick ing was the main cause of violence and corruption in Colombia was thus shortsighted. Illicit activities were as much a consequence of these problems as their cause. Hence, more was needed to build a better Colombia than reducing drug supplies. It was imperative to build the Colombian state and nation. Whereas elsewhere in Latin America, the state was built prior to attempts to construct a nation, Colombia had completed neither state-building nor nation-building (Zinecker 2002: 54, 64).

While the absence of a strong state and nation allowed the US to wield significant influence over Colombian politics and policies, coercion had a negative effect on Colombia. One could certainly argue that US military aid supported state-building, since US aid allowed Colombia to defend itself against violent non-state actors, and that this form of state-building was a precondition for nation-building. However, instead of strengthening the Colombian state and society, US coercive drug policies rather weakened both state and society. This is particularly obvious when looking at the Samper presidency. The US decision to decertify Colombia in 1996 and 1997 undermined Samper's credibility (few foreign heads of state and government were ready to meet with Samper) and Colombia's economy, which was conducive to an expansion of illicit activities. Moreover, decertification demoralized many Colombian citizens and alienated them from their government (Shifter 1999: 18).

Samper's weak international and national standing allowed the US to extract many concessions from Colombia in the fight against drugs. To prove its credibility, the Samper administration began an unprecedented fumigation campaign, as described in the Chapter 3. The Samper administration also extradited many Colombian citizens to the US. As one US government official said: "The good thing about Samper was that we could do whatever we wanted on the drug front. The extradition issue was another instance when we moved the 'goal posts back' in order to see how far we could push Samper on the drug stuff" (quoted in Crandall 2002a: 125). But by the late 1990s, many US officials had come to understand that by weakening the Colombian state, the US had inadvertently reinforced guerilla groups and paramilitaries (Crandall 2002a: 131). The FARC, for example, had become more popular among peasants who saw their livelihood destroyed by fumigation.

Coercion continued under Plan Colombia and the Andean Regional Initiative. These programs were more significant in scale than previous programs. But similar to earlier programs, they exacerbated the root causes of Colombia's problems, i.e. a delegitimized state and societal disintegration. Under pressure from US policy-makers who focused on drugs instead of peace, Bogotá was unable to pursue its own priorities. As one US embassy official said: "The US and Colombia have different priorities. Colombia has peace as a priority. We have narcotics" (quoted in Cooper 2001). US and Colombian government official assured their respective audiences that the Colombian state was being strengthened. However, as discussed further above, it is doubtful whether Plan Colombia and the Andean Regional Initiative had positive lasting effects in terms of drug supplies reduction, a curbing of violence, and more political stability. Rather, US coercive policies undermined state legitimacy and democracy.

What was bad for the Colombian state was equally bad for Colombia's society. State-building refers to the creation of bureaucratic structures that penetrate a society and protect a country's citizens. Nation-building goes deeper. It aims at the creation of a national community that is economically, ethnically, and socially integrated and that can solve conflicts through peaceful means as groups develop loyalties toward the state. A lack of clear rules where and when fumigation was to take place, as well as open-field experiments with ever more destructive herbicides (Vargas 2002: 31), not only weakened the state by alienating Colombians from their government, but also impeded nation-building by driving more humans into misery. Moreover, laws clearly favored the privileged, such as the law which exempted high school graduates from military service in combat units.

Violence continued during Plan Colombia and the Andean Regional Initiative, with six unarmed civilians dying for every armed combatant killed (WOLA 2002: 9). The number of Colombians fleeing from violence in rural areas reached staggering levels. As stated in a report of the Norwegian Refugee Council, up to 250,000 persons were uprooted in 2005, many of them as a result of fighting between paramilitaries and guerillas over drug trafficking routes. These refugees were at the center of one of the world's greatest humanitarian disasters: With up to 3.7 million internally displaced persons, Colombia ranked second only behind Sudan (Norwegian Refugee Council 2006: 10). And although the Colombian government claimed that its counter-insurgency campaign was successful, the UN reported for 2003 that out of 189 coca growing municipalities, guerilla groups were still present in 162 and paramilitary groups in 86 (United Nations Office on Drugs and Crime 2004a: 39). Three years later, the war continued, with guerillas, paramilitaries, and traffickers maintaining a strong presence in many parts of Colombia.

US drug policies were not the sole reason for Colombia's problems. After all, the Colombian state and society had been weak long before drugs began to dominate US–Colombian relations. Moreover, even if the US had invested more efforts into nation-building, it would have been difficult to achieve this objective, given the multiple challenges facing Colombia. But in any case, the US did not even attempt to help with building the Colombian nation. After Vietnam, Somalia, Haiti, Bosnia, Kosovo, Afghanistan and Iraq, US policy-makers refrained from nation-building. In fact, the whole topic of nation-building was off-limits in Washington at this point (Carpenter 2003: 87). What matters here is to emphasize the link between US drug policies and a weak Colombian state and society. A delegitimized state and a disintegrated society have enabled the drug industry to thrive in Colombia, and as long as state and societal weakness continue to persist, fumigation and other anti-drug measures are likely to merely displace the illicit drug industry (Friesendorf 2005a). The US thus kept in motion a vicious circle whereby militarized drug policies fuel violence and other problems. This leads to an increase in illicit activities, and thus to renewed coercive efforts to reduce drug supplies (Jelsma 2001). As Marc Chernick said in a Congressional hearing in June 2004:

> [P]eace will take more than battling the FARC or pushing coca cultivation into different corners of the country. It will ultimately require a negotiated settlement and the construction of a legitimate state presence that provides services, administers justice, promotes economic development and provides security. Current policy prioritizes security. It is a necessary but insufficien formula. Progress in confronting political violence, terrorism, and drug trafficking will only be made when the broader concerns are addressed and the illegal armed actors are re-incorporated into the political system after more than a half century of war.
>
> (Congress 2004: Testimony of Marc W. Chernick)

Hence, explanations of displacement that focus on poverty and geography are incomplete. To arrive at a more complete picture of displacement, one must take into account the fact that Colombia is characterized by a peculiar blend of political, economic, and social conditions. In combination, these conditions weaken the Colombian state and society and enable illicit activities. By applying its coercive powers in Colombia, the US additionally weakened the Colombian state and nation and thus contributed to the displacement of the drug industry.

Black boxes and alternative explanations

Attempts to analyze the drug industry are hampered by empirical black boxes, including unreliable figures for the land area used for coca and poppy cultivation. Coca is harvested more than once a year, and eradication is spread over several months, which means that cultivation levels are constantly changing. Keeping track of these changes with the help of reconnaissance airplanes and satellites is difficult. Fields are often draped in clouds, illicit crops are mixed with licit ones or grown in shade, and peasants and drug entrepreneurs reduce the size of illicit fields and thus the likeliness of detection. With poppy cultivation, data collection is even more difficult than with coca, since poppy grows at high altitudes where cloud coverage is more frequent.

In addition, data collection is complicated by the fact that peasants sometimes temporarily abandon their fields to recommence cultivation when the danger of eradication recedes. As mentioned further above, Peru saw a reduction of coca cultivation in 2003, although no forced eradication was undertaken during that year. A temporary abandonment of fields may explain this reduction. Hence, 2003 might not have been as great a success story as the US and Peruvian governments wished. To mention another problem pertaining to the collection of data, US satellites cannot detect newly planted coca bushes. Hence, figures may underestimate cultivation. Moreover, "the true extent of the displacement of coca cultivation is not [. . .] known since neither State Department nor UN estimates of coca cultivation accurately measure the number of coca fields planted outside primary coca producing areas" (Marsh 2004: 7–8). Lastly, and as mentioned above, peasants and traffickers try to increase the yield of coca leaves. Thus, less land used for cultivation does not necessarily translate into lower cocaine production levels. John Walsh (2004: 10) summarizes these data problems succinctly:

> The difficulties in measuring the land area under drug crop cultivation are compounded when estimating the size of the crop harvest and amount of finished drug produced. Such estimates are shaped by numerous factors which may vary by locale and over time, and about which verifiabl information is very limited. The State Department itself points out that the actual size of the crop harvest each year can hinge upon "small changes in factors such as soil fertility, weather, farming techniques, and disease." [. . .] Productivity (yield of leaves per bush) also varies over the plant's life, and the number of harvests per year varies by type of coca – factors that can have a dramatic impact on harvest estimates.

Due to these data-collection problems, as well as different data-gathering methods, official data on illicit crop cultivation is often contradictory. The above analysis used US government figures. UN estimates provide a somewhat different picture. While the UN reported a 30 percent drop in Colombian coca cultivation between December 2001 and December 2002, the US estimated that the drop was only 15 percent (Forero 2003). Similarly, according to a United Nations report published in March 2003, Peruvian coca cultivation was 46,700 hectares in 2002, a mere 1 percent increase when compared to the 46,200 hectares cultivated in 2001 (United Nations Office on Drugs and Crime 2003b: 4). However, the US Department of State (2003: Peru) writes that cultivation increased by 8 percent in 2002, contradicting the lower UN estimate. Moreover, figures are not always consistent. In the March 2003 report referred to above, the UN estimated Peruvian coca cultivation in 2002 at 46,700 hectares, but in another report, the UN provides an estimate of 52,500 hectares for the same year (United Nations Office on Drugs and Crime 2003c: 8). To complicate matters further, sometimes there are no figures at all. For 2003, for example, the Department of State (2004: Peru) reported that there were "no confirmed estimates as to the amount of opium poppy under cultivation in Peru." If the size of illicit cultivation is unknown, assessments of the impact of anti-drug policies on illicit cultivation are sketchy at best.

Even if figures were more accurate, they would still have to be interpreted. Similarly to the gathering of data, the interpretation of data is tricky and thus the subject of political and scientific controversy. Looking at the reasons behind high Peruvian coca prices in 2001, the Department of State (2002: Peru) writes that prices remained high "possibly in response to coca leaf shortfalls in Bolivia, and unmet demand in Colombia." Yet high prices have even more complex causes. Whereas Peru's drug czar Vega Llona attributed high prices to increased trafficking as a result of the suspension of the ABDP as well as a proliferation of small trafficking groups, the US embassy said that slow coca eradication was behind high prices. Independent observers widened the debate by referring to structural faults of AD and increasing demand on the international drug market (Rojas 2003: 8; McClintock and Vallas 2003: 166; Marshall 2001). Similar uncertainty governed the reasons for the decline in Colombian coca cultivation in 2002. The UN tried to explain this decline by referring to a variety of factors:

> Forced eradication was beyond doubt the key reason [...]. Nonetheless, other factors such as the practice of abandonment of fields and voluntary eradication seemed to have played a role as well. The armed conflict, which was fuelled by narcotics production, deteriorated the security situation in the country to a point that it prevented in some parts of the country the farmers from even cultivating coca. Moreover, a recovery of the prices of some key farm products, such as cocoa and sugar cane in 2002, seemed to have reduced the incentives for farmers to switch to coca cultivation.
>
> (United Nations Office on Drugs and Crime 2003a: 17

This quote reveals the difficulty of assessing the relative explanatory power of factors driving drug industry displacement. Did coca cultivation increase in department A due to a fighting between paramilitaries and rebels in department B, leading to the forced displacement of peasants to department A, or due to US-sponsored fumigation campaign in department B? A specialist in low-intensity warfare would say that the increase in cultivation was a consequence of fightin between paramilitaries and rebels, whereas an activist opposing coercive US drug policies would cite fumigation as a cause of the displacement of people and coca. The exact ratio of influences motivating peasants to migrate to department A would remain unknown unless a significant number of peasants were systematically interviewed about their motivation to migrate.

Similarly, little is known about drug entrepreneurs and the way they anticipated state policies. As shown above, some of Colombia's neighbors saw an increase in illicit activities even before the push into southern Colombia in December 2000. Did this increase result from traffickers' sensing future pressures and opportunities, or was it due to indigenous factors unrelated to the incipient Plan Colombia? There is not only a lack of knowledge about traffick ers' responses to anti-drug policies, but also about the traffickers themselves. In 2003–2004, the number of trafficking groups, or "baby cartels," operating in Colombia was estimated at 82 (Independent Commission 2004: 27). The Colombian government knew little about their activities and internal structure, which became clear in September 2004 when the head of Colombia's judicial police told a reporter that the Colombian government did not even know the names of the major traffickers (Molinski 2004)

Covert operations pose additional problems. A former US Special Forces member who had served in the Andes explained the frequent use of covert operations as follows: "The use of covert operations keeps down the size of the known U.S. footprint in trouble areas, where we want to keep a low profile (quoted in Tamayo 2001b). Inferring to the scope of covert operations from budgets does not lead far, since it is not known how the Pentagon spends its money in Colombia and how much money the CIA spends there.

Not only the US armed forces and intelligence services operate in the shadows and thus beyond public scrutiny, private contractors do so as well. As a US official said to a journalist in the late 1990s: "Of course they have to keep it secret. They're up to a lot of things that they shouldn't be" (quoted in Robberson 1998). In his attempt to investigate the activities of contractors, the same US journalist encountered obstacles. Officials of two private security companies operating in Colombia told him they were not allowed to discuss their activities. Similarly, a colleague of the journalist who had tried to talk to Dyncorp pilots at a Colombian air base was told that another attempt to talk to Dyncorp personnel would lead to his banishment from the US embassy (Robberson 1998).

In addition to empirical black boxes, the heuristic explanation of drug industry displacement offered in this chapter is challenged by an alternative explanation. One could argue that even without Plan Colombia and the Andean Regional Initiative, illicit activities would have spread across Colombia and to neighboring countries. According to this alternative explanation, US-sponsored anti-drug policies were not necessary for the displacement of the drug industry, since peasants would have escaped the violence and economic insecurity anyway, which would have dispersed illicit crop cultivation. Moreover, non-state armed groups would have fostered coca and poppy cultivation even in the absence of coercive US drug policies. Along the same lines, one could argue that illicit activities would have increased in neighboring countries anyway as Colombian drug entrepreneurs would have tried to expand their fiel of operations.

However, this alternative, counter-factual explanation cannot convince. To be sure, drug market dynamics can result from factors other than law enforcement. The displacement of the illicit drug industry within Colombia and to neighboring states was not only a result of Plan Colombia and the Andean Regional Initiative. However, the analysis above cites ample evidence showing that US-sponsored anti-drug initiatives exacerbated the displacement of the drug industry. In Colombia, there is a close link between anti-drug operations on the one hand and a displacement of people and illicit crops on the other hand. US drug policy was not the only cause of displacement, but it aggravated the problem. While many Colombian farmers would most likely have had to resettle elsewhere out of fear of guerillas, paramilitaries, and traffickers even in the absence of anti-drug operations, these operations, and most importantly fumigation, increased the pressure on peasants to move across the country in the search for physical and economic security.

Regarding the increase in illicit activities in neighboring countries, it is likely that this increase would have been smaller in the absence of Plan Colombia and the Andean Regional Initiative. Colombia would have probably further consolidated its position as the world's leading coca producer and as South America's leading poppy producer. As shown above, the country offered a perfect mix of conditions enabling illicit activities, and there is little reason to believe that drug entrepreneurs would have seen a need to cross Colombia's borders in the absence of state pressure. Although the motivations of non-state actors to cross national borders are obscure, there are indications that Colombian military and police operations motivated some drug entrepreneurs, as well as many peasants, to cross Colombia's borders.

Conclusion

This case study examined a crucial period in the history of US foreign drug policies: the early twenty-first century. In the framework of Plan Colombia and the Andean Regional Initiative, US policy-makers invested unprecedented sums of money into attempts to reduce domestic drug problems in the US by reducing the amount of drugs coming into the US from Colombia.

In the late 1990s, the Colombian conflict worsened. Rebels and paramilitaries committed numerous attacks against Colombian and foreign individuals and companies. Moreover, non-state armed groups increased the size of land used for coca cultivation and became increasingly involved in all stages of the illicit drug industry. Colombia seemed to be on the verge of collapse. This impression caused significant concern in Washington since the Colombian conflict was seen as undermining several US security interests. To improve the situation, the Clinton administration first had to improve its relationship with the Colombian government, a relationship that had suffered under the US decision to decertify Colombia in 1996 and 1997. By the end of the decade, US policy-makers had come to understand that ostracizing the Colombian government had been counterproductive. As a consequence, the Clinton and Pastrana administrations worked toward a rapprochement, leading to an increase in US aid.

As part of Plan Colombia, the US invested an initial sum of over one billion dollars into counter-drug efforts in the Andes. The main beneficiary of this huge aid flow was the Colombian military. Whereas during the 1990s the Colombian police had been the main recipient of US aid, US policy-makers now placed their hopes on the Colombian military, despite ardent criticism voiced by observers and policy-makers in South America, Europe, and the US. Observers were concerned about the impact of aerial fumigation and other coercive drug policies on human rights, the environment, and the legitimacy of the Colombian state. To buttress support for Plan Colombia and to counter the Vietnam analogy, the White House presented Plan Colombia as an anti-drug program only. However, it was clear that counter-drug and counter-insurgency were inseparable since rebels controlled many coca cultivation zones.

While Plan Colombia was implemented, coca cultivation spread geographically as farmers migrated from the most heavily sprayed zones to other parts of Colombia. In addition, Colombia's neighbors experienced an increase in illicit activities after the push into Southern Colombia. In Venezuela, Brazil, and Ecuador, new coca fields sprang up, and traffickers made their presence more strongly felt. In Peru, an increase in coca cultivation was aggravated by a concomitant increase in poppy cultivation.

Under the Andean Regional Initiative, the program that replaced Plan Colombia from fiscal year 2002, coercion continued to mark US drug policies toward Colombia, and there were even signs of escalation. Following 9/11, US policymakers saw the fight against Colombian non-state armed groups as part of the global US "war on terror" and thus allowed the use of US aid in counter-insurgency operations. With Alvaro Uribe, who became Colombian President in mid-2002 and who ruled out making any concessions to rebels, Washington developed a close relationship leading to record levels of fumigation, arrests, and extraditions. To support their claims of success, the Bush and Uribe administration referred to an increase in the number of rebels killed or captured, territories freed of rebel control, a decline in the number of civilians killed, and a decline in coca cultivation.

However, official claims of success warrant caution because Colombian coca cultivation remained relatively stable and because the Andean Regional Initiative was accompanied by a geographical expansion of coca (as well as poppy) cultivation. While coca cultivation decreased in some departments, other departments saw increases in cultivation, or even first-time cultivation. Hence, there is a clear correlation between US-sponsored drug policies and the displacement of coca cultivation within Colombia.

Moreover, US-sponsored drug policies continued to pose problems for Colombia's neighbors. Illicit activities increased in Brazil, Ecuador, and Venezuela, despite an increase in US aid granted under the Andean Regional Initiative. However, the feared massive import of violence and drugs from Colombia did not materialize. Although new coca fields were discovered and although traffickers expanded their activities across borders, coca cultivation levels in these countries continued to be low and drug trafficking has probably not greatly surpassed previous levels. In Peru and Bolivia, the increase in coca cultivation was more significant

To better understand and explain the displacement of the illicit drug industry within Colombia and to neighboring states, the chapter then referred to US policy selectivity, flexible responses by peasants and drug entrepreneurs to state pressure, and weak law enforcement capacities of drug-producing and transit states.

US drug policies were selective in several ways. In its decision to direct the initial thrust of Plan Colombia toward Colombia's southern coca regions, the US enabled the displacement of coca cultivation to other parts of the country.

Moreover, due to a focus on military programs and a neglect of non-coercive strategies, fumigation did not achieve sustainable results. Lastly, US drug policies were selective in that Washington failed to devise regional strategies against a regional problem. Instead, the US preferred to pursue several bilateral strategies. Bilateralism allowed the US to exert significant influence over South American states, but was ineffective in preventing a spillover of drugs across borders.

The analysis also showed that both peasants and traffickers responded innovatively to Plan Colombia and the Andean Regional Initiative. Destroyed coca plants were replanted, the yield of coca fields was increased, fields became smaller, and coca was grown in shade, mixed with licit crops, and planted in ever-remoter regions. Moreover, traffickers become more efficient in the conversion of coca leaves into cocaine, and they evaded law enforcement pressure through the frequent recourse to violence and corruption. In addition, they induced peasants in neighboring countries to grow coca and poppy by providing technical advice and cash loans.

With regard to the capacities of South American countries to implement anti-drug laws, weak law enforcement was a particularly acute problem in Colombia because the government did not control significant parts of the national territory. Lacking the necessary manpower, training and equipment, ranging from telephones to helicopters, the Colombian security forces were unable to defeat non-state armed groups, whose mobility led to a spread of coca cultivation across the country. Adverse geographic and climatic conditions hampered law enforcement as well. The governments of other countries were similarly weak, which helps to explain an increase in illicit activities in these countries. Bolivia is a special case, however. During the period analyzed, the country saw a significan increase in coca cultivation in the Yungas region, which was partly a consequence of a weak government. But unlike in other countries, the Colombian conflict seems to have had a relatively minor impact on Bolivia. Hence, the increase in Bolivian coca cultivation was not a side effect of US-sponsored anti-drug operations in Colombia.

Contingent conditions are important, too. Colombia offered a mix of political, economic, and social conditions that allowed drug production and trafficking to thrive. Both the Colombian state and the Colombian nation have traditionally been weak. While state and society were weak even before the implementation of US coercive drug policies in South America, these policies have further weakened state and society. Since state and societal weakness is conducive to the displacement of the drug industry across the country, Plan Colombia and the Andean Regional Initiative contributed to the displacement of the drug industry.

The chapter also looked at empirical black boxes and alternative explanations for the displacement of the drug industry. There is a lack of knowledge about the size of land used for illicit crop cultivation, the yield of coca crops, the way peasants and drug entrepreneurs responded to anti-drug operations, and the structure of Colombian drug trafficking. Moreover, due to the secrecy regarding covert operations and the activities of private contractors, little is known about the way the US and Andean governments implemented their joint anti-drug operations. Moreover, and as a consequence of these empirical black boxes, assessing the relative weight of causal factors behind the displacement of the drug industry is challenging.

Due to these empirical and analytical difficulties, the alternative explanation for the displacement of the drug industry that claims that the displacement would have taken place even in the absence of Plan Colombia and the Andean Regional Initiative is hard to refute beyond doubt. Nevertheless, there is significant evidence showing that these anti-drug programs, in combination with the other elements constituting the initial causal mechanism, acted as a catalyst for the displacement of the drug industry within Colombia and to neighboring states, with the exception of Bolivia. If it had not been for Plan Colombia and the Andean Regional Initiative, displacement might still have occurred, but not along the same spatial and temporal lines.

5 Drug industry displacement and side effects of foreign policy

This book set out to explain the link between the displacement of the illicit drug industry and US international drug policies. The first chapter described drug problems and drug policies, showing that the thrust of US foreign drug policy has been on supply-side eradication and interdiction. It argued that drug policy scholars do not pay enough attention to displacement and that IR scholars neglect side effects of foreign policy. To alleviate these shortcomings, a causal mechanism was developed that served as a heuristic explanation of displacement and that was applied to three empirical cases.

How can we explain worsening drug problems during a period of unprecedented US anti-drug efforts? This chapter argues that although displacement has resulted from various factors, US foreign policy has been a major driving factor behind displacement. Since displacement is a catalyst for drug-related problems, the US has worsened these problems. In a nutshell, the fact that we are living in a world of drugs is partially a consequence of coercive US drug policies.

The initial causal mechanism provides a plausible explanation of displacement. But more empirical information about the illicit drug industry is needed to formulate a more fine-grained mechanism. No matter how scholars research displacement, they should take into account the fact that temporally and spatially contingent factors influence displacement. With regard to the theorization of side effects, scholars must acknowledge the limits of law-based theorizing and accept contingency and complexity as crucial prerequisites for analyzing the link between foreign policy and change in international affairs.

Results

This book has looked at three major US international initiatives against drugs. These were undertaken at different times and focused on different countries. Moreover, while the first case study examined a US initiative aimed at reducing the supply of heroin, the second and third case studies dealt with historical periods during which the main thrust of US foreign drug policy was on cocaine.

The first case study examined US efforts in the early 1970s to reduce the supply of heroin from the Mediterranean to the US, and the impact of these efforts on Southeast Asia and Mexico. After US security policies had helped create a thriving illicit drug industry in Marseille, the Corsican French Connection became the main supplier of heroin to the US and retained this position for over 20 years. But in the early 1970s, the Connection was destroyed, and Turkey, where most of the opium used for heroin production came from, banned poppy cultivation.

Nixon's victory was only temporary, however. In Southeast Asia, the US had turned a blind eye to their anti-Communist proxies' drug deals. This circumstance, together with heroin consumption among GIs in Vietnam and other factors, led to a regional drug boom in Southeast Asia. The withdrawal of US troops from Vietnam and the disruption of Mediterranean heroin exports, shortly after, coincided with a global expansion of the Southeast Asian heroin industry. But while Southeast Asia never managed to dominate the US market, Mexico had established a near-monopoly by the mid-1970s. Hence, displacement is much more obvious with regard to Mexico than Southeast Asia. In Mexico, displacement occurred simultaneously with, and after, the Nixon initiative. Then again, Southeast Asia already had a thriving drug industry at the time of the Nixon initiative, and the region did not conquer the US heroin market.

The selective way in which the US implemented its drug policies, the adaptive capacities of the illicit drug industry, and the unwillingness and/or inability of Southeast Asian countries and Mexico to reduce drug supplies were all crucial for explaining the massive geographic shift in this illicit sector in the early 1970s. Moreover, numerous contingent and background conditions influ enced the displacement process. Since many of these contingent developments occurred before and simultaneously with the Nixon initiative against France and Turkey, the Nixon initiative was not a sufficient cause of displacement. Rather, a confluence of developments led to displacement

Empirical black boxes obscure the link between US foreign drug policies and displacement, and they make it difficult to refute alternative explanations for displacement beyond any doubt. However, these alternative explanations are not very convincing. Increasing economic interdependence or prohibition would most likely have led to *some kind* of restructuring process. Yet it is unlikely that displacement would have occurred along *the same*, or even along *similar*, temporal and spatial lines if the French Connection had not been dismantled and if Turkey had not banned poppy production. Without the Nixon initiative, the diversification and restructuring process would most probably have taken longer and would have involved more countries.

The second case study examined US efforts from the late 1980s to 2001 to reduce the amount of cocaine coming into the US from South America through the ABDP, the interdiction of small airplanes used for drug trafficking. During the program's initial phase, interdiction was rather haphazard. Then, in 1995, air interdiction entered into a new phase, and possibly dozens of airplanes flyin between Peru, Bolivia, and Colombia were interdicted. Simultaneously, coca cultivation surged in Colombia and declined in Peru, cocaine production increased in Peru and Bolivia, and trafficking routes and methods became more diverse. By the time the ABDP was suspended in 2001, the structure of the region's drug industry was much more complex than before the program.

But did the ABDP *cause* these changes in the structure of the South American coca/cocaine industry? The answer is yes and no. A confluence of factors led to displacement. Displacement was enabled by a selective application of US pressure, although it is also important to note that coca cultivation increased in Colombia despite a large US-sponsored aerial fumigation program in Colombia. In addition, traffickers were able to minimize the impact of aerial interdiction by diversifying trafficking routes, using sophisticated technology as well as simple, yet efficient means of transport, and reducing their dependency on coca from remote places. Displacement was also enabled by state weakness resulting from insurgency, a lack of funding, and corruption. In addition, numerous contingent conditions and complex interaction effects made the South American cocaine industry fuzzier. Since some of these contingencies and interaction effects are not, or only indirectly, related to decisions made in Washington, displacement was not simply a side effect of US foreign drug policy.

Black boxes further underline the need to go beyond a simple notion of causality. The number of airplanes interdicted, the amount of coca and cocaine produced, and the main actors involved in the drug business are all relatively obscure, leading to diverse assessments of the ABDP. The view held by many policy-makers that the program was a huge success is untenable because air interdiction was not the sole reason for the decline in Peruvian coca cultivation, total cultivation remained stable due to the Colombian coca boom, aerial drug smuggling continued, and the ABDP contributed to an increase in Peruvian and Bolivian cocaine production. Moreover, the ABDP did not alleviate US drug problems (Walsh 2004; Tokatlián 2003: 24). Yet an alternative view on displacement, according to which there is no causal link between displacement and the ABDP, is equally implausible. Although the displacement of coca cultivation from Peru to Colombia, the diversification of trafficking routes, and the verticalization of the Peruvian and Bolivian drug industries resulted from a confluenc of factors, US-sponsored air interdiction was one of these. The South American drug industry would probably have changed even in the absence of air interdiction. But displacement would have been slower and would have occurred along different geographical lines.

The third case study focused on drug displacement within Colombia and to other South American countries in the early twenty-first century. During the 1990s, strong rebel groups, US economic interests, and ever-increasing drug supplies led Washington to improve relations with the Colombian government and increase military aid. To counter criticism from the left (which feared the human rights implications of military aid) and the right (which feared that Clinton was dragging the US into a Vietnam-like military adventure), the White House presented Plan Colombia as a counter-drug plan instead of a counter-insurgency operation. Within a few years, the US had invested billions of dollars into the Plan and its successor program, the Andean Regional Initiative, with the bulk of the funding benefiting the Colombian armed forces

During the "push into Southern Colombia" in late December 2000, US-supported Colombian security forces destroyed large coca plantations and forced the FARC into retreat. However, these were Pyrrhic victories, since they came at the cost of drug displacement across Colombia and, although to a limited extent, to other countries. Moreover, and partly because of this displacement, US-sponsored operations against coca fields, drug laboratories, and traffickers did not reduce total South American coca production – despite a significant escalation of US involvement in Colombia after 9/11, when the administration of George W. Bush merged the campaigns against drugs, terrorism, and insurgency.

Displacement was partly driven by the local application of US-sponsored law enforcement pressure, the focus on coercion instead of more sustainable strategies, and a preference for bilateralism. Moreover, traffickers, rebels, paramilitaries, and farmers evaded law enforcement through innovative behavior. Displacement was further enabled by state weakness, manifesting itself particularly in a lack of territorial control and weak security forces in Colombia who battled against strong insurgent groups. For various domestic reasons, the freedom of maneuver of other governments was also limited. Regarding contingent conditions, the drug industry has been thriving in Colombia for so long due to the country's weak state and society, and US coercive drug policies further weakened the state and society.

Despite black boxes that make it difficult to determine the exact ratio of stimuli behind displacement, the available evidence shows that Plan Colombia and the Andean Regional Initiative contributed to displacement. Although violence and poverty would have led to some displacement anyway, US drug policies functioned as a catalyst for the displacement of the drug industry within Colombia, and, with the exception of Bolivia, to other South American countries. It is unlikely that coca (and poppy) cultivation would have spread as fast, and along similar geographical lines, across the country and the region in the absence of US foreign drug policy.

Solving the puzzle of worsening drug problems and US coercion

This book began with a conundrum: Why have drug problems become worse simultaneously with significant US attempts to reduce illicit drug supplies? It was argued that explaining displacement would help to solve this puzzle, since a displacement of drugs means a displacement of drug-related problems.

All three case studies showed that US foreign policy contributed significantl to displacement. Although US foreign policy was not sufficient for changing the structure of the drug industry, Washington's efforts were necessary for affecting the changes observed.[1] If it had not been for US foreign policy, displacement would most likely have occurred as well, but along different temporal and spatial lines. Hence, the three case studies underscore Washington's role in fostering destructive change.

This does not mean that all instances of displacement in the past were a result of US initiatives against drugs. Displacement can occur even without US pressure on peasants, traffickers, or governments. The drug industry is constantly in flux, with new peasant groups engaging in illicit cultivation, new drug entrepreneurs entering the market, and new trafficking routes evolving. But when Washington decides to intervene, it is likely to push drugs from one place to another – as well as all the problems that accompany the illicit drug industry. Given the priority Washington has been according to drug supply reduction over recent decades, it is safe to say that many instances of displacement – not only the three analyzed in this book – have been co-created by shortsighted US drug policies.

Displacement is bad both for the US and for the countries in which the US tries to reduce illicit drug supplies through eradication and interdiction. It is bad for the US because displacement guarantees a relatively stable, and often increasing, supply of illicit drugs, leading to the loss of billions of dollars invested into anti-drug initiatives. It is bad for cocaine and heroin producing and transit countries because displacement inevitably aggravates violence, corruption, human rights abuses, environmental destruction, the spread of AIDS, and other drug-related problems. US foreign policy has not been the only cause of displacement, and US-induced displacement has not been the only cause of drug-related problems. The drug trade itself causes significant harm (Youngers 2005: 339–340). However, by co-creating a world of drugs, US policies have had a detrimental impact on individuals, the environment, the economy, and political institutions.

Due to its focus on displacement, this book has largely neglected drug-related problems. However, the case studies did cite some negative consequences of displacement. In the early 1970s, the US pushed drugs around the globe and thus contributed to a globalization of drug problems, and it cooperated with repressive governments such as that of Burma, which diverted US anti-drug aid to counter-insurgency operations. The air interdiction program in the 1990s brought the US into league with the administration of Peruvian President Alberto Fujimori, "one of the most corrupt and authoritarian regimes in Peruvian history" (Rojas 2005: 222). Further, the ABDP was part of a coercive anti-drug strategy implemented in the 1990s that exacerbated weak state legitimacy, environmental destruction, and South American drug consumption. In Colombia in the early twenty-first century, aerial fumigation and anti-drug operations on the ground pitched the coalition of Colombian and US security forces against rebels, led to significant environmental destruction, and was accompanied by the migration of tens of thousands of Colombians to other parts of the country and also across Colombia's borders. Fumigation and military cooperation aggravated violence and poverty and thereby further undermined Colombian state legitimacy and social integration.

Given the dismal record of US international drug policies, one cannot ignore the issue of alternative policies. Before turning to this question in the last chapter, the following sections discuss the lessons learned from the empirical analysis for the theorization of displacement in particular and foreign policy side effects in general.

Theorizing the displacement of the drug industry

The initial causal mechanism helped to shed light on displacement in the three cases analyzed. Yet its usefulness goes beyond these three cases. Since the mechanism was applied to three different historical periods and regions, as well as to two types of drugs, the causal mechanism seems to be a general one, i.e. one that is applicable beyond the three cases. However, the case studies also reveal variation in the temporal and geographical patterns of displacement, as well as in the power of explanatory factors. The selective implementation of US foreign drug policy, for example, was shown to have facilitated displacement. But the second case study also underlined that coca cultivation increased in Colombia despite US-sponsored aerial fumigation.

Variation in the chronology of displacement and its underlying causality underline the need to gather more information on drugs, to study more cases of displacement in which the US was active or inactive, and to apply the causal mechanism to more cases in order to discover a more refined mechanism. This would counterbalance oversimplified views of displacement. Displacement is complex. In Mexico, the Nixon initiative was followed by a drug boom, but in Southeast Asia, the link between the Nixon initiative and displacement is much less obvious. Here, the effect of US foreign policy was more indirect: US Cold War policies had created the conditions that allowed Southeast Asia to eventually enter the global drug market. The second case study showed that incipient displacement occurred during a period in which US air interdiction was implemented unsystematically. And the third case revealed that although displacement was significant within Colombia, the effects of US drug policies on other South American countries were more muted. Hence, scholars must specify the intensity of displacement and the chronological sequence of events leading from a foreign policy initiative to displacement, and they must pay particular attention to antecedent conditions and policies that influence displacement

Analyzing displacement is theoretically and methodologically challenging and underlines the need to be more skeptical about social laws. This becomes clear when looking at the flexibility of the drug industry. The ability of many traffickers to avoid arrest or death is impressive. They anticipate political and drug market changes, avoid raw material shortages, diversify trafficking routes, and employ new drug producing and smuggling methods. Generally, the drug industry adapts to law enforcement better than states adapt to changes in drug markets.[2] Michael Kenney (2002: xiii) argues that this adaptive behavior reflect the ability of trafficking organizations to learn, i.e. "to alter their organizational structures and behavior in response to information and experience, store this knowledge in practices, procedures and performance programs, and select and retain innovations that produce satisfactory outcomes."[3]

The way a trafficking group adapts to law enforcement pressure depends on the group's financial resources, its ability to avoid internal strife, its integration into a national or ethnic community, or simply chance. A sudden draught destroying poppy plants, the death of a prominent trafficker, or the decision of a political leader to improve his international image by instituting a law enforcement campaign can destroy a trafficking group. The French Connection was unable to survive the onslaught of security forces, whereas many South American traffickers continued aerial smuggling despite the US-sponsored interdiction program. Hence, the drug industry changes its form when put under pressure, but the adaptive responses depend on too many factors to predict the responses precisely.

All three case studies underlined the impact of contingent factors on displacement. In the early 1970s, displacement occurred not least due to domestic political changes in France and Turkey, US post-World War II containment strategies in Southeast Asia, and the withdrawal of US troops from Vietnam. In the 1990s, displacement was exacerbated by an array of changes ranging from a disintegrating Peruvian insurgency movement to a worsening Colombian civil war. In the early twenty-first century, the drug industry was on the move within Colombia, not least because of a weak state and society that reflect a uniquely violent history.

These developments indicate that there is always going to be a war, coup d'état, draught, or fungus influencing displacement, but that nobody can say who is going to fight whom, which group will topple which government, where the rain will stop falling, and which fungus will attack illicit crops where. Exact predictions of displacement ("In the next five years, Pakistan will see an explosion of drug production and trafficking") are therefore impossible. Developments on drug markets are too complex to be compatible with deterministic predictions of the if–then type – except of the most banal type. There is little doubt, for example, that a US initiative against drugs will contribute to displacement. Yet the exact nature of displacement can be extrapolated neither from the empirical past nor from theory.

Contingent factors also obstruct the development of "softer," probabilistic scenarios ("If the poppy eradication program in Afghanistan works, and if Islamabad fails to control tribal areas in Pakistan, then drug production may well increase significantly in Pakistan"). Theorizing change in a probabilistic fashion means defining the conditions under which change occurs. Yet the diversity of factors that can influence phenomena such as displacement hampers attempts to define scope conditions under which change is likely to occur. Whether Pakistan will attract more drug production and trafficking depends on the ability of the Iranian government to prevent large-scale poppy cultivation in Iran, the stance toward drugs taken by religious leaders in Pakistani tribal zones, and many other conditions.

Contingencies thus highlight the need to go beyond a simplified notion of displacement. The popular metaphor of a "balloon effect" is misleading (for a critique, see Friesendorf 2005b). Displacement results from various factors that may coincide, occur randomly, interact with one another, and/or be historically contingent. Washington has indeed squeezed the balloon and failed to burst it. But it is not only US foreign policy that makes drug producers shift their operations. Moreover, in a balloon, the amount of air or water is constant. Sometimes, a similar phenomenon can be observed in the case of the drug trade, for example, in the 1990s, when a decrease in Peruvian and Bolivian coca cultivation was almost perfectly compensated by increasing Colombian cultivation. More often, however, displacement increases total drug supplies.

Contingencies do not imply that displacement must be treated agnostically. It may be possible to limit the range of contingencies, or to define different categories of contingencies, particularly if the analyst studies only one region or historical period.[4] But the larger the temporal and geographical focus, the less likely it is to define contingencies precisely. Research designs must therefore leave room for the unexpected, and empirical research must allow for accidents, coincidences, and randomness.

Black boxes also undermine law-based theorizing. The identity of drug traffickers, the origins of drugs smuggled to the US, the size of the drug industry, reasons for changing drug prices, details about anti-drug operations, and the relative weight of explanatory factors are just some of the black boxes identified in this book. They show that our empirical knowledge of the drug industry is relatively small – which should caution researchers against oversimplifying the mechanisms of displacement.

Arriving at more fine-grained explanations means abandoning a perspective that only looks at the macro level. It is important, for example, to understand better how traffickers assess risks and deal with law enforcement. Interviews with traffickers can unearth information about their business behavior, which would help to explain displacement (for interesting examples of works along this path, see Zaitch 2002; Kenney 2002). If the aim of terrorism researchers is to "Know thy enemy," drug policy researchers must also better comprehend their protagonists. Moreover, in order to understand better why drugs shift to country A and not to country B, it is crucial to examine geographical factors as well (Allen 2002; Chouvy 2002). Alternatively, researchers could focus on the implementation of prohibition regimes in different countries and across different criminalized activities (Nadelmann 1990; Thoumi 2002b). To better understand actors and structures, IR scholars can benefit from the knowledge of experts of one particular country, region, or public policy. IR scholars should integrate different strands of thought into their theories. Eclectic approaches are needed that draw insights from various disciplines, theories within specific disciplines, and various methodologies (Katzenstein and Okawara 2001/2002).[5]

No matter how scholars deal with contingent factors and black boxes, and regardless of how they strike the balance between a micro and a macro perspective, displacement research must be at least as much of a hermeneutic endeavor as one informed by the standard techniques of positivist science. Applying John Stuart Mill's method of difference and agreement and other approaches of controlled variation poses significant problems. As shown in this book, researchers are faced with unreliable data, phenomena such as corruption that are difficult to operationalize, and complex, or even enigmatic, causal chains (on complex and enigmatic causal chains, see Bennett and George 2001).

The limits of positivism and the merits of interpretation are illustrated by the difficulty of assessing the relative weight of explanatory factors in complex scenarios (Elman and Elman 2001: 23; Jervis 1997: 40). In some cases it is obvious that factor A was more important than factor B for creating outcome C. In other cases, researchers can only describe the different elements leading to the outcome, show how they are related, and evaluate their aggregate impact. The displacement of coca cultivation and drug production in Colombia, for example, was not only due to Plan Colombia and the Andean Regional Initiative, but was also a consequence of the migration of people escaping from rebels and paramilitaries.[6] While it may be possible to show whether law enforcement or rebel and paramilitary activity was the main driving force behind displacement in a particular area of Colombia at a particular time, analyzing displacement across the country and over a period of several years yields less precise results.

The next section, which looks at side effects of foreign policy in general, further underlines the need to go beyond the search for social laws and take into account complexity and contingency.

Theorizing side effects of foreign policy

Often, political change and crucial events have taken IR scholars by surprise. Of course, few people anticipated the end of the Cold War or 9/11. But scholars would have been better prepared for the end of the Cold War and 9/11 if they had had less faith in structural balance-of-power theories that neglect domestic politics and the catalytic role of individuals such as Michael Gorbachev, and if they had earlier abandoned a state-centric perspective that eclipses the presence of violent non-state actors such as al-Qaida in international affairs (Bernstein *et al.* 2000: 52; Leheny 2002). Drug policy scholars can cite many other cases of scholarly neglect, such as the silence of theory-informed IR journals on the violence that has been engulfing Colombia in recent decades

The search for social laws, preferably parsimonious ones, prevents IR scholars from analyzing outcomes that result from a complex constellation of factors and actors and that do not occur along linear causal paths. As Gunther Hellmann and Harald Müller (2003: 377) point out, "linear causality, still the ideal of much of our theoretical and empirical work, might not be good enough to explain events that move in vicious feedback circles, jumps, chaos-like trajectories or law-exempt singularities." Similarly, Robert Jervis (1997: 125) argues that a

> change in an element or relationship often alters others, which in turn affect the original one. We then are dealing with cycles in which causation is mutual or circular rather than one-way, as it is in most of our theories. [. . .] [It] is difficult for observers to assign responsibility and for actors to break out of reinforcing patterns that seem to come from everywhere and nowhere. The actors' behavior collectively causes and explains itself.

Taking complexity into account is particularly pertinent when looking at criminalization. When states decide to forbid specific activities and use their police or military forces to enforce criminal laws, they inevitably set in motion a flurry of attempts to circumvent state control. The history of US drug control provides clear lessons. But more recent examples can be cited as well. Since the 1990s, the trafficking of women and girls for the purpose of sexual exploitation has been booming in Europe, particularly in Southeast Europe, not least because of the presence of tens of thousands of peacekeepers in the region, many of whom have purchased sexual services (Mendelson 2005). States have responded to these developments by enacting laws against sex trafficking and investing more resources into implementing these laws. This has pushed the sex industry underground and made it more complex. Flats have replaced large brothels as the places where trafficked women and girls are kept; traffickers have adopted flexible, networked forms of cooperation; and they use mobile phones rather than landlines (Vandenberg 2005: 75).

Cases of terrorism and insurgency also reveal that state pressure increases the complexity of a foreign policy problem. The global US "war on terror" and the invasion of Afghanistan have transformed, not destroyed, al-Qaida. Before 9/11, the organization had a fairly hierarchical structure. In 2004, Bruce Hoffmann (2004: 423) wrote that "Al Qaeda has survived the military onslaught directed against it in Afghanistan [. . .] and has reconfigured itself. [. . .] It is now a more diffuse and amorphous ideological movement inspiring like-minded affiliate and associates that pose new, different, and more complex challenges." Similarly, Iraqi insurgents have learned fast and have improved the effectiveness of their attacks against US forces since the end of major US military operations in Iraq was announced in May 2003 (Hoffmann 2006: 113). Explaining these developments means acknowledging complexity.

Historians are arguably more prepared to accept complexity than political scientists. For political scientists, complexity is a problem equated with overdetermination (the positing of more causes for an outcome than are needed to explain it) and equifinality (the fact that different paths can lead to the same outcome). Political scientists therefore focus on primary causes and leave secondary causes to historians. Historians, in contrast, have little faith in attempts to establish testable relationships between variables, to identify necessary and sufficient conditions, and to weigh explanatory factors. Historians are also more willing than political scientists to provide explanations based on multiple causation (Elman and Elman 2001: 20–23).

Defending themselves against the charge of offering "shopping-list" explanations, historians say that explanatory factors cannot be isolated from their context. They "find political scientists' insistence on isolating a few fundamental causes acting independently bemusing because causality is complex, and things often happen because variables are mutually reinforcing, intersecting at particular moments in space and time" (Elman and Elman 2001: 23). Some historians even defend the notion of "total history," or accounts that include all aspects of the phenomenon that is to be explained (Levy 2001: 54–55). Since historians emphasize the interconnection of events, sequences, and processes, they are reluctant to engage in variable-based theorizing. John Lewis Gaddis (2001: 312, emphasis in the original) writes: "Trained to be sensitive both to timescape *and* landscape, we fail to see how any variable (apart from perhaps God) can be truly independent."

The charge of many political scientists that historians provide over-determined explanations is based on a conflation of over-determination and multi-causality. Over-determined explanations posit several factors that are individually sufficient for an outcome. Multi-causal explanations focus on a set of factors that are jointly sufficient for an outcome. Most historians would deny that single explanatory factors are sufficient for explaining outcomes, arguing that outcomes result from combinations of factors. For example, US anti-drug initiatives, weak law enforcement, or flexible responses by traffickers are not individually sufficient causes for drug industry displacement. Rather, it is the *combination* of these factors that leads to displacement. Hence, this book, like many works by historians, provides a multi-causal explanation. If one explanatory factor had been absent, the outcome would have been different.

The divide between history and political science is unfortunate. Jack Levy (1997: 33) writes that history "is too important to leave to the historians, and theory is too important to leave to the theorists." This book tries to strike a balance between context and parsimony. On the one hand, the case studies have examined contingencies, multi-causality, and complex interactions of explanatory factors, and have thus sacrificed as little history as possible to theoretical parsimony. On the other hand, they have bracketed aspects that seemed to be of secondary relevance for displacement.

Whether students of foreign policy side effects argue on a higher level of explanation (i.e. a more theoretical level) or a lower one (i.e. a more empirical level) depends on the empirical subject-matter and the research question. In any case, process tracing and mechanism-based theorizing are appropriate for all analyses of foreign policy side effects, given that they can accommodate complexity and contingency.

Process tracing helps to narrow the gap between history and political science, and it is a suitable method for addressing the conditions that allowed an event to happen. Process tracing is similar to historical methods such as genetic or sequential explanation that show in detail how one event leads to another (Levy 2001: 69, 76; Bennett and George 2001: 138). For Andrew Bennett and Alexander George (2001: 144), process tracing "has many advantages for theory development and theory testing, some of them unique. It can identify paths to an outcome, point out variables that were left out in the initial comparison of cases, check for spuriousness, and permit causal inference on the basis of a few cases or even a single case."

In this book, process tracing has helped to reveal factors contributing to displacement, similarities and differences in chronologies, and similarities and differences in causal paths. Process tracing has thus contributed to the theorization of displacement and, generally, of foreign policy side effects. The approach taken in this book thus counterbalances the dominance of positivism in IR, or what Timothy McKeown calls the "statistical worldview," as well as the positivist tendency toward testing theories at the expense of constructing theories (McKeown 1999: 183–186).[7]

As a complement of process tracing, mechanism-based theorizing is crucial for analyzing foreign policy side effects. One can develop "small" causal mechanisms that refer to the smallest link between explanatory factors, or, as in this book, "big" mechanisms that include several explanatory factors and that cover large social phenomena (Bennett and George 2001: 140). Moreover, mechanisms can be variable-based, but also about rules, enabling conditions, or catalysts (as in the present work). Finally, scholars can trace mechanisms that are linear and which posit causal processes unfolding in a chronological sequence, or chaotic ones that allow for randomly appearing, interacting, and reinforcing causal factors (the mechanism in this book represents the latter type).

Complexity and contingency impose limits on law-based, predictive theorizing. Attempts by political scientists to establish laws by looking at an event as a class of events lead many to eschew complexity. Jack Levy (2001: 55) writes:

> The preference for parsimony derives from the goal of theorizing about relationships between classes and events rather than explaining individual events, and the belief that theoretical generalization must be based on models that are considerably less complex than the world they aim to represent. The more complex and nuanced an explanation, the less likely that it will "travel well" across cases.

Political scientists working in the nomothetic research tradition formulate "if–then" relationships and social laws. For historians, in contrast, complex phenomena "such as a war, a revolution, and the rise of a parliament, are too rich in detail and too different from other members of its class to be subsumed under any covering law. [. . .] Individual events are not simply instances, but the main theme" (Elman and Elman 2001: 15 and 16). Here, historians have something in common with military strategists who acknowledge the impact of contingency on the outcomes of human interaction. For Carl von Clausewitz, as interpreted by Alan Beyerchen (1992/1993: 73, italics in the original), "the core cause of analytical unpredictability in war is the *very nature of interaction* itself." A historian pressed to defend the idiographic approach could argue that law-based theorizing has led nowhere. Indeed, the observation that democracies do not fight each other seems to be the only law-like phenomenon discovered by researchers, and there are doubts even about the validity of this "law" (Bernstein *et al.* 2000: 44; Levy 2001: 82). The difficulties of generalization, the historian would argue, are not surprising, given the contingent nature of history.

The surprising turns of history result not least from the fact that human behavior is often erratic. This limits the ability of analysts to predict how the targets of foreign policies, whether presidents or criminals (or both), respond to foreign policies. Chance should also nurture skepticism of variable-based explanations. "It is actors and not variables who do the acting" (Hedström and Swedberg 1998: 24). Conceiving of actors as variables is misleading when explaining foreign policy, and particularly foreign policy side effects, since the researcher will then be examining both a foreign policy initiator and a target. In other words, the researcher examines complex patterns of human interaction. When structural theories such as neo-realism or Marxism, which overstate the constraints imposed on human behavior by structure, are combined with positivist methodologies, which reduce human beings to variables, accounts are likely to be particularly simplistic.

As an alternative to social laws, this book proposes causal mechanisms. Mechanisms still allow for generalization – but in a probabilistic fashion. A foreign policy will lead to change, but temporally and spatially contingent conditions will influence the nature of change. No foreign policy has a zero effect, and analysts might be able to define a range of possible scenarios of foreign policy outcomes (see Bernstein *et al.* 2000). Nevertheless, complexity and contingency mean that one cannot predict the exact outcome, the sequence of events leading to an outcome, or the causal process underlying this sequence. As this book has shown, foreign policy outcomes, chronologies, and causal processes can vary significantly. This variation could not have been deduced from theoretical assumptions, but became apparent only in the course of the empirical research.

Hence, generalizations must leave room for surprise and chance. No two wars are ever the same. The same holds true for terrorist attacks or the evolution of new drug smuggling routes. There is no formula for life, as evolutionary biologists would confirm. Human beings are the product of historical contingency, similar to other forms of life whose creation cannot be couched into variables. To use the examples of John Lewis Gaddis (2001: 320), historical chance makes it "hard to find the independent variables for Neanderthals, kangaroos, or pumpkins." And there certainly is no formula for social life. Or what are the independent variables of Colombian paramilitaries?

6 Alternatives to the US war on drugs

This book has shown that US efforts to reduce the illicit supply of cocaine and heroin through interdiction and eradication are ineffective and sometimes counterproductive. Moreover, US drug policy has a harmful effect on human rights, human health, democratic accountability, and the environment, to mention just a few negative repercussions of Washington's coercive stance. Given the ineffectiveness and "collateral damage" of US foreign drug policies, it is essential to consider alternative policies.

Harm reduction on the drug production side

The question of how to deal with potentially dangerous substances such as cocaine and heroin has been controversial for a long time. Two extreme views define the boundaries of the debate

Some argue that the production, trade, and consumption of cocaine and heroin should be legalized. "Legalizers" do not represent a monolithic bloc. Whereas some argue that people should have complete discretion over how they produce and consume drugs, others advocate a regulatory model that allows for tight state controls.[1] The main advantage of legalization would be the sudden disappearance of the illicit drug industry due to a sudden drop in drug prices and, subsequently, a steep reduction of profit margins. Yet legalization, or rather the commercialization of cocaine and heroin, would probably come at the cost of higher drug prevalence, i.e. the total number of users, and consumption, that is the total amount of cocaine and heroin consumed (MacCoun and Reuter 2001: chapter 14; *The Economist* 2001b: 15–16).[2]

On the opposite side of the debate, policy advocates plead for maintaining a coercive course against drugs, or even promote an increase in police, military, and intelligence operations against drug producers and consumers. People adhering to this view argue that although coercive drug policies have not solved drug problems, those problems would be worse if it had not been for coercion. This book underlines that this argument is flawed, given that supply-side eradication and interdiction co-creates negative side effects.

Over recent years, both legalizers and reformers (for whom legalization is too radical an option) have promoted principles of harm reduction. Promoters of harm reduction argue that governments should reduce the harmful effects of drugs on individuals, societies, and polities, instead of pursuing coercive policies that aggravate harm. Advocates promote the decriminalization of the possession of small amounts of drugs for personal use (in order to allow police to focus on other things and treat illicit drugs on a par with alcohol and cigarettes, which after all kill many more people than illicit drugs); the introduction of needle exchange programs (in order to reduce the spread of HIV/AIDS exacerbated by the sharing of contaminated needles); and the distribution of drugs to users and addicts in state-controlled facilities (in order to reduce drug-related crime and deaths from overdosing).

Although the advantages of harm reduction are most obvious with regard to drug consumption, the same principles can also be applied in regions that not only consume illicit drugs, but also produce coca and poppy, cocaine base paste and opium, and cocaine and heroin. Indeed, on the drug production side, harm reduction is a viable alternative paradigm to policies aiming at short-term reductions of illicit coca and poppy cultivation. As researchers of the Transnational Institute (2002: 8) write:

> If the international community could finally recognize the narrowness of the margins for policy intervention in terms of global supply reduction and accept the fact that the phenomenon of drug-linked crop cultivation is here to stay as long as demand exists, countries and AD donors could be relieved of the pressure to comply with reduction targets and deadlines. [. . .] More realistic and flexible time frames allowing for the gradual reduction over a period of several years and greater compatibility with local rural development plans are essential.

Particularly in South America, development aid has often been coupled with tight eradication deadlines. But since aid has often arrived late, has been insufficient, and has not provided coca and poppy farmers with a sustainable source of income, many farmers have faced the choice of either risking starvation by eradicating illicit crops, or exposing themselves and their families to the violence and health risks that often come along with fumigation and manual eradication.

A more gradual eradication based on dialog with the involved communities, as well as the provision of development aid that reduces farmers' dependency on illicit crops, would thus be advantageous (Deutsche Gesellschaft für Technische Zusammenarbeit 2001). Harm reduction would help avoid the negative effects of eradication on people and the environment. Moreover, insofar as AD succeeds in reducing farmers' dependency on illicit crops, it would make these communities less vulnerable to drug traffickers and mitigate the pressure on farmers to migrate in search of income.

Measures for improving the living conditions in coca and poppy producing regions include land reform; providing farmers with access to credit and technical assistance; improving public infrastructure (roads, schools, hospitals); fostering a dialog between peasants, NGOs, governments, and international organizations; permitting peasants to continue planting illicit crops on a small scale until an economic alternative is available; allowing peasants to provide the opium or coca products needed for drug maintenance facilities and hospitals in the US, Europe and elsewhere; and endorsing the export of coca products that have been consumed and traded for hundreds of years (Independent Commission 2004; Senlis Council 2005).

More far-ranging strategies are needed as well. Industrialized countries must open their markets to licit agricultural products from poor countries, while poor countries must be protected from cheap imports, even if that means introducing tariffs; more money must be made available for AD; and debt relief is needed to allow the governments of poor countries to help rural populations (Youngers 2005: 364–365).

These examples show that the future of drug policies hinges on the ability of states to pursue development and trade policies that reduce economic inequalities between and within countries. Since it is far from certain that the international political economy will create more economic and social equality in the future, drug problems will not simply go away. Another reason why they are likely to stay is that poverty and inequality are not the only determinants of the drug industry, as shown by the fact that illicit drugs are not produced on a large scale in some of the world's poorest countries. To reduce drug supplies in countries such as Colombia, the state and nation need to be rebuilt. Although this is a long-term and complex task, harm reduction would be a step in the right direction.

Harm reduction would still allow governments to arrest traffickers, prevent the diversion of precursor chemicals into illicit channels, stop traffickers from acquiring weapons, and act against money laundering. To be sure, these measures can have negative side effects. Gathering intelligence on traffickers often violates the privacy of innocent citizens, and measures against the diversion of precursor chemicals or money laundering can impose extra costs on licit economic transactions. However, operations against traffickers, smugglers of precursor chemicals, or money launderers arguably have more positive than negative effects. The reverse is true with regard to the use of security forces against coca and poppy farmers. Law enforcement is still needed, and due to their material capacities and know-how, US security forces will remain the world's preeminent sponsor of law enforcement operations for the time being. But Washington should use coercive means in more effective and humane ways to avoid human rights violations, an erosion of democratic control of armed forces, and other negative side effects of supply-side eradication and interdiction.

Specifically, the US should not promote the use of foreign militaries for law enforcement operations; the US military should not train local police forces; all authority for foreign military support should reside with the State Department; US police assistance should increase the transparency and accountability of police forces; cooperation with foreign security forces should be made conditional upon the protection of human rights; and US drug laws, as well as drug laws advocated by the US abroad, must be compatible with international human rights standards (Youngers 2005). Moreover, US decision-makers should avoid the use of martial language. Speaking of the need to "win the fight" against "narco-terrorists" feeds the illusory hope of victory and prevents a sober analysis of the political, economic, and social causes and consequences of the illicit drug industry.

While coercive drug policies carry risks and have limits, the same holds true for harm reduction. AD, for example, is no panacea for reducing drug supplies. In fact, the historical record of AD is ambiguous. One review of two decades of UN-sponsored socioeconomic development programs in 11 countries shows that these programs have contributed little to reducing drug supplies (Farrell 1998). The UN has shifted from crop substitution to more sophisticated approaches, and some projects have been successful. But projects were confined to relatively small areas, and they contributed to pushing illicit cultivation to adjacent areas. A reduction in poppy cultivation in Thailand, for example, was followed by increasing heroin use in Thailand and more opium production in neighboring Burma (Tullis 1995: 179). AD can also facilitate illicit activities through modernization programs that make farmers reluctant to leave coca-growing areas or that benefit traffickers (Clawson and Lee 1998: 233–238; Tullis 1995: 163

Most assessments of AD are not very uplifting. Examining the examples of Pakistan, Thailand, and Peru, Martin Jelsma shows that reductions in drug supplies in these countries cannot be clearly attributed to AD. Rather, "increases and decreases of illicit cultivation obey largely to the workings of the illicit drug economy and its driving forces like demand patterns [. . .], price trends, traffick ing routes and composition of entrepreneurial structures and geopolitical developments especially around armed conflicts. The margins to intervene in this through AD or eradication are very small" (Jelsma 2002: 10). Indeed, many attempts by international donors to reduce illicit cultivation failed, despite considerable sums of money invested.[3] One could say that this is because AD was not properly decoupled from coercion and because the planning and implementation of AD projects was flawed. To be sure, gross mistakes have been made (for examples, see Léons 1997; Lupu 2004; Vellinga 1998: 17–18). But the fact remains that AD faces significant political and economic obstacles, even if planned and implemented properly.

The main factor limiting the effectiveness of AD is the relative profitabilit of coca and poppy. If a truckload of pineapples can earn a farmer as little as $10, competition with traffickers becomes difficult[4] And even if the price of licit crops were raised, traffickers could easily pay more to peasants, since coca and poppy are a low-cost factor. Although many peasants are willing to trade income losses for more security, they will not stop illicit cultivation if that puts their economic survival at risk. Another problem in the past was that peasants have not been able to supply international traders with licit agricultural products according to agreed schedules, and that the quality of products was not always satisfactory.[5] Worse still, after many bad experiences, farmers have little confi dence in AD.

Although more information is now available, many projects of governments, international organizations, and NGOs still disappoint. Observers write, for example, that it "is not the cocaleros who have benefited the most from alternative development schemes, but the consultants and technical staff involved in them, both nationally and internationally" (Transnational Institute 2004: 11). Often, donors fail to find formulas for helping people either in the short term or in the long term. A leader of a Peruvian coca grower's association once said: "Bridges and roads are fine, but tell me how I am supposed to eat a bridge or a road" (quoted in Hall 2003).

While AD can be improved by learning from the past, the "tremendous geographical, political, economic and social complexity of the coca-growing valleys posits serious challenges for any alternative development program" (Rojas 2003: 11). The drug industry will continue to thrive as long as there is demand, which poses significant problems to anti-drug efforts, whether coercive or non-coercive. And demand is here to stay. Drug consumption seems to be a feature of human life, maybe with one exception mentioned by Francisco Thoumi (1995: 289, fn 1): "Anthropologist Billie Jean Isbell has commented to me that only the traditional Eskimo society did not consume [psychoactive drugs], principally because they did not have any products to use. However, they had a time during the winter during which they could psyche themselves and 'run amok.'" Although cocaine and heroin consumption patterns have changed over the last 100 years and will change in the future, demand for these two drugs will not go away.

Given the limits of AD, why should states continue to invest in it? AD remains important for several reasons. Many people depend on these programs, and a withdrawal of funds would mean abandoning these beneficiaries. Moreover, although AD cannot quickly and significantly reduce drug supplies, and although it may sometimes be conducive to drug industry displacement, it mitigates the violence, corruption, and other problems that have befallen drug-producing regions.[6] Furthermore, AD, if decoupled from eradication, can undercut farmers' support for rebels in conflict-ridden areas and increase farmers' willingness to participate in drug control. "Alternative development projects offer a way to convince national public opinion that counternarcotics is not antipoor or antipeople" (Clawson and Lee 1998: 163). Last, and perhaps most importantly with regard to the future of drug control, citing the success stories of AD and other harm reduction strategies counterbalances a discourse that emphasizes the advantages of coercion.

Reforming UN drug control

This discourse has not only left its mark on US drug policy. It has also been a feature of UN drug control. A shift from coercion toward harm reduction, both in net drug producing and net drug consuming countries, hinges on the possibilities of reforming the multilateral drug control framework. The UN is the only body endowed with the legitimacy to change drug policies around the globe. Consequently, policy reformers have focused on the UN in their efforts to promote the principles of harm reduction. They regard the international drug control framework, which has been set up from the 1960s onward, as "a historical error" that has made drug problems worse (Jelsma and Metaal 2004: 1).

There are signs that the calls for reform have not gone unnoticed. Over the recent years, some governments have come to understand the limits and negative effects of coercion. Western European states, for example, have implemented various harm reduction programs in their national jurisdictions. Harm reduction on the production side has become popular as well, with agencies such as the German Society for Technical Cooperation (GTZ) at the forefront of innovative drug policies implemented in countries as diverse as Afghanistan, Laos, and Peru.

But although voices dissenting from punitive policies have weakened the global drug prohibition system, reform-minded countries and pressure groups have had limited success in changing UN drug control. At conferences such as the 1998 General Assembly Special Session on Drugs and the 2003 Mid-term Review, UN bodies responsible for drug control, or rather some of the governments represented in these bodies, affirmed their commitment to rather unrealistic drug reduction plans that undermine the credibility of the UN in the field of drug control (Jelsma 2003).

The UN's reputation was particularly tainted during the notorious reign of Pino Arlacchi lasting between 1997 and 2002. As UN Under-Secretary-General and executive director of the United Nations Office for Drug Control and Crime Prevention, Arlacchi was responsible for mismanagement and the dissemination of information that presented an overly positive picture of global drug problems, all of which alienated UN staff, donors, and the general public (Thoumi 2002a; European NGO Council on Drugs and Development 2001). While the reign of Arlacchi was a particularly bleak period in UN drug control, it indicated structural weaknesses of the system, such as an insecure revenue base, a mix of lowest-common-denominator agreements and no-tolerance declarations, the dominance of major donor countries, a heterogeneous staff, and the repetitive declarations of progress based on dubious indicators (see the contributions in Fazey and Bewley-Taylor 2003).

The UN drug control framework has become a straightjacket preventing the adoption of harm reduction and, more generally, a rational debate about the pros and cons of different strategies against drugs. The International Narcotics Control Board (INCB) has routinely criticized reform-minded countries such as Switzerland, Germany, and the Netherlands for experimenting with harm reduction strategies that can save the lives of drug users and reduce violence and AIDS, but which – according to the INCB – violate the spirit of international drug control laws. These governments thus found themselves under considerable international pressure. Switzerland, for example, has been criticized by the INCB in unusually strong terms compared to normal diplomatic parlance. However, Switzerland, Germany, and other rich industrialized countries, although they remain susceptible to diplomatic pressure, have continued along the path of harm reduction.

Poor net drug producing countries, in contrast, have much less room for maneuver. Although the legalization of coca products or a very gradual reduction of coca cultivation through AD might be beneficial for South American countries, it is difficult to systematically implement such policies because UN conventions regard coca first and foremost as a drug (Bewley-Taylor 2004: 485–486). Opponents of harm reduction have often equated this approach with the indiscriminate legalization of all drugs in order to delegitimize harm reduction.

To be sure, governments could change international drugs laws and thus loosen the straightjacket preventing a wider use of harm reduction. However, many governments support coercion. The biggest stumbling block for policy change is the fact that the US continues to shape UN drug policies and politics. International drug laws mirror the policy preferences of the US. Washington has played a pivotal role in the creation of the international drug control regime and has been using the UN to force other countries to respect the UN conventions and the verdicts of the INCB (for an example, see Martin 2001). In the early twenty-first century, Washington augmented its financial contributions to UN drug control, thus securing even more influence for US policy-makers over drug control projects and the UN bureaucratic apparatus (Jelsma and Metaal 2004: 7).

Given the entrenched US position, what can reform-minded countries do? They could ignore international drug laws, form a caucus within the UN, or try and change the UN drug control framework incrementally (Bewley-Taylor 2004). More generally, governments should acknowledge the limits of state action against drugs. In order to deal with contemporary transnational problems in effective and legitimate ways, there should be a shift from government to governance (Czempiel and Rosenau 1992; Krahmann 2005). That implies that governments disaggregate into their functionally differentiated parts (police, intelligence, military, or development agencies). These parts form transnational networks with their counterparts from other countries (Slaughter 2004). Moreover, governments draw on the problem solving capacities of international organizations, NGOs, and businesses. Although governments are likely to continue to dominate the formulation and implementation of drug policies, private actors have an important role to play. NGOs often know more about the conditions in coca and poppy growing regions than governments, and companies can provide the capital needed to create sustainable local and regional economies. In the past, drug policies have not only been too coercive, but also too state-centric. New actors must come to the fore to foster effective and fair policies.

What are the chances of changing the direction of international drug policy? The possibility of reform hinges significantly on US drug politics and policies, given the country's preeminent position in drug control and world politics. Unfortunately, the prospects for change in this area are not bright.

Reforming US drug control

The first chapter briefly discussed the domestic motives behind coercive US drug policies. Authors examine opportunistic politics, an entrenched drug war bureaucracy, and the popular public view of drug supply as a criminal phenomenon. These domestic conditions in the US are likely to shape Washington's drug policies for the time being, and will continue to hamper the efforts of drug policy reformers to promote harm reduction. Pushing for policy reform has been made even more arduous by the "war on terror," which has been conducive to the establishment of a "national security state" in the US (Andreas and Price 2001) and which has given new impetus to US-led global policing (Andreas and Nadelmann 2006).

Washington's coercive international drug policies have aggravated global drug problems. The combination of prohibition, which drives up drug prices and thus creates economic opportunities for suppliers around the world, and supply-side eradication and interdiction, which is conducive to the displacement of the drug industry, has proven destructive. Alfred McCoy (2004: 30) writes:

> Over the past 30 years, the U.S. war on drugs, in alliance with the United Nations, has simply served to push production, processing, and smuggling of illicit drugs back and forth across the globe's three critical traffickin regions – between Turkey and Laos in the Asian opium zone, from Bolivia to Colombia in the Andes coca belt, and from southern Florida to northern Mexico along the U.S. border. At each turn in these many shifts, consumption, production, and corruption have ratcheted upward. In sum, we can speak [. . .] of a stimulus of prohibition.

US policy-makers could argue that a worsening of global drug problems is an acceptable cost for improving drug problems in the US. However, there is no such improvement, as the General Accounting Office confirmed in 1998: "Despite long-standing efforts and expenditures of billions of dollars, illegal drugs still flood the United States. Although U.S. and host-nation counternarcotics efforts have resulted in the arrest of major drug traffickers and the seizure of large amounts of drugs, they have not materially reduced the availability of drugs in the United States" (quoted in Transnational Institute 2003a: 22).

This book has focused on international, not domestic anti-drug policies. However, at the same time as the US was undertaking significant international efforts, there was an escalation in domestic law enforcement as well. One domestic consequence of punishing not only big traffickers and small dealers, but also drug consumers, is an explosion of drug-related arrests and incarcerations. Between 1980 and 2002, the number of people behind bars in the US for drug offences has increased elevenfold, from fewer than 42,000 to more than 480,000 (Walsh 2004: 7). Minorities are particularly affected.

US policy-makers could now argue that incarceration and other coercive domestic drug policies are effective. After all, drugs fetch the highest profi margins on US streets, which makes it logical to focus on street dealers and consumers.[7] However, this rationale underestimates the costs of prisons, security forces, health costs through the spread of AIDS, costs of drug-related crime, as well as the aggravation of racial and economic inequalities and other negative repercussions of domestic coercion. Moreover, domestic law enforcement is less cost-efficient than drug treatment

No matter whether we look at coercive domestic or international strategies, putting pressure on drug producers, traffickers, and consumers is less cost-effi cient than investing in harm reduction measures. John Walsh (2004: 18) summarizes the results of drug policy research as follows:

> By contrast with supply-side drug control, the effectiveness of drug treatment in reducing drug use is supported by three decades of scientifi research and clinical practice. [. . .] Moreover, the reductions in drug use achieved through treatment bring corresponding reductions in crime and the spread of disease, meaning that the benefits of treatment far exceed its costs. A landmark 1994 study in California found that every dollar invested in treatment saved the state's taxpayers seven dollars in future costs, primarily by preventing crime. [. . .] Compared to alternative strategies, treatment is also an exceptionally cost-effective way to reduce drug consumption. In 1994, RAND found that as a means of reducing cocaine consumption, treatment for heavy cocaine users is 23 times more effective than drug crop eradication and other source-country programs, 11 times more effective than interdiction, and three times more effective than mandatory minimum sentencing.[8]

Despite these obvious financial (as well as moral) advantages of changing the course of US domestic and international drug policy, the repressive momentum is surprisingly persistent. Given the immunity of ineffective and harmful policies to rational and moral criticism, the *cui bono*-question is pertinent. Most drug policy researchers would probably subscribe to the view of Peter Dale Scott (2003: 100) that the drug war has become "a bureaucratic habit: a habit in which failure, predictably, becomes a case for escalation." After decades of coercive drug policies that have yielded questionable results, advocates of coercion resemble World War I and Vietnam War generals who viewed failure not as resulting from flawed policies, but from a lack of determination. Whoever dares to voice dissent will be accused of defeatism (Bertram *et al.* 1996).

As Barbara Tuchman (1984) reminds us, Washington escalated the Vietnam War despite clear signs of failure. Most policy-makers were simply reluctant to admit defeat. The drug war continues because many bureaucrats and policy-makers do not see that the initial war strategy failed to take into account the realities of the global drug industry. These advocates of coercion are "true believers" (Gordon 1994: 161). Others continue along the same old path even if they know better. But vested interests are at stake. Bureaucracies who want more money, politicians who want more votes, and media corporations who want more viewers or readers all benefit from a perpetuation and escalation of drug problems and coercive drug policies. One US senator made his priorities clear when he said: "I have no doubt that what we are doing on the war on drugs is not working. But I also have no doubt that if I say it and come out in favor of legalizing some drugs [. . .] I will lose my next election" (quoted in Naim 2005: 62).

Yet the instrumentalization of drug problems by bureaucracies, politicians, and the media can only partly explain the puzzling persistence of failed policies. Successive US administrations have been able to ignore criticism from scientists, human rights groups, and libertarians concerned about individual freedom because coercive drug policies strike a cord with large segments of the US population. The drug war is not only fought in the Colombian jungles and in the inner cities of the US, but also in peoples' heads. Sara Manaugh (2000: 9) writes that the "drug war [. . .] performs a ritual of persuasion that serves to constitute and reinforce a set of uniquely American ideals and truths." This essentially non-utilitarian process of identity construction is a formidable psychological barrier to policy reform. After all, criticism of US drug policies can easily be perceived and portrayed as criticism of the American way of life.

An additional, and more straightforward, psychological explanation for the implicit or explicit support for coercive drug policies among bureaucrats, policy-makers, and the public is frustration. The perpetuation and escalation of US domestic and international drug policies reflects a deeply felt disappointment at the failure to put an end to illicit activities, despite the fact that the political, military, economic, and normative capacities of the US clearly outmatch the capacities of other countries. A senior US military officer in 1997 implicitly expressed this frustration as follows: "Previous 'failures' do not preclude future successes. [The difficulty of measuring the effectiveness of anti-drug programs] is not a justifiable reason to reward the drug traffickers with an additional degree of freedom to conduct criminal activity" (quoted in Transnational Institute 2003a: 23). Ted Dalen Carpenter (2004) aptly describes the impact of this can-do attitude on US international drug policies:

> Each new initiative in Washington's international campaign to stem the supply of illegal drugs is launched with great fanfare. During the early phase, isolated examples of success are touted as evidence that the overall strategy is working. Ultimately, though, reality intrudes and it becomes clear that the drug supply is as plentiful as ever. Thrown on the defensive, drug warriors admit that the task has proven more difficult than anticipated but argue that if we stay the course, success is just around the corner. When such predictions prove faulty often enough, the existing initiative is quietly buried and a new one is launched with the appropriate fanfare.

This cycle of policy perpetuation and escalation means that side effects will stay with us as long as there is no fundamental reorientation of US international drug policy, whether toward legalization (a highly improbable option) or harm reduction (an option that would meet with less, though still significant, domestic opposition).

This book has focused on one of these side effects – the displacement of the illicit drug industry – and argued that displacement aggravates global drug problems. Future research can provide a full-circle argument, showing how the displacement of the drug industry leads to policy perpetuation and escalation. In the language of IR theory, agents and structures mutually constitute each other. Over the last 100 years, and particularly since the early 1970s, an agent (the US) has been co-creating a structure (a world of drugs), which in turn has undermined the perceived security of the US, triggering new foreign policy initiatives, and so on. Political resolve to maintain the repressive thrust of US international drug policy, in combination with public support for policy continuity and escalation, leads to a vicious circle in which US coercive policies contribute to displacement, which aggravates drug problems, which lead to calls for more coercion.

Given the bureaucratic, political, and psychological obstacles to policy reform, it will be hard to break out of this vicious circle. Nevertheless, drug policy reformers and researchers should continue to point out the ineffectiveness and "collateral damage" of drug policies that focus too much on coercion and too little on the social, economic, and normative root causes of drug production, trafficking, and consumption. Much can be gained, and little lost, from attempts to change policy. And there is much to be lost, and little to be gained, if US drug policy does not change.

In late 2003, US Secretary of Defense Donald Rumsfeld reportedly said with regard to the worsening violence in Iraq: "We know we're killing a lot, capturing a lot, collecting arms. We just don't know yet whether that's the same as winning" (quoted in Loeb 2003). Events in Iraq subsequently showed that it was not the same as winning. Similarly, seizing a lot of drugs, capturing a lot of traffickers, and collecting a lot of arms is not the same as winning the drug war. Nevertheless, policies that lead to human-rights violations, less democracy, environmental destruction, and other negative effects continue to find political, bureaucratic, and popular support, with no real change in policy direction in sight.

The lessons of history are not always obvious. In the case of drug policy, however, they are fairly simple. Time alone will prove whether Aldous Huxley's (1959: 308) statement still remains valid: "That men do not learn very much from the lessons of history is the most important of all the lessons that history has to teach."

Annex I

Maps

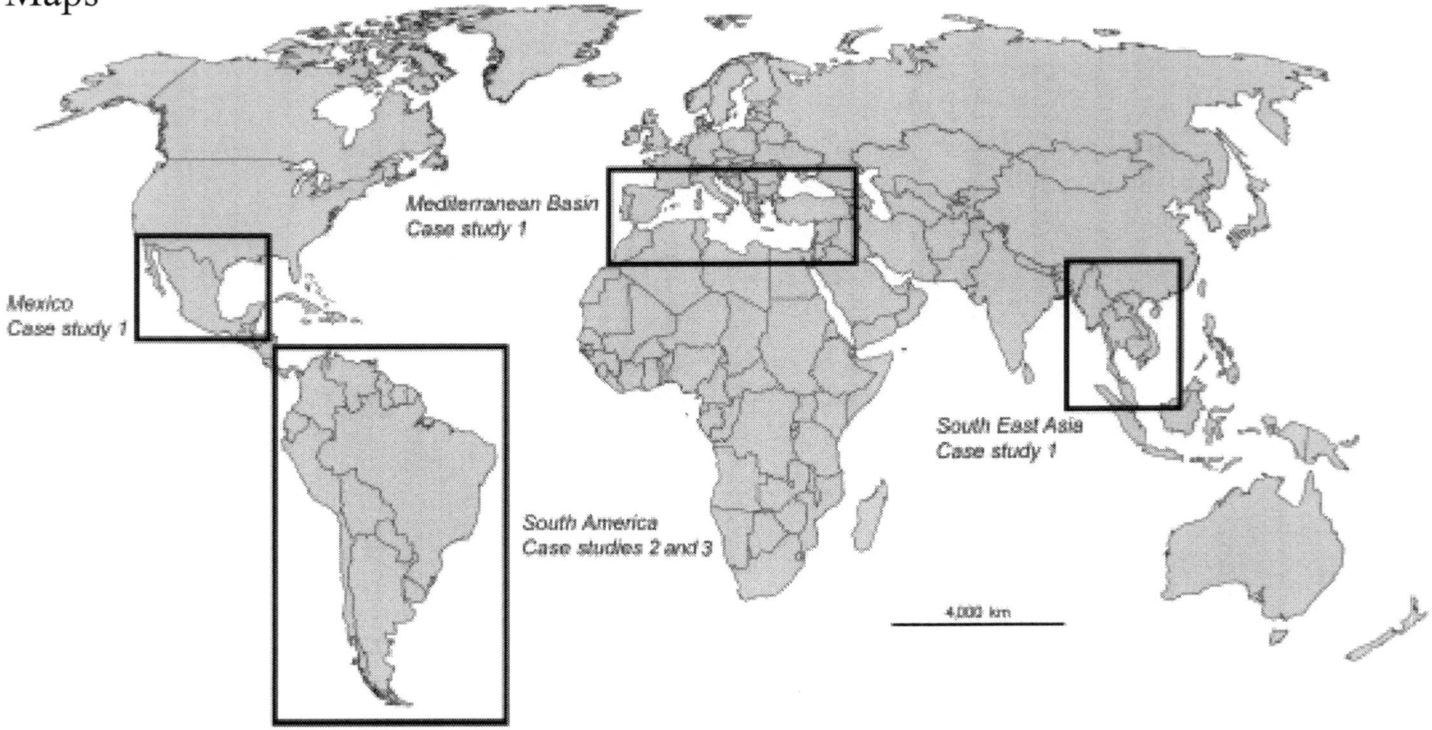

Map 1 Case studies (source: Bertrand Lefebvre, reproduced with kind permission).

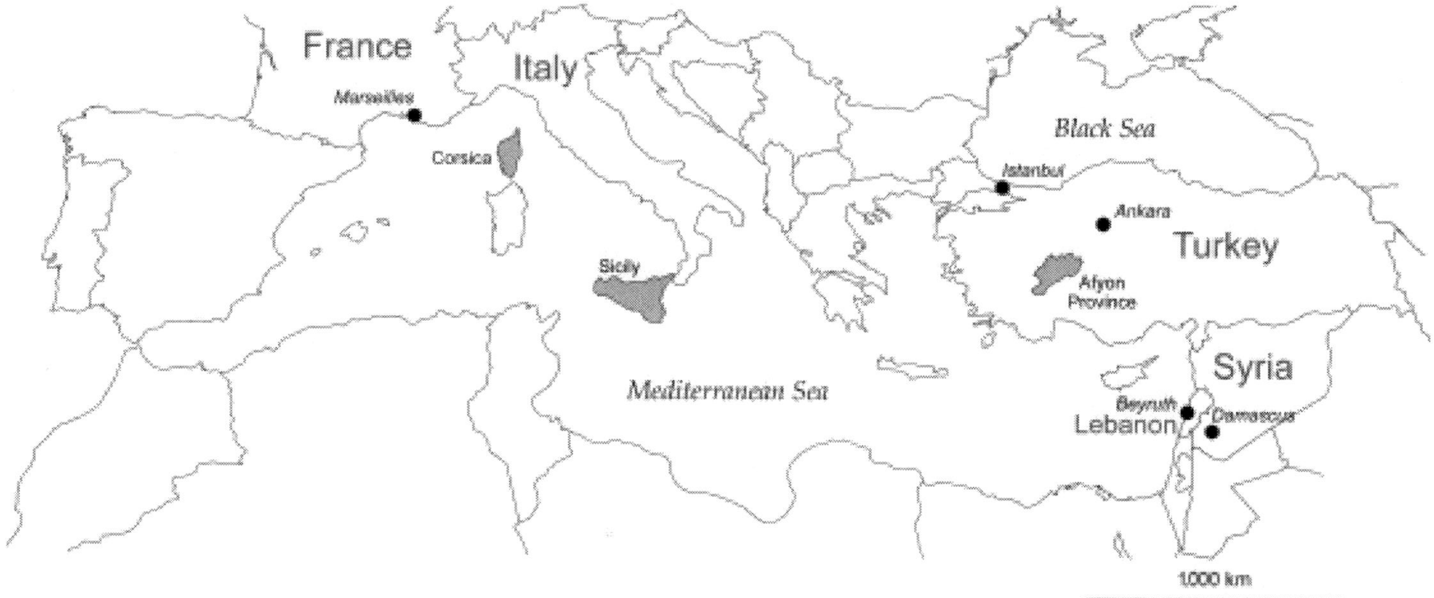

Map 2 The Mediterranean Basin (source: Bertrand Lefebvre, reproduced with kind permission).

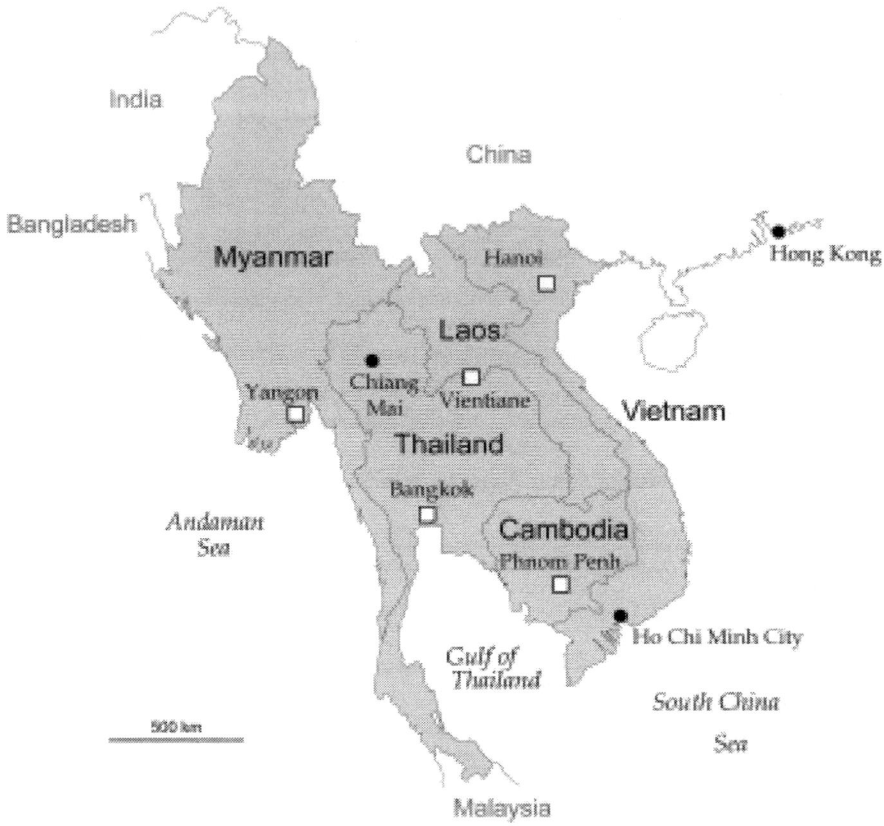

Map 3 Southeast Asia (source: Bertrand Lefebvre, reproduced with kind permission).

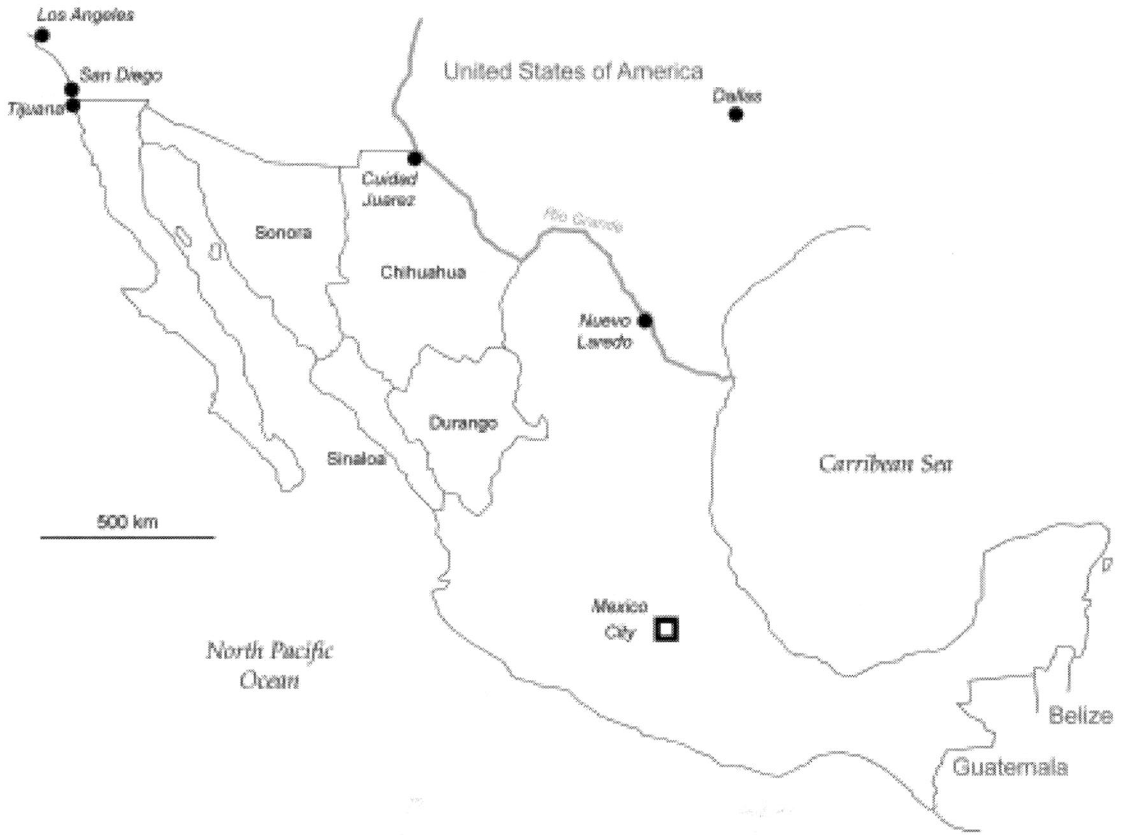

Map 4 Mexico (source: Bertrand Lefebvre, reproduced with kind permission).

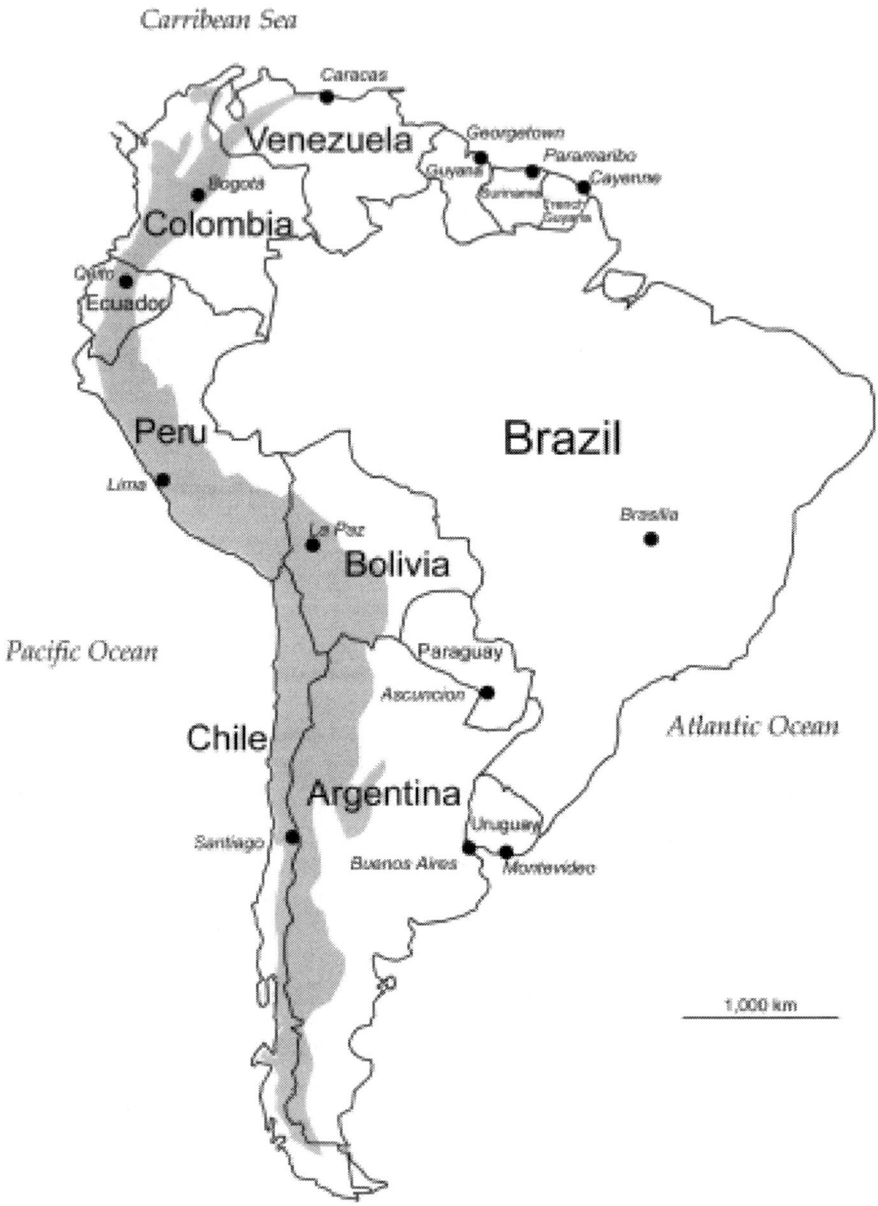

Map 5 South America (source: Bertrand Lefebvre, reproduced with kind permission).

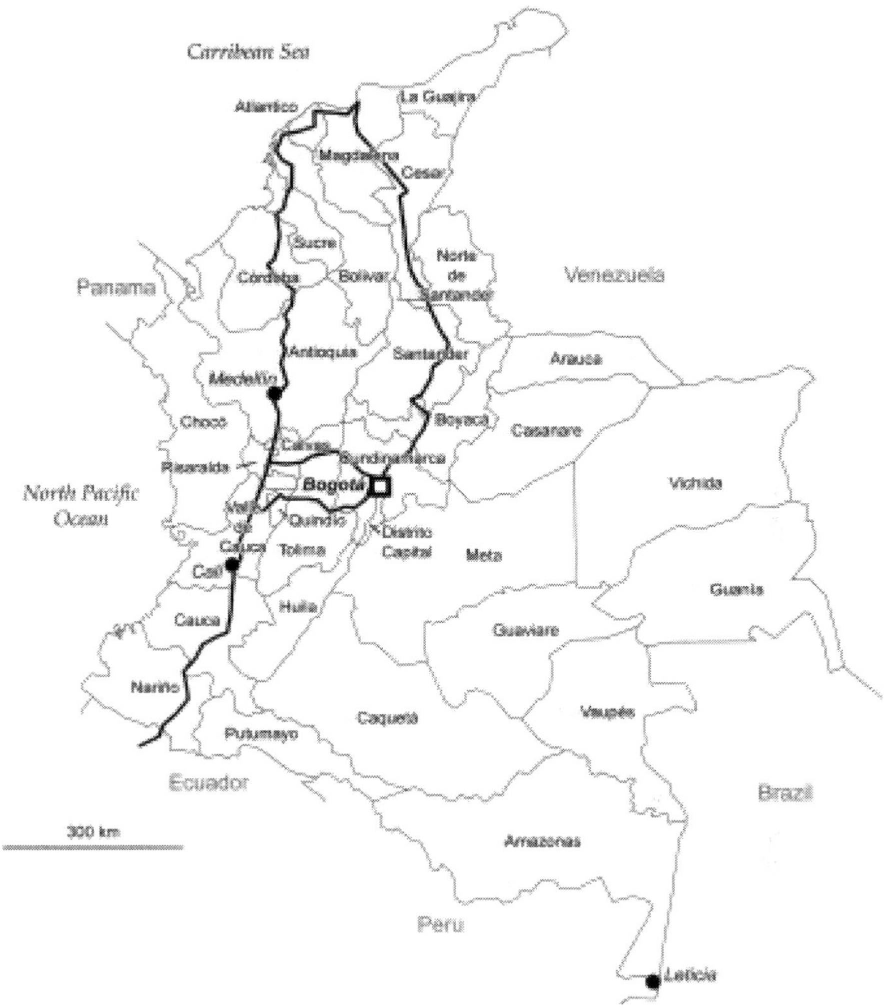

Map 6 Colombia (source: Bertrand Lefebvre, reproduced with kind permission).

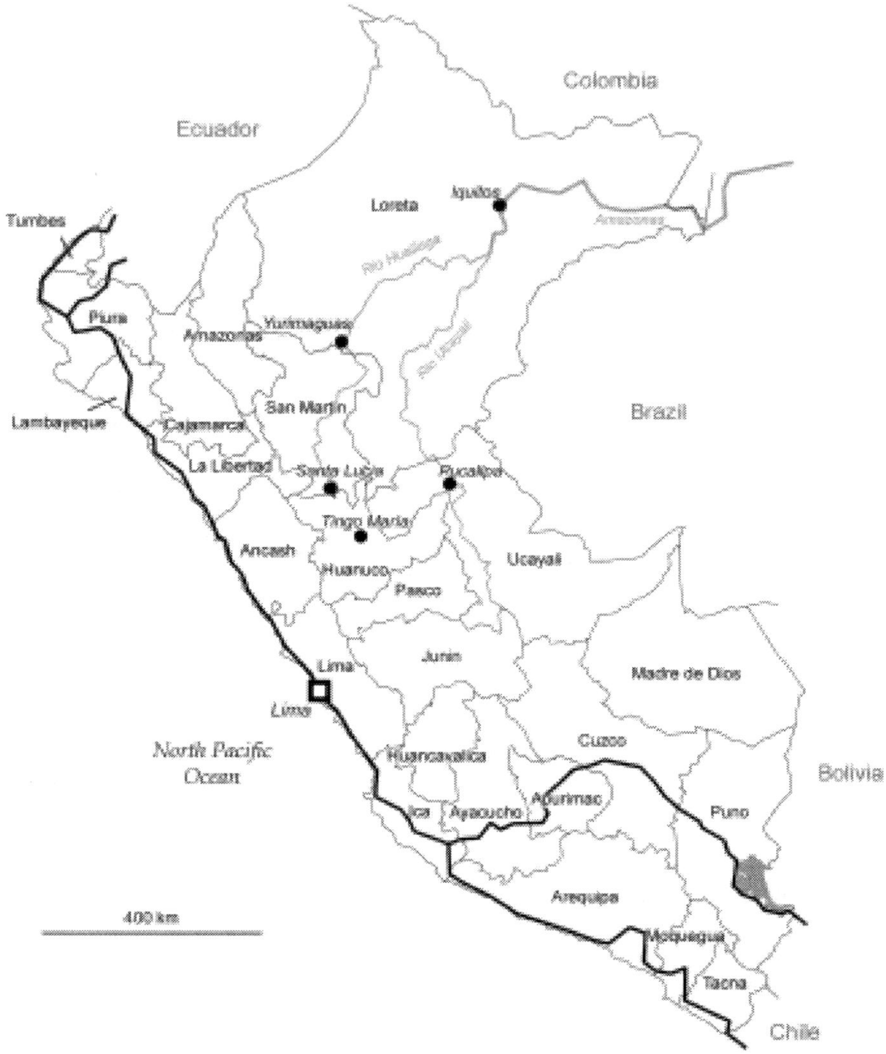

Map 7 Peru (source: Bertrand Lefebvre, reproduced with kind permission).

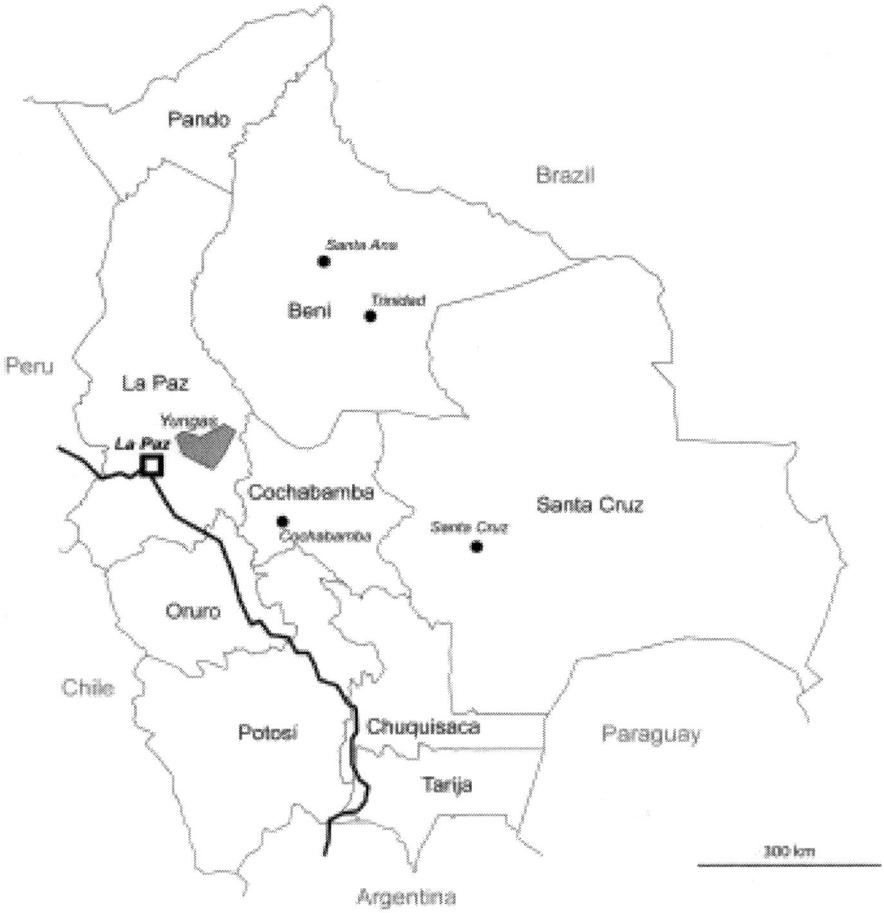

Map 8 Bolivia (source: Bertrand Lefebvre, reproduced with kind permission).

Annex II

Charts

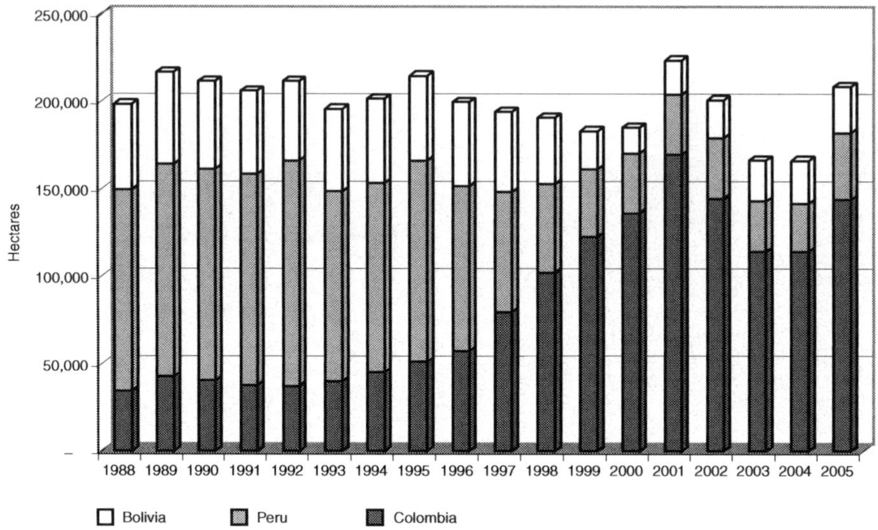

Chart 1 Andean coca cultivation, 1988–2005 (source: State Department International Narcotics Control Strategy Reports. Chart produced by the Center for International Policy (www.ciponline.org) and reproduced here with kind permission).

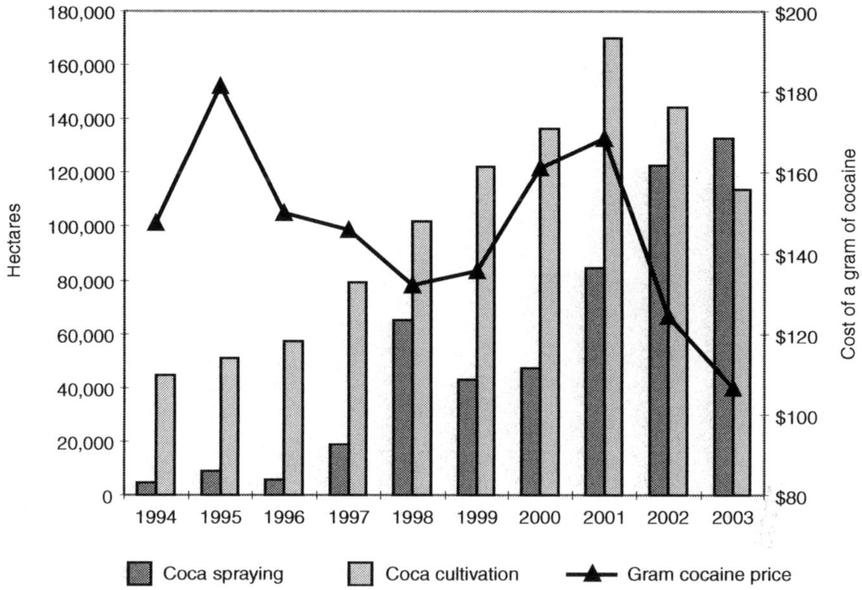

Chart 2 Colombian coca cultivation and fumigation, and retail cocaine prices in the US, 1993–2003 (source: Produced by the Center for International Policy (www.ciponline.org) and reproduced here with kind permission).

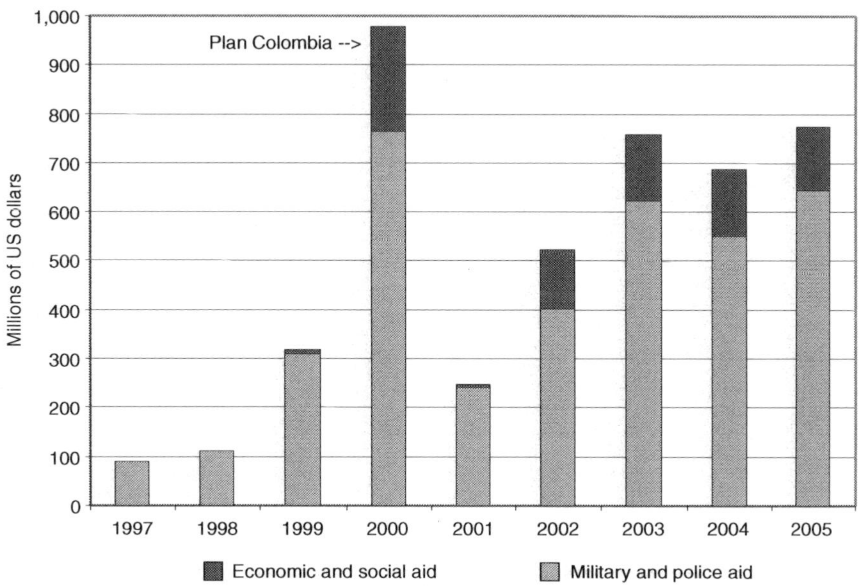

Chart 3 US aid to Colombia, 1997–2005 (source: Produced by the Center for International Policy (www.ciponline.org) and reproduced here with kind permission).

Notes

1 US drug policy and drug industry displacement

1 This book refers to the drug industry in the singular. This is not meant to deny important differences between the production, trade, and consumption of cocaine, on the one hand, and the production, trade, and consumption of heroin, on the other.
2 This book refers to US dollars throughout.
3 Coercion is here defined as "the use of threatened force, and at times the limited use of actual force to back up the threat, to induce an adversary to behave differently than it otherwise would" (Byman and Waxman 2002: 30).
4 One might object to the terms "drug consuming," "drug producing," and "transit" states for several good reasons. First, the distinction between consuming and producing/transit states is blurred. Western European countries, for example, are important drug transit points, and consumption is widespread in traditional producing countries. Second, a state in which coca and poppy grow should not automatically be labeled a drug-producing state, since coca and poppy cultivation are not the same as cocaine and heroin production. Third, precursor chemicals often originate from industrial plants owned by companies based in industrialized countries. Fourth, substantial shares of drug revenues are laundered in consuming countries with good banking facilities. These differentiations are important, and the terms "drug consuming," "drug producing," and "transit" states are only used as a matter of convenience.
5 This work analyses cocaine and heroin and does not refer to cannabis or synthetic substances.
6 The document is available online at www.fas.org/irp/offdocs/nsdd/nsdd-221.htm (accessed March 27, 2006).
7 On recent changes to the certification process see Ledebur (2005: 146)
8 Author interviews with representatives of the EU, Germany, and Switzerland in Rabat, August 2002.
9 US states spend an additional estimated $20 billion a year on drug control, mainly on coercive programs.
10 US drug policies arguably yield positive results as well. For example, they foster police cooperation even with "rogue states" such as Iran or Cuba. However, the negative effects probably outweigh the positive ones, although what is positive and negative is in the eye of the beholder. The arms industry might see a civil war as positive, and some might see international police cooperation as problematic, since it leads to information exchange beyond parliamentary control.
11 The first edition of the book was published in 1972, the second in 1991, and the third in 2003.
12 Patrick Baert (1991) offers a typology of side effects (or what he calls "unintended consequences"), according to which side effects can have an effect on the policy initiator, on the policy target, or on both; be desirable, undesirable, or neutral from the

point of view of the policy initiator; fulfill, frustrate, or have a neutral effect on the original intention; and be intended or unintended. The classic treatise on "unanticipated consequences" is an article by Robert Merton (1936). Robert Jervis (1997: 10) argues that the term "side effect" is misleading since "there is no criterion other than our own desires that determines which effects are 'main' and which are 'side'." Hence, he implicitly argues that scholars must analyze intentions. However, if it is implausible that an outcome called a "side effect" by an analyst was the main effect intended by an actor, and if analyzing intentions renders a research design and the empirical account overly fuzzy, speaking of side effects is justified

13 For a discussion of classical and modern social scientists' writings on side effects and unintended consequences, see Boudon 1982; Daase 2001: 14–15; Greshoff *et al.* 2003.

14 For interesting exceptions, see Daase *et al.* (2002), who use risk theory to explain policy side effects; Cortell and Peterson (2001), who explain unintended consequences of institutional change; and Lischer (2003), who explains how humanitarian assistance can exacerbate conflict

15 Prediction is not limited to the future. It sounds paradoxical, but laws also purport to predict the past. Applying a law to various temporal and spatial contexts that played no role in its formulation, and seeing whether the predictions derived from the law are true, is crucial for assessing the validity of the law (Levy 2001: 62–63).

2 Targeting Turkey and the French Connection: the early 1970s

1 The main source on this period is McCoy (1991), although his arguments do not go unchallenged. Meyer and Parssinen (1998: conclusion) criticize what they regard as conspiracy theorizing. However, they do not offer an alternative reading, but essentially confirm that the US cooperated with drug entrepreneurs. For criticism of McCoy see also Yawnghwe (1993) and Walker (1992: 208).

2 I thank Jörg Friedrichs for his comments on this point.

3 On the causes of this policy reversal see Brundage and Mitchell (1977), Spain (1975), Stavrou (1974), and Bölükbasi (1988: 173–175). I thank Claude Nicolet for drawing my attention to the latter source and for providing me with archive material that shows how the US tried to force Turkey not to lift the ban, and how the US responded to the ban's eventual revocation.

4 Consumption increased since opium dealers sold their drugs on regional markets and since governments began to implement the US-instigated global prohibition regime. Anti-drug laws led to, among others, the closure of opium dens, as a consequence of which many drug users switched from opium to heroin. Between 1950 and 1961, all state opium monopolies of mainland Southeast Asia were abolished and the opium trade largely prohibited. See Westermeyer 1982; McCoy 2000: 203.

5 According to a slightly different interpretation proposed by DEA analysts, Chinese syndicates had performed a product test on GIs. This implies that traffickers had thought of expanding their activities already before the withdrawal of US troops. The impressive results encouraged them to expand their activities and venture onto US territory. See McCoy 1991: 391–392.

6 Bresler (1980: 85), however, writes that the number of agents increased shortly after Nixon promised drug supply reductions in June 1971.

7 Rangoon also employed the helicopters for counterinsurgency operations, which entailed human rights violations and were sometimes directed against tribes who were not involved in drugs.

8 Many projects were implemented through the United Nations Fund for Drug Abuse Control (UNFDAC), the predecessor of the United Nations Drug Control Program. The UNFDAC was created in 1973. It allowed the US to distribute funds under a multilateral banner.

9 US officials had already identified Amsterdam as Europe's distribution center for Asian heroin in March 1972, as Chiu chau began making regular heroin deliveries to Western Europe (Bresler 1980: 13, 134–135; McCoy 1991: 392).
10 Operation Condor formed part of *La Campaña Permanente*, the successor program of Operation Cooperation, which replaced Operation Intercept.
11 However, in the late 1970s, Southeast Asia supplied about a third of the US heroin market. Hence, the region continued to pose a problem. See Van Wert 1982: 132.
12 I thank James Robinson for his comments on this point.
13 I thank Andreas Wenger for his comments on this point.

3 Targeting smugglers flying over the Andes: the 1990s

1 See, among others, a CIA report issued in February 1988 that describes the lack of success of Operation Blast Furnace. Available online at www.drugpolicy.org/docUploads/bigwood_blast_furnace.pdf (accessed March 30, 2006).
2 See the original document online at www.fas.org/irp/offdocs/nsdd/nsdd-221.htm (accessed March 30, 2006).
3 The subordination of drug control to other US foreign policy goals is discussed in a 1988 report issued by a subcommittee of the Senate Foreign Relations Committee (Congress 1988). The report summarizes the results of a two-year investigation begun by Senator John Kerry (D-MA) in early 1986. It confirmed that White House strategies were frequently at odds with drug policies.
4 The discussion between US officials representing various departments is documented in a briefing book of the National Security Archive (Evans 2001a)
5 Operation Laser Strike was begun at different times in different countries. In Bolivia, it was implemented in June and July 1996.
6 One of these countries was Brazil. As a matter of fact, Operation Laser Strike was an important step in the involvement of Brazil's armed forces in drug control (Brener 1997: 17). In 1998, Washington welcomed the Brazilian government's decision to adopt a shoot-down policy against suspected trafficking airplanes flying over the Amazon region. After all, this vast space had become a convenient alternative for traffickers who found the Andean route too dangerous
7 In the early twenty-first century, a Truth and Reconciliation Commission appointed by the Peruvian government found that between 1980 and 2000, the Shining Path insurgency had led to the death of 69,000 Peruvians. Shining Path was responsible for most of the deaths, but security forces and citizen militias had murdered many people as well (Independent Commission 2004: 9).
8 For a different interpretation of the impact of the border conflict on aerial trafficking see Rojas (2005: 197).
9 To be fair, not all US officials have subscribed to this view. In an interview with the author of this study on August 28, 2003, a senior official at the Narcotics Affairs Section (NAS) of the US Embassy in Lima said that the causes of declining Peruvian coca cultivation in the 1990s were complex and not only a result of the Air Bridge Denial Program.
10 During his trial, Chavez accused Montesinos of complicity in the trade, saying that he had paid Montesinos a lot of money for protecting his operations (Rojas 2005: 200, 208).
11 Author interview with senior official of the NAS, August 28, 2003, Lima. Author interview with senior official of the NAS, September 2, 2003, La Paz
12 I thank Theo Roncken for his comments on this point.
13 Operation Support Justice IV began in Colombia in November 1992 and in Peru in January 1993.

4 Targeting the Colombian drug industry: the early twenty-first century

1 The job was dangerous indeed. Between 1998 and October 2004, 11 employees, US and other foreign nationals, working for US companies contracted by the Pentagon to implement the anti-drug program, were killed (*New York Times* 2004).

2 Colombian–Venezuelan relations were far from smooth during the period analyzed here. For example, Colombian authorities accused the Venezuelan government of providing arms and sanctuary to members of the FARC and ELN (Millett 2002: 7–8).

3 The names of US anti-drug programs are often confusing. From 1999 to 2000, the US implemented Plan Colombia. From 2001, the US anti-drug program in the Andes was named the Andean Regional Initiative. This Initiative encompassed a previous program named the Andean Counterdrug Initiative, as well as other programs. In its fiscal year 2004 budget, the US government again used the name Andean Counterdrug Initiative. The present book, however, refers to the successor program of Plan Colombia as the Andean Regional Initiative.

4 To be sure, the failure to adopt regional policies against drugs also resulted from the inability of South American states to work together.

5 Author interview with senior official of the Narcotics Affairs Section (NAS), US Embassy, August 28, 2003, Lima.

6 This interpretation was corroborated in author interviews with US and German Embassy officials (interview with a senior US drug control official on September 2, 2003 at the US Embassy, La Paz; interview with a senior German diplomat on September 2, 2003 at the German Embassy, La Paz). As the German diplomat said, "Plan Colombia is not a big topic here."

7 Author interview, NAS, US Embassy in La Paz, September 2, 2003.

8 I thank Francisco Thoumi for discussing these issues with me at a conference in Berlin in October 2002.

5 Drug industry displacement and side effects of foreign policy

1 Lawrence Gooberman (1974: 199) argues that complexity poses limits to a type of theorizing that tries to discern necessary and sufficient conditions. Instead of looking at public policies as necessary or sufficient for creating an outcome, they should be regarded as contributories to the outcome.

2 Author interview with senior official of the NAS, US Embassy, August 28, 2003, Lima. See also Riley 1996: 194–195.

3 In their ability to learn from experience, smuggling networks are similar to terrorist networks such as al-Qaida (Kenney 2005).

4 I thank Andrew Bennett for his comments on this point.

5 On the need for analytical eclecticism for the study of transnational organized crime, see Nordstrom (2000: 39–40).

6 Kathryn Ledebur (2005) argues that side effects are more visible in some countries than in others. In Bolivia, human rights abuses can be more directly attributed to US foreign policy than in Colombia, where strong non-state forces are present. On the challenge of weighing factors contributing to foreign policy outcomes, see also Byman and Waxman (2002: 122).

7 One could argue that the use of methodologies such as process tracing is distinct from theory development. However, innovative theorizing requires the use of innovative methodologies. Broadening the ontology of IR has methodological consequences.

6 Alternatives to the US war on drugs

1 I thank Peter Andreas for his comments on this point.

2 Drug legalization would have different effects on different groups. In the US, legalization might benefit poor inner-city neighborhoods by reducing levels of crime, but could lead to more drug consumption among suburban middle and upper-middle classes. The fact that the latter groups are politically influential makes legalization an unlikely policy option (Thoumi 1995: 283–284). Legalization would have asymmetric effects on drug producing countries as well. Colombia, for example, might benefit from a reduction of violence, whereas Bolivia might be worse off, since the drug industry generates an important share of the national income.

3 In Peru, donors spent around $190 million between 1987 and 1996 to wean farmers away from coca. The effect of these investments in terms of coca reduction was arguably negligible (Transnational Institute 2002: 11). In the Bolivian Chapare region alone, more than $200 million were invested between 1989 and 1996, transforming it into one of the country's most developed regions. Yet coca cultivation continued unabated (Vellinga 1998: 11; Thoumi 2002b: 365). It must be said, however, that the share of AD funding that directly reached farmers has been relatively small and that living conditions continue to be precarious.

4 Author interview with Bolivian coca farmer who had migrated from the Chapare to the Yungas, conducted in the vicinity of Coroico (Yungas), September 19, 2003.

5 Author interview with a senior diplomat at the German Embassy in La Paz, September 2, 2003.

6 Certainly, if AD does not reduce drug supplies, one could argue that AD funds can be used in better ways to improve development in drug producing countries (Farrell 1998: 396).

7 Peter Reuter (2001) argues in favor of domestic law enforcement when he writes that arresting street dealers can limit drug supply *and* demand, since many dealers are also drug consumers.

8 To be sure, treatment is no panacea, as many drug users drop out of programs or relapse after completing a program.

Bibliography

Adams, D. (2005) "GAO: Data Too Fuzzy to Measure Drug War," *St. Petersburg Times*, Florida, December 24.

Allen, C.M. (2002) "An Industrial Geography of Cocaine," Unpublished Ph.D. Thesis, University of Cincinnati, Cincinnati, OH.

Anderson, M.B. (1999) *Do No Harm: How Aid Can Support Peace – or War*, Boulder, CO: Lynne Rienner.

Andreas, P. (1999) "When Policies Collide: Market Reform, Market Prohibition, and the Narcotization of the Mexican Economy," in H.R. Friman and P. Andreas (eds) *The Illicit Global Economy and State Power*, Lanham, MD: Rowman & Littlefield, pp. 125–142.

—— (2004) "Illicit International Political Economy: The Clandestine Side of Globalization," *Review of International Political Economy* 11(3): 641–652.

—— (2005) "Criminalizing Consequences of Sanctions: Embargo Busting and Its Legacy," *International Studies Quarterly* 49(2): 335–360.

Andreas, P. and Nadelmann, E.A. (2006) *Policing the Globe: Criminalization and Crime Control in International Relations*, New York and Oxford: Oxford University Press.

Andreas, P. and Price, R. (2001) "From War Fighting to Crime Fighting: Transforming the American National Security State," *International Studies Review* 3(3): 31–52.

Andreas, P. and Youngers, C. (1989) "U.S. Drug Policy and the Andean Cocaine Industry," *World Policy Journal* 6(3): 529–562.

Anthony, R.W., Crane, B.D., and Hanson, S.F. (2000) *Deterrence Effects and Peru's Force-Down/Shoot-Down Policy: Lessons Learned for Counter-Cocaine Interdiction Operations*, Alexandria, IN: Institute for Defense Analyses, April.

Arquilla, J. and Ronfeldt, D. (eds) (2001) *Networks and Netwars: The Future of Terror, Crime, and Militancy*, Santa Monica, CA: RAND.

Arrieta, C.G., Orjuela, L.J., Palacio, E.S., and Tokatlián, J.G. (1993) *Narcotrafico en Colombia: Dimensiones Políticas, Económicas, Jurídicas e Internacionales*, Bogotá, Colombia: Ediciones Uniandes y Tercer Mundo Editores.

Baert, P. (1991) "Unintended Consequences: A Typology and Examples," *International Sociology* 6(2): 201–210.

Bagley, B.M. (1988) "The New Hundred Years War? US National Security and the War on Drugs in Latin America," *Journal of Interamerican Studies and World Affairs* 30(2–3): 161–186.

—— (2001) "Drug Trafficking, Political Violence and U.S. Policy in Colombia in the 1990s," *Working Paper*, February 7, Center for Latin American Studies, University of California, Berkeley. Available online at www.clas.berkeley.edu:7001/Events/conferences/Colombia/workingpapers/working_paper_bagley.html (accessed April 27, 2006).

Basov, S., Jacobson, M., and Miron, J.A. (2001) "Prohibition and the Market for Illegal Drugs: An Overview of Recent History," *World Economics* 2(4): 133–157.

Baum, D. (1997) *Smoke and Mirrors: The War on Drugs and the Politics of Failure*, Boston, MA: Little, Brown and Company.

Bellis, D.J. (1981) *Heroin and Politicians: The Failure of Public Policy to Control Addiction in America*, Westport, VA: Greenwood Press.

Bennett, A. and George, A.L. (1997a) "Research Design Tasks in Case Study Methods," Paper presented at the Belfer Center for Science and International Affairs, Harvard University, October 17–19.

—— (1997b) "Process Tracing in Case Study Research," Paper presented at the Belfer Center for Science and International Affairs, Harvard University, October 17–19.

—— (2001) "Case Studies and Process Tracing in History and Political Science: Similar Strokes for Different Foci," in C. Elman and M.F. Elman (eds) *Bridges and Boundaries: Historians, Political Scientists, and the Study of International Relations*, Cambridge, MA and London: The MIT Press, pp. 137–166.

Bernstein, S., Lebow, R.N., Stein, J.G., and Weber, S. (2000) "God Gave Physics the Easy Problems: Adapting Social Science to an Unpredictable World," *European Journal of International Relations* 6(1): 43–76.

Bertram, E., Blachman, M., Sharpe, K., and Andreas, P. (1996) *Drug War Politics: The Price of Denial*, Berkeley, CA: University of California Press.

Bewley-Taylor, D.R. (1999) *The United States and International Drug Control, 1909–1997*, London: Continuum.

—— (2004) "Harm Reduction and the Global Drug Control Regime: Contemporary Problems and Future Prospects," *Drug and Alcohol Review* 23(4): 483–489.

Beyerchen, A. (1992/1993) "Clausewitz, Nonlinearity, and the Unpredictability of War," *International Security* 17(3): 59–90.

Block, A.A. (1989) "European Drug Traffic and Traffickers Between the Wars: The Policy of Suppression and Its Consequences," *Journal of Social History* 23(2): 315–337.

Blum, V. (2006), "US Charges 50 Colombian Guerillas in Drug-Smuggling," *Fort Lauderdale Sun-Sentinel*, Florida, March 23.

Bölükbasi, S. (1988) *The Superpowers and the Third World: Turkish–American Relations and Cyprus*, Lanham, MD: University Press of America.

Booth, M. (1998) *Opium: A History*, New York: St. Martin's Press.

Boudon, R. (1982) *The Unintended Consequences of Social Action*, London: Macmillan Press.

Bowden, M. (2001) *Killing Pablo: The Hunt for the Richest, Most Powerful Criminal in History*, London: Atlantic Books.

Brener, J. (1997) "Radical Maneuvers," in Transnational Institute, The Bolivian Documentation and Information Center, and Inforpress Centroamericana (eds) *Democracy, Human Rights, and Militarism in the War on Drugs in Latin America*, Guatemala: Inforpress Centroamericana.

Bresler, F.S. (1980) *The Trail of the Triads: An Investigation into International Crime*, London: Weidenfeld and Nicolson.

Brock, L. and Albert, M. (1995) "Entgrenzung der Staatenwelt," *Zeitschrift für Internationale Beziehungen* 2(2): 259–285.

Brouet, O. (1991) *Drogues et Relations Internationals: Du Phénomène de Société à la Narcodiplomatie*, Brussels, Belgium: Editions Complexe.

Brundage, W.H. and Mitchell, W.A. (1977) "Toward an Understanding of Opium Poppy Production in Turkey," *Journal of Asian and African Studies* 12(1–4): 259–267.

Bruun, K., Pan, L., and Rexed, I. (1975) *The Gentlemen's Club: International Control of Drugs and Alcohol*, Chicago, IL and London: The University of Chicago Press.

Byman, D. and Waxman, M. (2002) *The Dynamics of Coercion: American Foreign Policy and the Limits of Military Might*, Cambridge: Cambridge University Press.

Calvani, S., Guia, E., and Lemahieu, J. (1997) "Drug Resistance Rating: An Innovative Approach for Measuring a Country's Capacity to Resist Illegal Drugs," *Third World Quarterly* 18(4): 659–672.

Canby, P. (2004) "Latin America's Longest War," *The Nation*, July 29.

Carnwath, T. and Smith, I. (2002) *Heroin Century*, London: Routledge.

Carpenter, T.G. (2003) *Bad Neighbor Policy: Washington's Futile War on Drugs in Latin America*, New York: Palgrave Macmillan.

—— (2004) "Yet Another Drug War Failure," *Cato Daily*, August 13, The Cato Institute, Washington, DC. Available online at www.cato.org/dailys/08-13-04-2.html (accessed April 27, 2006).

Cederstav, A. and Puentes, A. (2004) "The Plan Colombia Aerial Eradication Program for Illicit Crops – An Analysis of the 2003 Department of State Certification to Congress," *Research Report*, Oakland, CA: Asociación Interamericana para la Defensa del Ambiente and Earthjustice, February 26.

Center for International Policy (2006) "Colombian Coca Cultivation in 2005," *Press Release*, April 15, Washington, DC. Available online at ciponline.org/colombia/060415coca.pdf (accessed April 22, 2006).

Central Intelligence Agency (CIA) (1998) "Changing Drug Trade in the Americas: Intelligence Report," Washington, DC: DCI Crime and Narcotics Center, February 23.

Charles, R.B. (2003) "Challenges for U.S. Policy Toward Colombia: Is Plan Colombia Working?," Testimony, Assistant Secretary of State for International Narcotics and Law Enforcement Affairs, Committee on Foreign Relations, United States Senate, October 29, Washington, DC.

Chepesiuk, R. (1999a) *Hard Target: The United States War Against International Drug Trafficking, 1982–1997*, Jefferson, MO: McFarland.

—— (1999b) *The War on Drugs: An International Encyclopedia*, Santa Barbara, CA: ABC-Clio.

Chouvy, P. (2002) *Les Territoires de l'Opium: Conflits et Trafics du Triangle d'Or et du Croissant d'Or*, Geneva: Olizane.

Claudio, A. (1992) "Heroin: The Colombian Cartels Diversify," *Low Intensity Conflict and Law Enforcement* 1(1): 3–13.

Clawson, P.L. and Lee, R.W. (1998) *The Andean Cocaine Industry*, New York: St. Martin's Press.

Coffin, P. (1998) "Coca Eradication," *Foreign Policy in Focus* 3: 29.

Common Sense for Drug Policy (2001) *Drug War Facts by Topic*, Washington, DC.

Comptroller's Office (2005) "En los Últimos 20 Años: Narcotraficantes Realizaron Gigantesca Contrareforma Agraria," *Colombian Government Press Bulletin*, June 9. Available online at www.contraloriagen.gov.co:8081/internet/cartelera/Archivos/1516/info_noticia.jsp?id=1516 (accessed April 15, 2006).

Congress (1974) *Turkish Opium Ban Negotiations*, Committee on Foreign Affairs, United States House of Representatives, 93rd Congress, 2nd Session, July 16, Washington, DC.

—— (1988) *Drugs, Law Enforcement and Foreign Policy*, Report prepared by the Subcommittee on Terrorism, Narcotics and International Operations, Committee on Foreign Relations, United States Senate, 100th Congress, 2nd Session, December, Washington, DC.

—— (2002) *U.S. Policy Toward Colombia*, Hearing, Subcommittee on the Western Hemisphere, Committee on International Relations, United States House of Representatives, 107th Congress, 2nd Session, April 11, Washington, DC.

—— (2003) *Colombia and the Andean Initiative on Narcotics*, Debate, United States House of Representatives, 108th Congress, 1st Session, July 8, Washington, DC. Available online at www.airportmonitor.org/documents/cr/03/jy/08/cr08jy03-110.html (accessed April 27, 2006).

—— (2004) *The War Against Drugs and Thugs: A Status Report on Plan Colombia Successes and Remaining Challenges*, Hearing, Committee on Government Reform, United States House of Representatives, 108th Congress, 2nd Session, June 17, Washington, DC.

Connolly, W.E. (1999) "Drugs, the Nation, and Freelancing: Decoding the Moral Universe of William Bennett," in P. de Greiff (ed.) *Drugs and the Limits of Liberalism: Moral and Legal Issues*, Ithaca, NY: Cornell University Press, pp. 173–190.

Cooper, M. (2001) "Plan Colombia," *The Nation*, March 19.

Cortell, A.P. and Peterson, S. (2001) "Limiting the Unintended Consequences of Institutional Change," *Comparative Political Studies* 34(7): 768–799.

Cottam, M.L. and Marenin, O. (1999) "International Cooperation in the War on Drugs: Mexico and the United States," *Policing and Society* 9(3): 209–240.

Courtwright, D.T. (2001) *Forces of Habit: Drugs and the Making of the Modern World*, Cambridge, MA: Harvard University Press.

Craig, R.B. (1978) "La Campaña Permanente: Mexico's Antidrug Campaign," *Journal of Interamerican Studies and World Affairs* 20(2): 107–131.

Crandall, R. (2002a) *Driven by Drugs: U.S. Policy Toward Colombia*, Boulder, CO: Lynne Rienner.

—— (2002b) "Clinton, Bush and Plan Colombia," *Survival* 44(1): 159–172.

Crawford, G. and Reuter, P. (1988) *Simulation of Adaptive Response: A Model of Drug Interdiction*, Santa Monica, CA: RAND.

Cusack, J.T. (1974) "Response of the Government of France to the International Heroin Problem," in L.R.S. Simmons and A.A. Said (eds) *Drugs, Politics, and Diplomacy: The International Connection*, Beverly Hills, CA: Sage, pp. 229–256.

Czempiel, E. and Rosenau, J.N. (eds) (1992) *Governance Without Government: Order and Change in World Politics*, Cambridge: Cambridge University Press.

Daase, C. (1991) "Drogenkrieg oder Droge Krieg? Der US-amerikanische Kampf gegen das Rauschgift," in H. Birckenbach, U. Jäger, and C. Wellmann (eds) *Jahrbuch Frieden 1991: Ereignisse, Entwicklungen, Analysen*, Munich: C.H. Beck, pp. 70–78.

—— (1999) *Kleine Kriege – Große Wirkung: Wie unkonventionelle Kriegführung die internationale Politik verändert*, Baden-Baden: Nomos.

—— (2001) *Paradoxien internationaler Risikopolitik: Das Problem nicht-intendierter Konsequenzen politischer Steuerung*, Unpublished manuscript, Free University Berlin.

Daase, C., Feske, S., and Peters, I. (eds) (2002) *Internationale Risikopolitik: Der Umgang mit neuen Gefahren in den internationalen Beziehungen*, Baden-Baden: Nomos.

Darling, J. (1999) "U.S. is Losing War on Drugs in Colombia," *Los Angeles Times*, August 8.

Dawisha, A. (1977) "Perceptions, Decisions and Consequences in Foreign Policy: The Egyptian Intervention in the Yemen," *Political Studies* 25(2): 201–226.

Department of State (Annually) *International Narcotics Control Strategy Report*, Washington, DC.

Dessler, D. (1991) "Beyond Correlations: Toward a Causal Theory of War," *International Studies Quarterly* 35(3): 337–355.

Deutsche Gesellschaft für Technische Zusammenarbeit (GTZ) (2001) *Drogen und Entwicklung in Lateinamerika: Strategien, Erfahrungen und Projektbeispiele aus der Arbeit der GTZ*, Eschborn.

Dietrich, I. (2002) "Alternative Entwicklung in Peru – ein Erfolgsmodell?," *Entwicklung und ländlicher Raum* 36(3): 25–27.

Dorn, N. and South, N. (1993) "After Mr Bennett and Mr Bush: US Foreign Policy and the Prospects for Drug Control," in F. Pearce and M. Woodiwiss (eds) *Global Crime Connections: Dynamics and Control*, Houndsmill, Basingstoke: Macmillan, 72–90.

Drug Enforcement Administration (DEA) (1998) *Statement by Thomas A. Constantine*, Subcommittee on the Western Hemisphere, Peace Corps, Narcotics, and Terrorism, Committee on Foreign Relations, United States Senate, February 26, Washington, DC.

Dunning, T. and Wirpsa, L. (2004) "Oil and the Political Economy of Conflict in Colombia and Beyond: A Linkages Approach," *Geopolitics* 9(1): 81–108.

Dupont, A. (1999) "Transnational Crime, Drugs, and Security in East Asia," *Asian Survey* 39(3): 433–455.

DuPont, R.L. (1978) "The Drug Abuse Decade," *Journal of Drug Issues* 8(2): 173–187.

Durlacher, J. (2000) *Heroin: Its History and Lore*, London: Carlton Books.

El Comercio (2003) "Las Drogas Representan el Segundo Problema Más Importante del País," Lima, Peru, August 27.

Elman, C. and Elman, M.F. (2001) "Negotiating International History and Politics," in C. Elman and M.F. Elman (eds) *Bridges and Boundaries: Historians, Political Scientists, and the Study of International Relations*, Cambridge, MA and London: The MIT Press, pp. 1–36.

Elster, J. (1989) *Nuts and Bolts for the Social Sciences*, Cambridge: Cambridge University Press.

—— (1990) "Merton's Functionalism and the Unintended Consequences of Action," in J. Clark, C. Modgil, and S. Modgil (eds) *Robert Merton: Consensus and Controversy*, London: Falmer Press, pp. 129–135.

Emdad-ul Haq, M. (2000) *Drugs in South Asia: From the Opium Trade to the Present Day*, Houndsmill, Basingstoke: Macmillian.

Epstein, E.J. (1977) *Agency of Fear: Opiates and Political Power in America*, New York: G.P. Putnam's Sons.

European NGO Council on Drugs and Development (2001) "Drugs and Development," *Newsletter*, No. 27, May, Antwerp, Belgium.

Evans, M.L. (2001a) "Shootdown in Peru: The Secret U.S. Debate over Intelligence Sharing With Peru and Colombia," *A National Security Archive Electronic Briefing Book*, April 23. Available online at www.gwu.edu/~nsarchiv/NSAEBB/NSAEBB44/ (accessed April 25, 2006).

—— (2001b) "U.S. Drug Policy and Intelligence Operations in the Andes," *Foreign Policy in Focus*, Policy Brief 6: 22.

—— (2002) "War in Colombia: Guerillas, Drugs and Human Rights in U.S.–Colombia Policy, 1988–2002," *A National Security Archive Electronic Briefing Book*, 3 May. Available online at www.gwu.edu/~nsarchiv/NSAEBB/NSAEBB69/ (accessed April 25, 2006).

Fabricio, R. (1997) "Giant Flying Radar Station Helps US in War Against Drugs," *The Miami Herald*, March 3.

Farah, D. (1998) "A Tutor to Every Army in Latin America: U.S. Expands Latin American Training Role," *Washington Post*, July 13.

Farrell, G. (1998) "A Global Empirical Review of Drug Crop Eradication and United

Nations' Crop Substitution and Alternative Development Strategies," *Journal of Drug Issues* 28(2): 395–436.

Fazey, C. and Bewley-Taylor, D. (eds) (2003) "The United Nations Conventions on Illicit Drugs: Is Change Possible?," *The International Journal of Drug Policy* 14: 2 (Special Issue).

Felbab-Brown, V. (2004) "The Coca Connection: The Impact of Illicit Substances on Militarized Conflicts," Unpublished manuscript, April, Security Studies Program, Department of Political Science, Massachusetts Institute of Technology.

Filippone, R. (1994) "The Medellin Cartel: Why We Can't Win the Drug War," *Studies in Conflict and Terrorism* 17(4): 323–344.

Forero, J. (2003) "U.N. Sees Progress in U.S. Effort on Colombian Coca," *New York Times*, September 18.

—— (2006) "Commanders Recast Old Militias of Colombia as Syndicates for Drugs and Extortion," *New York Times*, March 6.

Franco, G.H. (2004) "Battling Narcoterrorism: The Peruvian Experience in the Ucayali," *Orbis* 48(3): 505–516.

Friesendorf, Cornelius (2001) *Der internationale Drogenhandel als sicherheitspolitisches Risiko: Eine Erklärung der deutschen und US-amerikanischen Gegenstrategien*, Münster, Germany: LIT.

—— (2005a) "Drogen, Krieg und Drogenkrieg: Die USA und Kolumbien im aussichtslosen Kampf?," *WeltTrends* 13(49): 47–59.

—— (2005b) "Squeezing the Balloon? United States Air Interdiction and the Restructuring of the South American Drug Industry in the 1990s," *Crime, Law and Social Change* 44(1): 35–78.

Friman, R.H. (1996) *NarcoDiplomacy: Exporting the U.S. War on Drugs*, Ithaca, NY: Cornell University Press.

—— (2003) "Caught Up in the Madness? State Power and Transnational Organized Crime in the Work of Susan Strange," *Alternatives* 28(4): 473–489.

Gaddis, J.L. (2001) "In Defense of Particular Generalizations: Rewriting Cold War History, Rethinking International Relations Theory," in C. Elman and M.F. Elman (eds) *Bridges and Boundaries: Historians, Political Scientists, and the Study of International Relations*, Cambridge, MA and London: The MIT Press, 301–326.

General Accounting Office (GAO) (1997) *Long-Standing Problems Hinder U.S. International Efforts*, February, GAO/NSIAD-97-75, Washington, DC.

—— (1998a) *An Overview of U.S. Counterdrug Intelligence Activities*, June, NSIAD-98-142, Washington, DC.

—— (1998b) *U.S. Counternarcotics Efforts in Colombia Face Continuing Challenges*, February, GAO/NSIAD-98-60, Washington, DC.

—— (2000) *U.S. Assistance to Colombia Will Take Years to Produce Results*, October, GAO-01–26, Washington, DC.

—— (2004a) *U.S. Nonmilitary Assistance to Colombia is Beginning to Show Intended Results, But Programs Are Not Readily Sustainable*, July, GAO-04-726, Washington, DC.

—— (2004b) *Aviation Program Safety Concerns in Colombia Are Being Addressed, But State's Planning and Budgeting Process Can Be Improved*, July, GAO-04-918, Washington, DC.

George, A.L. (2000) "The Role of Force in Diplomacy: A Continuing Dilemma for U.S. Foreign Policy," in W.H. Brands (ed.) *The Use of Force After the Cold War*, College Station, TX: Texas A & M University Press, 59–92.

George, A.L. and Bennett, A. (2005) *Case Studies and Theory Development in the Social Sciences*, Cambridge, MA and London: MIT Press.

Gilboa, E. (1995/96) "The Panama Invasion Revisited: Lessons for the Use of Force in the Post Cold War Era," *Political Science Quarterly* 110(4): 539–562.

Gillon, S.M. (2000) *"That's Not What We Meant to Do": Reform and Its Unintended Consequences in Twentieth-Century America*, New York: Norton.

Goldsmith, A. (2003) "Fear, Fumbling and Frustration: Reflections on Doing Criminological Fieldwork in Colombia," *Criminal Justice* 3(1): 103–125.

González, G. and Tienda, M. (eds) (1989) *Retos de las Relaciones Entre México y Estados Unidos: México y Estados Unidos en la Cadena Internacional des Narcotráfico*, Mexico City: Comisión Sobre el Futuro de las Relaciones México–Estados Unidos.

Gooberman, L.A. (1974) *Operation Intercept: The Multiple Consequences of Public Policy*, New York: Pergamon Press.

Gootenberg, P. (ed.) (1999) *Cocaine: Global Histories*, London and New York: Routledge.

Gordon, D.G. (1994) *The Return of the Dangerous Classes: Drug Prohibition and Policy Politics*, New York: Norton.

Government Accountability Office (2005) *Air Bridge Denial Program in Colombia Has Implemented New Safeguards, But Its Effect on Drug Trafficking Is Not Clear*, September, GAO-05-970, Washington, DC.

Grande, E. and Risse, T. (2000) "Bridging the Gap: Konzeptionelle Anforderungen an die politikwissenschaftliche Analyse von Globalisierungsprozessen," *Zeitschrift für Internationale Beziehungen* 7(2): 235–266.

Gray, M. (1998) *Drug Crazy: How We Got into this Mess and How We Can Get Out*, New York: Random House.

Greshoff, R., Kneer, G., and Schimank, U. (eds) (2003) *Die Transintentionalität des Sozialen: Eine vergleichende Betrachtung klassischer und moderner Sozialtheorien*, Wiesbaden: Westdeutscher Verlag.

Gutierrez, P.R. (2000) "Colombia: The War on Drugs," *Fort Lauderdale Sun-Sentinel*, Florida September 17.

Haftendorn, H., Keohane, R.O., and Wallander, C.A. (eds) (1999) *Imperfect Unions: Security Institutions Over Time and Space*, Oxford: Oxford University Press.

Hall, K.G. (2003) "Cocaine Production Increases in Peru as U.S. Pressures Colombian Growers," *Knight Ridder*, June 10.

Hedges, M. (2001) "Colombian Cartels Moving into Peru," *Houston Chronicle*, July 24.

Hedström, P. and Swedberg, R. (1998) "Social Mechanisms: An Introductory Essay," in P. Hedström and R. Swedberg (eds) *Social Mechanisms: An Analytical Approach to Social Theory*, Cambridge: Cambridge University Press, pp. 1–31.

Hellmann, G. and Müller, H. (2003) "Editing (I)nternational (R)elations: A Changing World," *Journal of International Relations and Development* 6(4): 372–389.

Hempel, C.G. (1942) "The Function of General Laws in History," *Journal of Philosophy* 39(1): 35–48.

—— (1965) *Aspects of Scientific Explanation and Other Essays in the Philosophy of Science*, New York: Free Press.

Hill, C. (2003) *The Changing Politics of Foreign Policy*, Houndsmill, Basingstoke: Palgrave Macmillan.

Hoffman, B. (2004) "Al Qaeda and the War on Terrorism: An Update," *Current History* 103(677): 423–427.

—— (2006) "Insurgency and Counterinsurgency in Iraq," *Studies in Conflict and Terrorism* 29(2): 103–121.

Hoffmann, K. (1995) "Eine konfliktbeladene 'unheilige Allianz': Guerilla und Drogenhandel in Peru," *Nord-Süd aktuell* 9(4): 577–589.

Hollis, M. and Smith, S. (1990) *Explaining and Understanding International Relations*, Oxford: Clarendon Press.

Howard, S.P. (2001) "The Military War on Drugs: Too Many Assets, Too Few Results," *Research Report*, Monterey, CA: Naval Postgraduate School.

Huxley, A. (1959) "A Case of Voluntary Ignorance," in *Collected Essays*, New York: Harper & Row, pp. 308–318.

Inciardi, J.A. (1981) *The Drugs–Crime Connection*, Beverly Hills, CA: Sage.

Independent Commission (2004) *Andes 2020: A New Strategy for the Challenges of Colombia and the Region*, Washington, DC: Council on Foreign Relations.

Independent Task Force (1997) *Rethinking International Drug Control: New Directions for U.S. Policy*, Washington, DC: Council on Foreign Relations.

Inglis, B. (1975) *The Forbidden Game: A Social History of Drugs*, London: Hodder and Stoughton.

International Drug Report (1976) "Mexico Opens New Attack on Narcotic Traffic Crackdown Follows U.S. Criticism on Laxity," *International Narcotic Enforcement Officers Association* 17: 2.

Isacson, Adam (2004) "The State Department's Data on Drug Crop Cultivation," *Press Release*, Center for International Policy, March 22, Washington. Available online at ciponline.org/colombia/040322coca.pdf (April 22, 2006).

—— (2005) "The U.S. Military in the War on Drugs," in C.A. Youngers and E. Rosin (eds) *Drugs and Democracy in Latin America: The Impact of U.S. Policy*, Boulder, CO and London: Lynne Rienner, pp. 15–60.

—— (2006) "Did Plan Colombia Work? A Look at the Numbers," Democracy Arsenal. Guest Posting, January 18. Available online at www.democracyarsenal.org/2006/01/did_plan_colomb.html (accessed April 11, 2006).

Isikoff, M. and Vistica, G. (2000) "Fighting the Other Drug War: Is a $1.3 Billion Colombia Aid Package Smart Policy?," *Newsweek*, April 3.

Itzkowitz, G. (1996) *Contingency Theory: Rethinking the Boundaries of Social Thought*, Lanham, MD: University Press of America.

Jaffe, J.H. (2002) "One Bite of the Apple: Establishing the Special Action Office for Drug Abuse Prevention," in D.F. Musto (ed.) *One Hundred Years of Heroin*, Westport, VA: Auburn House, 43–53.

Jelsma, M. (2001) *Vicious Circle: The Chemical and Biological 'War on Drugs'*, Amsterdam, The Netherlands: Transnational Institute.

—— (2002) "Alternative Development and Drug Control: A Critical Assessment," Paper presented at the Conference on "The Role of Alternative Development in Drug Control and Development Cooperation," January 7–12, Feldafing, Germany

—— (2003) "Drugs in the UN System: The Unwritten History of the 1998 United Nations General Assembly Special Session on Drugs," *The International Journal of Drug Policy* 14(2): 181–195.

Jelsma, M. and Metaal, P. (2004) "Cracks in the Vienna Consensus: The UN Drug Control Debate," *WOLA Drug War Monitor*, January, Washington, DC: Washington Office on Latin America

Jervis, R. (1997) *System Effects: Complexity in Political and Social Life*, Princeton, NJ: Princeton University Press.

Johnson, T. (1999) "U.S. Diplomat Tries to Allay Invasion Fear in Colombia," *The Miami Herald*, August 11.

Joyce, E. (1997) "EU Drug Policy in the Andes: International Cooperation and the Politics of Illicit Cocaine Supply," Unpublished DPhil Thesis, University of Oxford.

Kaldor, M. (1999) *New and Old Wars: Organized Violence in a Global Era*, Cambridge: Polity.

Kaplan, J. (1983) *The Hardest Drug: Heroin and Public Policy*, Chicago, IL and London: The University of Chicago Press.

Katzenstein, P.J. and Okawara, N. (2001/2002) "Japan, Asian-Pacific Security, and the Case for Analytical Eclecticism," *International Organization* 26(3): 153–185.

Kay, B.H. (1999) "Violent Opportunities: The Rise and Fall of 'King Coca' and Shining Path," *Journal of Interamerican Studies and World Affairs* 41(3): 97–127.

Kenney, M.C. (2002) "Outsmarting the State: A Comparative Case Study of the Learning Capacity of Colombian Drug Trafficking Organizations and Government Drug Enforcement Agencies," Unpublished Ph.D. Thesis, University of Florida, Gainesville, FL.

—— (2005) "State Led Prohibition Regimes and the Challenge of Dismantling Illicit Non-State Networks," in E. Krahmann (ed.) *New Threats and New Actors in International Security*, New York: Palgrave, pp. 69–90.

King, G., Keohane, R.O. and Verba, S. (1994) *Designing Social Inquiry: Scientific Inference in Qualitative Research*, Princeton, NJ: Princeton University Press.

King, R. (1972) *The Drug Hang-Up: America's Fifty-Year Folly*, New York: Norton.

Kotler, J. (2001) "U.S. Official Sees Long Road Ahead in Colombia Drug War," *San Diego Union Tribune*, April 8.

Krahmann, E. (2005), "Security Governance and Networks: New Theoretical Perspectives in Transatlantic Security," *Cambridge Review of International Affairs* 18(1): 15–30.

Krauss, C. (1999) "Peru's Drug Successes Erode as Traffickers Adapt," *New York Times*, August 19.

—— (2000) "Neighbors Worry About Colombian Aid," *New York Times*, August 24.

Krüger, H. (1980) *The Great Heroin Coup: Drugs, Intelligence and International Fascism*, Boston, MA: South End Press.

Kunnes, R. (1972) *The American Heroin Empire: Power, Profits, and Politics*, New York: Dodd, Mead & Company.

Kurki, M. (2002) "Causes of a Divided Discipline: A Critical Examination of the Concept of Cause in International Relations Theory," *Working Paper*, Global Politics Network. Available online at www.globalpolitics.net (accessed April 26, 2006).

Labrousse, A. (1992) "La Culture du Pavot Dans le District de Dir (Pakistan): Economie Paysanne, Productions Illicites et Alternatives de Développement Dans le Contexte d'un Conflit Regional," *Revue Tiers Monde* 33(131): 623–644.

—— (2000) *Drogues: Un Marché de Dupes*, Paris: Editions Alternatives.

—— (ed.) (2003) *Dictionnaire Géopolitique des Drogues: La Drogue Dans 134 Pays – Productions, Traffics, Conflits, Usages*, Brussels, Belgium: de boeck.

Labrousse, A. and Koutouzis, M. (1996) "Narcotrafic: Une Guerre Perdue d'Avance?," *Politique Internationale*, 73 (Autumn): 313–328.

Lamberti, M. and Lamour, C. (1973) *Die Opium-Mafia*, Frankfurt/Main, Germany: Suhrkamp.

Latin America Working Group Education Fund, Center for International Policy, and Washington Office on Latin America (2005) *Erasing the Lines: Trends in U.S. Military Programs With Latin America*, December, Washington, DC.

Lebow, R.N. and Risse-Kappen, T. (1996) "Introduction: International Relations Theory and the End of the Cold War," in R.N. Lebow and T. Risse-Kappen (eds) *International Relations Theory and the End of the Cold War*, New York: Columbia University Press, pp. 1–21.

Ledebur, K. (2005) "Bolivia: Clear Consequences," in C.A. Youngers and E. Rosin (eds) *Drugs and Democracy in Latin America: The Impact of U.S. Policy*, Boulder, CO and London: Lynne Rienner, pp. 143–184.

Lee, R.W. (1989) *The White Labyrinth: Cocaine and Political Power*, New Brunswick, Canada: Transaction Publishers.

—— (2002) "Perverse Effects of Andean Counternarcotics Policy," *Orbis* 46(3): 537–554.

Lee, R.W. and Thoumi, F.E. (1999) "The Political–Criminal Nexus in Colombia," *Trends in Organized Crime* 5(2): 59–84.

Leheny, D. (2002) "Symbols, Strategies, and Choices for International Relations Scholarship After September 11," *International Organization*, Dialog-IO, Spring, 57–70.

Léons, M.B. (1997) "After the Boom: Income Decline, Eradication, and Alternative Development in the Yungas," in M.B. Léons and H. Sanabria (eds) *Coca, Cocaine, and the Bolivian Reality*, Albany, NY: State University of New York Press, pp. 139–168.

Lessmann, R. (2000) "Amerikanisierung und Militarisierung: Die auswärtige Drogenpolitik der USA," in P. Rudolf and J. Wilzewski (eds) *Weltmacht ohne Gegner: Amerikanische Aussenpolitik zu Beginn des 21. Jahrhunderts*, Baden-Baden: Nomos, pp. 335–362.

Levy, J.S. (1997) "Too Important to Leave to the Other: History and Political Science in the Study of International Relations," *International Security* 22(1): 22–33.

—— (2001) "Explaining Events and Developing Theories: History, Political Science, and the Analysis of International Relations," in C. Elman and M.F. Elman (eds) *Bridges and Boundaries: Historians, Political Scientists, and the Study of International Relations*, Cambridge, MA, and London: The MIT Press, pp. 39–110.

Lintner, B. (1999) *Burma in Revolt: Opium and Insurgency since 1948*, Chiang Mai, Thailand: Silkworm Books.

Lischer, S.K. (2003) "Collateral Damage: Humanitarian Assistance as a Cause of Conflict," *International Security* 28(1): 79–109.

Loane, G. and Moyroud, C. (eds) (2001) *Tracing Unintended Consequences of Humanitarian Assistance: The Case of Sudan*, Baden-Baden: Nomos.

Loeb, V. (2003) "Rumsfeld Seeks Better Intelligence on Iraqi Insurgents," *Washington Post*, December 11.

Lupsha, P.A. (1981) "Drug Trafficking: Mexico and Colombia in Comparative Perspective," *Journal of International Affairs* 35(1): 95–115.

Lupsha, P.A. and Schlegel, K. (1980) "The Political Economy of Drug Trafficking: The Herrera Organization (Mexico and the United States)," *Working Paper*, No. 2, Albuquerque, NM: University of New Mexico.

Lupu, N. (2004) "Towards a New Articulation of Alternative Development: Lessons From Coca Supply Reduction in Bolivia," *Development Policy Review* 22(4): 405–421.

Mabry, D.J. (1989) "Narcotics and National Security," in D.J. Mabry (ed.) *The Latin American Narcotics Trade and U.S. National Security*, New York: Greenwood Press, pp. 3–9.

McAllister, W.B. (1999) *Drug Diplomacy in the Twentieth Century: An International History*, London: Routledge.

McClintock, C. (1988) "The War on Drugs: The Peruvian Case," *Journal of Inter-american Studies and World Affairs* 30(2–3): 127–142.

McClintock, C. and Vallas, F. (2003) *The United States and Peru: Cooperation at a Cost*, New York and London: Routledge.

MacCoun, R.J. and Reuter, P. (2001) *Drug War Heresies: Learning from Other Vices, Times, and Places*, Cambridge: Cambridge University Press.

McCoy, A.W. (1974) "The Politics of the Poppy in Indochina: A Comparative Study of Patron–Client Relations Under French and American Administrations," in L.R.S. Simmons and A.A. Said (eds) *Drugs, Politics, and Diplomacy: The International Connection*, Beverly Hills, CA: Sage, pp. 112–158.

—— (1991) *The Politics of Heroin: CIA Complicity in the Global Drug Trade*, 2nd edn, Chicago, IL: Lawrence Hill.

—— (1996) "Heroinhandel und internationale Politik: Ein Vergleich zwischen Südostasien und Südwestasien," in A. Labrousse and A. Wallon (eds) *Der Planet der Drogen: Analyse einer kriminellen Weltmacht*, Frankfurt/Main, Germany: Fischer, pp. 251–263.

—— (1999) "Lord of the Drug Lords: One Life As Lesson for US Drug Policy," *Crime, Law and Social Change* 30(4): 301–331.

—— (2000) "Coercion and Its Unintended Consequences: A Study of Heroin Traffickin in Southeast and South West Asia," *Crime, Law and Social Change* 33(3): 191–224.

—— (2003) *The Politics of Heroin: CIA Complicity in the Global Drug Trade (Afghanistan, Southeast Asia, Central America, Colombia)*, 3rd edn, Chicago, IL: Lawrence Hill.

—— (2004) "The Stimulus of Prohibition: A Critical History of the Global Narcotics Trade," in M.K. Steinberg, J.J. Hobbs, and K. Mathewson (eds) *Dangerous Harvest: Drug Plants and the Transformation of Indigenous Landscapes*, New York and Oxford: Oxford University Press, pp. 24–111.

McDermott, J. (2006) "Peru's Guerillas Back on Warpath in Alliance with Drug Barons," *Daily Telegraph*, March 20.

MacDonald, S.B. (1988) *Dancing on a Volcano: The Latin American Drug Trade*, New York: Praeger.

McKeown, T.J. (1999) "Case Studies and the Statistical Worldview: Review of King, Keohane, and Verba's Designing Social Inquiry: Scientific Inference in Qualitative Research," *International Organization* 53(1): 161–190.

McWilliams, J.C. (1990) "The History of Drug Control Policies in the United States," in J.A. Inciardi (ed.) *Handbook of Drug Control in the United States*, London: Greenwood Press, pp. 29–50.

—— (1991) "Through the Past Darkly: The Politics and Policies of America's Drug War," *Journal of Policy History* 3(4): 356–392.

Malinowska-Sempruch, K., Hoover, J., and Alexandrova, A. (2003) "Unintended Consequences: Drug Policies Fuel the HIV Epidemic in Russia and Ukraine," April, Paper for Consideration by the UN Commission on Narcotic Drugs and National Governments, Published by the Open Society Institute.

Manaugh, S.L. (2000) "Without Reason: Drug War Politics in the United States," Unpublished Ph.D. Thesis, University of California, Berkeley, CA.

Marsh, B. (2004) "Going to Extremes: The U.S.-Funded Aerial Eradication Program in Colombia," *Research Report*, March, Washington, DC: The Latin America Working Group Education Fund.

Marshall, C. (2001) "Peru Set to Be Drug Leader," *BBC News*, February 17.

Marshall, J. (1993) "Drugs and United States Foreign Policy," in R. Hamowy (ed.) *Dealing with Drugs: Consequences of Government Control*, San Francisco, CA: Pacific Research Institute for Public Policy, pp. 137–176

Martin, S.T. (2001) "U.S. Versus Them: U.S. Policy Not Limited to Borders," *St. Petersburg Times*, Florida, July 29.

Massing, M. (2000) *The Fix*, Berkeley, CA: University of California Press.

Mendel, W.W. (1992) "Illusive Victory: From Blast Furnace to Green Sweep," *Military Review*, December: 74–87.

Mendel, W.W. and Munger, M.D. (1997) "The Drug Threat: Getting Priorities Straight," *Parameters*, Summer: 110–124.

Mendelson, S.E. (2005) *Barracks and Brothels: Peacekeepers and Human Trafficking in the Balkans*, Washington, DC: Center for Strategic and International Studies.

Menzel, S.H. (1996) *Fire in the Andes: U.S. Foreign Policy and Cocaine Politics in Bolivia and Peru*, Lanham, MD: University Press of America.

—— (1997) *Cocaine Quagmire: Implementing the U.S. Anti-Drug Policy in the North Andes–Colombia*, Lanham, MD: University Press of America.

Merton, R.K. (1936) "The Unanticipated Consequences of Purposive Social Action," *American Sociological Review* 1(6): 894–904.

Meyer, K. and Parssinnen, T. (1998) *Webs of Smoke: Smugglers, Warlords, Spies, and the History of the International Drug Trade*, Lanham, MD: Rowman & Littlefield

Millett, R.L. (2002) "Colombia's Conflicts: The Spillover Effects of a Wider War," *Agenda Paper*, Miami, FL: The North–South Center, University of Miami.

Mittelman, J.H. and Johnston, R. (1999) "The Globalization of Organized Crime, the Courtesan State, and the Corruption of Civil Society," *Global Governance* 5(1): 103–126.

Molinski, D. (2004) "New Wave of Colombia Drug Kingpins Emerges," *Associated Press*, September 22.

—— (2006) "Air Assault Targets Drug Crops," *Miami Herald*, February 18.

Mora, F.O. (1996) "Victims of the Balloon Effect: Drug Trafficking and U.S. Policy in Brazil and the Southern Cone of Latin America," *The Journal of Social, Political and Economic Studies* 21(2): 115–140.

Morales, E. (1989) *Cocaine: White Gold Rush in Peru*, Tucson, AZ: The University of Arizona Press.

Morrison, S. (1997) "The Dynamics of Illicit Drugs Production: Future Sources and Threats," *Crime, Law and Social Change* 27(2): 121–138.

Moynihan, D.P. (2002) "One Hundred Years of Heroics," in D.F. Musto (ed.) *One Hundred Years of Heroin*, Westport, VA: Auburn House, pp. 23–38.

Murphy, M.F. and Steele, R.H. (1971) "The World Heroin Problem," *Report of Special Study Mission*, Committee on Foreign Affairs, United States House of Representatives, Washington, DC.

Musto, D.F. (1999) *The American Disease: Origins of Narcotic Control*, 3rd edn, New York and Oxford: Oxford University Press.

Musto, D.F. and Korsmeyer, P. (2002) *The Quest for Drug Control: Politics and Federal Policy in a Period of Increasing Substance Abuse, 1963–1981*, New Haven, CT: Yale University Press.

Nadelmann, E.A. (1990) "Global Prohibition Regimes: The Evolution of Norms in International Society," *International Organization* 44(4): 479–526.

—— (1993) *Cops Across Borders: The Internationalization of US Criminal Law Enforcement*, University Park, PA: Pennsylvania State University Press.

Naim, M. (2005) "Broken Borders," *Newsweek*, October 24, pp. 56–62.

National Drug Intelligence Center (2004) *National Drug Threat Assessment 2004*, March, Department of Justice, Washington, DC.

—— (2006) *National Drug Threat Assessment 2006*, January, Department of Justice, Washington, DC.

National Narcotics Intelligence Consumers Committee (1998) *The Supply of Illicit Drugs to the United States, 1997 Report*, November, Washington, DC.

Nations, R. (1976) "An Uphill Battle in Thailand," *Far Eastern Economic Review* 92(18) (April 30).

Naylor, T.R. (1995) "From Cold War to Crime War: The Search for a New 'National Security' Threat," *Transnational Organized Crime* 1(4): 37–56.

Network of Reform Groups (1999) *The Effective National Drug Control Strategy*, Washington, DC.

Newsday (1973) *The Heroin Trail: The First Journalistic Investigation to Trace Heroin Traffic From Turkey to France to Its Ultimate Customer – the Young American Addict!*, New York: Signet.

New York Times (2004) "Congress Approves Doubling U.S. Troops in Colombia to 800," October 11.

Nieves, R.J. (1998) "Colombian Cocaine Cartels: Lessons From the Front," *Trends in Organized Crime* 4(3): 13–26.

Nordstrom, C. (2000) "Shadows and Sovereigns," *Theory, Culture and Society* 17(4): 35–54.

Norwegian Refugee Council (2006) *Internal Displacement: Global Overview of Trends and Developments in 2005*, The Internal Displacement Monitoring Centre, March, Geneva.

Nussbaum, B. (1972) "Narcotics: The Asian Connection," *Far Eastern Economic Review* 77(34) (August 19).

Nye, J.S. (2002/2003) "Limits of American Power," *Political Science Quarterly* 117(4): 545–559.

Office of National Drug Control Policy (ONDCP) (Annually) *National Drug Control Strategy*, Washington, DC.

Painter, J. (1994) *Bolivia and Coca: A Study in Dependency*, Boulder, CO: Lynne Rienner.

Palmer, D.S. (1992) "Peru, the Drug Business and Shining Path: Between Scylla and Charybdis?," *Journal of Interamerican Studies and World Affairs* 34(3): 65–88.

Perl, R.F. (1992) "United States Andean Drug Policy: Background and Issues for Decisionmakers," *Journal of Interamerican Studies and World Affairs* 34(3): 13–35.

Phares, D. (1973) "The Simple Economics of Heroin and Organizing Public Policy," *Journal of Drug Issues* 3(2): 186–200.

Poret, S. (2003) "Paradoxical Effects of Law Enforcement Policies: The Case of the Illicit Drug Market," *International Review of Law and Economics* 22(4): 465–493.

President's Commission on Organized Crime (1986) *America's Habit: Drug Abuse, Drug Trafficking, and Organized Crime*, Report to the President and Attorney General, Washington, DC.

Priest, D. (1998) "Sidestepping Sanctions: U.S. Military Trains Foreign Troops," *Washington Post*, July 12.

Ramírez, M.C., Stanton, K., and Walsh, J. (2005) "Colombia: A Vicious Circle of Drugs and War," in C.A. Youngers and E. Rosin (eds) *Drugs and Democracy in Latin America: The Impact of U.S. Policy*, Boulder, CO and London: Lynne Rienner, pp. 99–142.

Reinarman, C. and Levine, H.G. (1994) "The Construction of America's Crack Crisis," in L. Böllinger (ed.) *De-Americanizing Drug-Policy: The Search for Alternatives for Failed Repression*, Frankfurt/Main, Germany: Peter Lang, pp. 49–87.

Renard, R.D. (1996) *The Burmese Connection: Illegal Drugs and the Making of the Golden Triangle*, Boulder, CO: Lynne Rienner.

Reuter, P. (1984) "The (Continued) Vitality of Mythical Numbers," *The Public Interest*, 75 (Spring): 135–147.

—— (1985) "Eternal Hope: America's Quest for Narcotics Control," *The Public Interest*, 79 (Spring): 79–95.

—— (1994) "The Limits and Consequences of U.S. Foreign Drug Control Efforts," in R.F. Perl (ed.) *Drugs and Foreign Policy: A Critical Review*, Boulder, CO: Westview Press, pp. 209–221.

—— (2001) "The Limits of Supply-Side Drug Control," *The Milken Institute Review*, First Quarter: 15–23.

Reuter, P. and Greenfield, V. (2001) "Measuring Global Drug Markets: How Good are the Numbers and Why Should We Care About Them?," *World Economics* 2(4): 159–173.

Reuters (1999) "US Drug Chief Says Colombia Is Everyone's Problem," August 11.

Riley, K.J. (1996) *Snow Job? The War Against International Cocaine Trafficking*, New Brunswick, Canada: Transaction Publishers.

Robberson, T. (1998) "U.S. Launches Covert Program to Aid Colombia," *Dallas Morning News*, August 19.

Rohter, L. (1999) "With U.S. Training, Colombia Melds War on Rebels and Drugs," *New York Times*, July 29.

—— (2000) "Narcotics and War Become Intertwined," *New York Times*, April 21.

Rojas, I. (2003) "The Push for Zero Coca: Democratic Transition and Counternarcotics Policy in Peru," *WOLA Drug War Monitor*, February, Washington, DC: Washington Office on Latin America

—— (2005) "Peru: Drug Control Policy, Human Rights, and Democracy," in C.A. Youngers and E. Rosin (eds) *Drugs and Democracy in Latin America: The Impact of U.S. Policy*, Boulder, CO and London: Lynne Rienner, pp. 185–230.

Roncken, T. (ed.) (1999) *The Drug War in the Skies: The U.S. "Air Bridge Denial" Strategy – the Success of a Failure*, Cochabamba, Bolivia: Acción Andina and Transnational Institute.

Rosenau, J.N. (1990) *Turbulence in World Politics: A Theory of Change and Continuity*, Princeton, NJ: Princeton University Press.

Ruiz, B. (2001) *The Colombian Civil War*, Jefferson, MO and London: McFarland.

Rydell, P.C. and Everingham, S.S. (1994) *Controlling Cocaine: Supply Versus Demand Programs*, Santa Monica, CA: RAND.

Schroeder, R.C. (1980) *The Politics of Drugs: An American Dilemma*, 2nd edn, Washington, DC: Congressional Quarterly Press.

Scott, P.D. (2003) *Drugs, Oil, and War: The United States in Afghanistan, Colombia, and Indochina*, Lanham, MD: Rowman & Littlefield

Scott, P.D. and Marshall, J. (1991) *Cocaine Politics: Drugs, Armies and the CIA in Central America*, Berkeley, CA: University of California Press.

Seccombe, R. (1995) "Squeezing the Balloon: International Drugs Policy," *Drug and Alcohol Review* 14(3): 311–316.

Senlis Council (2005) *Feasibility Study on Opium Licencing in Afghanistan for the Production of Morphine and Other Essential Medicines*, September 26, London.

Shifter, M. (1999) "Colombia on the Brink: There Goes the Neighborhood," *Foreign Affairs* 78(4): 14–20.
—— (2000) "The United States and Colombia: Partners in Ambiguity," *Current History* 99(634): 51–55.
Simmons, L.R.S. and Said, A.A. (1974) "The Politics of Addiction," in L.R.S. Simmons and A.A. Said (eds) *Drugs, Politics, and Diplomacy: The International Connection*, Beverly Hills, CA: Sage, pp. 3–48.
Slaughter, A. (2004) *A New World Order*, Princeton, NJ: Princeton University Press.
Smith, A. (1976 [1776]) *An Inquiry into the Nature and Causes of the Wealth of Nations*, Oxford: Clarendon Press.
Smith, C.E. (2000) *Inevitable Partnership: Understanding Mexico–U.S. Relations*, Boulder, CO: Lynne Rienner.
Smith, S. and Clarke, M. (1985) *Foreign Policy Implementation*, London: George Allen & Unwin.
Spain, J. (1975) "The United States, Turkey and the Poppy," *Middle East Journal* 29(3): 295–307
Stanton, J. (2001) "War on Drugs – U.S. Has No 'Exit Strategy,'" *National Defense Magazine* 85(570): 18–20.
Stares, P.B. (1996) *Global Habit: The Drug Problem in a Borderless World*, Washington, DC: Brookings Institute.
Stavrou, N.A. (1974) "The Politics of Opium in Turkey," in L.R.S. Simmons and A.A. Said (eds) *Drugs, Politics, and Diplomacy: The International Connection*, Beverly Hills, CA: Sage, pp. 214–228.
Stiles, K. (2002) "International Support for NGOs in Bangladesh: Some Unintended Consequences," *World Development* 30(5): 835–846.
Stokes, D. (2005) *America's Other War: Terrorizing Colombia*, London: Zed Books.
Strange, S. (1996) *The Retreat of the State: The Diffusion of Power in the World Economy*, Cambridge: Cambridge University Press.
Sunshine Project (2001) "Risks of Using Biological Agents in Drug Eradication: A Briefing Paper with Emphasis on Human Health," *Background Series*, No. 4, February, Hamburg.
Tamayo, J.O. (2001a) "Risks for U.S. Military in Andes Drug War," *Miami Herald*, May 22.
—— (2001b) "CIA's Andean Spying Under Attack," *Miami Herald*, May 20.
Tate, W. (1999) "Colombia's Role in the International Drug Industry," *Foreign Policy in Focus* 4: 30.
Tenner, E. (1996) *Why Things Bite Back: Technology and the Revenge of Unintended Consequences*, New York: Alfred A. Knopf.
The Economist (1998) "Colombia on the Brink," August 8.
—— (2001a) "The Struggle to Exterminate a Much-Loved Andean Shrub," May 23.
—— (2001b) "High Time: A Survey of Illegal Drugs," July 28.
—— (2002) "Drugs in the Andes: Spectres Stir in Peru," February 16.
—— (2003) "The Andean Drug Industry: The Balloon Goes Up," March 3.
The International Institute for Strategic Studies (2000) "US Anti-Narcotics Strategy: At War With Reality?," *IISS Strategic Comments* 6: 2.
Thoumi, F.E. (1994) "The Size of the Illegal Drug Industry," in B.M. Bagley and W.O. Walker (eds) *Drug Trafficking in the Americas*, New Brunswick, Canada: Transaction Publishers, pp. 77–94.
—— (1995) *Political Economy and Illegal Drugs in Colombia*, Boulder, CO: Lynne Rienner.

—— (2002a) "Can the United Nations Support 'Objective' and Unhampered Illicit Drug Policy Research? A Testimony of a UN Funded Researcher," *Crime, Law and Social Change* 38(2): 161–183.

—— (2002b) *El Imperio de la Droga: Narcotráfico, Economía y Sociedad en Los Andes*, Bogotá, Colombia: Planeta.

Tickner, A.B. (2003) "Colombia and the United States: From Counternarcotics to Counterterrorism," *Current History* 101(661): 77–85.

Tokatlián, J.G. (1995) *Drogas, Dilemmas y Dogmas: Estados Unidos y el Narcocriminalidad Organizada En Colombia*, Bogotá, Colombia: Tercer Mundo Editores.

—— (2003) "The United States and Illegal Crops in Colombia: The Tragic Mistake of Futile Fumigation," *Working Paper*, No. 3, June, Center for Latin American Studies, University of California, Berkeley, CA.

Toro, M.C. (1995) *Mexico's "War" on Drugs: Causes and Consequences*, Boulder, CO: Lynne Rienner.

Transnational Institute (2001) "Europe and Plan Colombia: Chronicle of a Commitment With an Uncomfortable Plan," *Debate Paper*, No. 1, Amsterdam, The Netherlands.

—— (2002) "Peru: From Virtual Success to Realistic Policies?," *Drug Policy Briefing*, No. 3, Amsterdam, The Netherlands.

—— (2003a) "Forward Operation Locations in Latin America: Transcending Drug Control," *Debate Paper*, No. 8, Amsterdam, The Netherlands.

—— (2003b) "Measuring Progress: Global Supply of Illicit Drugs, Progress Report as a Contribution to the Midterm Review of UNGASS," April, Amsterdam, The Netherlands.

—— (2004) "Coca or Death? Cocalero Movements in Peru and Bolivia," *Debate Paper*, No. 10, Amsterdam, The Netherlands.

Trebach, A.S. (1993) "The Need for Reform of International Narcotics Laws," in R. Hamowy (ed.) *Dealing with Drugs: Consequences of Government Control*, San Francisco, CA: Pacific Research Institute for Public Policy, pp. 101–136

Tuchman, B. (1984) *The March of Folly: From Troy to Vietnam*, New York: Alfred A. Knopf.

Tullis, L. (1991) "Beneficiaries of the Illicit Drug Trade: Political Consequences and International Policy At the Intersection of Supply and Demand," *Discussion Paper*, No. 19, Geneva: United Nations Research Institute for Social Development.

—— (1995) *Unintended Consequences: Illegal Drugs and Drug Policies in Nine Countries*, Boulder, CO: Lynne Rienner.

Turner, M.A. (1975) "The International Politics of Narcotics: The United States and Turkey," Unpublished Ph.D. Thesis, Kent State University.

United Nations Drug Control Programme (1997) *World Drug Report*, Oxford: Oxford University Press.

United Nations Office for Drug Control and Crime Prevention (2000) *World Drug Report*, Oxford: Oxford University Press.

United Nations Office on Drugs and Crime (2003a) *Colombia: Coca Survey for December 2002 and Semi-Annual Estimate for July 2003*, Vienna.

—— (2003b) *Peru: Coca Survey for 2002*, March, Vienna.

—— (2003c) *Global Illicit Drug Trends 2003*, Vienna.

—— (2004a) *Colombia: Coca Cultivation Survey for 2003*, June, Vienna.

—— (2004b) *Bolivia: Coca Cultivation Survey for 2003*, June, Vienna.

Vandenberg, M.E. (2005) "Trafficking in Armed and Post-Conflict Situations," in Sector Project Against Trafficking in Women (ed.) *Challenging Trafficking in Persons: Theoretical Debate and Practical Approaches*, Baden-Baden: Nomos, pp. 69–75.

Van Wert, J. (1982) "U.S.–Mexican Aerial Opium Eradication Program: A Summative Evaluation," Unpublished Ph.D. Thesis, University of Southern California.

Vargas, R. (1997) "Die ökonomischen und sozialen Auswirkungen einer Gangster-Wirtschaft: Drogengeschäft und Arbeitsplätze in Kolumbien," in B. Rütsche and P. Stirnimann (eds) *Drogen und dritte Welt: Plädoyer für eine neue Nord-Süd-Drogenpolitik*, Lucerne, Switzerland: Edition Exodus, pp. 62–73.

—— (1999) "The Impact of the U.S. Fumigation Program," in George Washington University and Washington Office on Latin America (eds) *Counter-Narcotics Policy and Prospects for Peace: Eradication and Alternative Development in Southern Colombia*, Seminar Report, 29 October, Washington, DC.

—— (2002) "The Anti-Drug Policy, Aerial Spraying of Illicit Crops and their Social, Environmental and Political Impacts in Colombia," *Journal of Drug Issues* 32(1): 11–60.

—— (2004) "Política Antidrogas En Colombia . . . Lejos del Éxito," *La Esquina Regional*, September/October. Available online at www.tni.org/archives/vargas/exito.htm (accessed April 22, 2006).

Vellinga, M.L. (1998) "Alternative Development and Supply Side Control in the Drug Industry: The Bolivian Experience," *European Review of Latin American and Caribbean Studies*, 64 (June): 7–26.

Wagner, R. (2000) "Kolumbiens illusionsloser Kampf gegen das Kokain," *Frankfurter Allgemeine Zeitung*, May 20.

Walker, W.O. (1991) *Opium and Foreign Policy: The Anglo–American Search for Order in Asia, 1912–1954*, Chapel Hill: The University of North Carolina Press.

—— (1993/94) "The Foreign Narcotics Policy of the United States Since 1980: An End to the War on Drugs?," *International Journal* 19(1): 37–66.

—— (ed.) (1992) *Drug Control Policy: Essays in Historical and Comparative Perspective*, University Park, PA: Penn State University Press.

—— (ed.) (1996) *Drugs in the Western Hemisphere: An Odyssey of Cultures in Conflict*, Wilmington, DE: Scholarly Resources.

Walsh, J.M. (2004) "Are We There Yet? Measuring Progress in the U.S. War on Drugs in Latin America," *WOLA Drug War Monitor*, December, Washington, DC: Washington Office on Latin America

Walters, J.P. (2004) "Colombia: Delivering Good Counter-Drug Results," *Statement*, Director of the Office of National Drug Control Policy, June 17, Committee on Government Reform, United States House of Representatives, Washington, DC.

Washington Office on Latin America (WOLA) (2002) "Taking Stock: Plan Colombia's First Year," *Colombia Monitor*, 1 (March).

Wellmann, H.R. (1974) "American Diplomacy and the International Narcotics Traffic, in L.R.S. Simmons and A.A. Said (eds) *Drugs, Politics, and Diplomacy: The International Connection*, Beverly Hills, CA: Sage, pp. 65–90.

Wendt, A.E. (1998) "On Constitution and Causation in International Relations," *Review of International Studies* 24 (Special Issue): 101–117.

—— (1999) *Social Theory of International Politics*, Cambridge: Cambridge University Press.

Westermeyer, J. (1982) *Poppies, Pipes, and People: Opium and Its Use in Laos*, Berkeley, CA: University of California Press.

White House (2002) "Coca Cultivation in Colombia 2001," *Press Release*, March 7, Office of National Drug Control Policy, Washington, DC

—— (2006) "2005 Coca Estimates for Colombia," *Press Release*, 14 April, Office of National Drug Control Policy, Washington, DC.

Wiant, J.A. (1985) "Narcotics in the Golden Triangle," *The Washington Quarterly* 8(4): 125–140.

Williams, J., Pacula, R., Chaloupka, F., and Wechsler, H. (2006) "College Students' Use of Cocaine," *Substance Use and Misuse* 41(4): 489–509.

Williams, P. (1995) "Transnational Criminal Organizations: Strategic Alliances," *The Washington Quarterly* 18(1): 57–72.

—— (1998) "The Nature of Drug-Trafficking Networks," *Current History* 97(618): 154–159.

Yawnghwe, C. (1993) "The Political Economy of the Opium Trade: Implications for Shan State," *Journal of Contemporary Asia* 23(3): 306–326.

Yee, A.S. (1996) "The Causal Effects of Ideas on Policies," *International Organization* 50(1): 69–108.

Young, S. (2000) *Maximizing Harm: Losers and Winners in the Drug War*, San Jose, CA: Writer's Showcase.

Youngers, C.A. (1995) "Fueling Failure: U.S. Drug Control Efforts in the Andes," April, *WOLA Briefing Series*, Washington, DC: Washington Office on Latin America

—— (2001) "Collateral Damage: U.S. Drug Control Efforts in the Andes," Paper presented at the Latin American Studies Association, Washington, DC, September 6–8.

—— (2005) "The Collateral Damage of the U.S. War on Drugs: Conclusions and Recommendations," in C.A. Youngers and E. Rosin (eds) *Drugs and Democracy in Latin America: The Impact of U.S. Policy*, Boulder, CO and London: Lynne Rienner, pp. 339–366.

Youngers, C.A. and Rosin, E. (2005) "The U.S. 'War on Drugs': Its Impact in Latin America and the Caribbean," in C.A. Youngers and E. Rosin (eds) *Drugs and Democracy in Latin America: The Impact of U.S. Policy*, Boulder, CO and London: Lynne Rienner, pp. 1–13.

Zaitch, D. (2002) *Trafficking Cocaine: Colombian Drug Entrepreneurs in the Netherlands*, The Hague, The Netherlands: Kluwer Law International.

Zimring, F.E. and Hawkins, G. (1992) *The Search for Rational Drug Control*, Cambridge: Cambridge University Press.

Zinecker, H. (2002) "Kolumbien – Wie viel Demokratisierung braucht der Frieden?," *HSFK-Report*, No. 2, Frankfurt/Main, Germany: Hessische Stiftung Friedens- und Konfliktforschung

Zirnite, P. (1997) *Reluctant Recruits: The U.S. Military and the War on Drugs*, Washington, DC: Washington Office on Latin America

—— (1998) "The Militarization of the Drug War in Latin America," *Current History* 97(618): 166–173.

Index

Tables are indicated by italic page numbers, figures, charts and maps by bold numbers

Afghanistan 6, 60
AIDS: and contaminated needles 6; as side effect of coercive drug policies 16
Air Bridge Denial Program (ABDP): assumptions based on 90; changes in trafficking routes and methods 102 claims of success 100–1; close cooperation with Andean states 91; coca cultivation move to Colombia from Peru 101; immunity for US personnel 98; impact on South American drug industry 117; impact on traffickers' ris 100; lack of governmental control over territory 110; number of planes forced or shot down or seized 114–15; number of smuggling flights prevented 115 organisations involved 90–1; radar stations 92–3; reaction of traffickers t 107–9; reduction of coca cultivation in Peru 103; shooting down of aircraft 96; shooting down of missionary family 103–4; verticalization of Peruvian and Bolivian drug markets 102
al-Qaida: compared to smuggling networks 203n5.3; complexity of after 9/11 175
Albright, Madeleine 130
alternative development (AD) 9, 182–3, 204n3
alternative explanations for displacement: ABDP no contribution to displacement 117–19; and black boxes 73; displacement as intended conscious plan 78; expansion of Mexican drug industry 73; increased international trade and movement of people 73–4; political engineering by US 74; prohibition 73; US anti-drug policies not necessary 161–2
Alvarez Machain, Humberto 87
Amsterdam, hub of European heroin distribution 56, 202n2.9
Andean coca cultivation (1988–2005) *98*, **198**
Andean Initiative 85, 92
Andean Regional Initiative: catalyst for displacement of drug industry 165; confusion about names of programs 203n4.3; effect on US drug problems 143; funding for Colombia's neighbors 136–7; gradual implementation of 146–7; merging of wars on drugs, terror and insurgency 137–8; violence under 157
Andreas, Peter 21
Anti Drug Abuse Act 81
anti-drug strategies 7, *8*, 9
Arlacchi, Pino 184
Autodefensas Unidas de Colombia (AUC) 129

Baert, Patrick 200n1.12
Bagley, Bruce 32, 133
"balloon effect" 20, 22; *see also* displacement of the drug industry
Banzer, Hugo 103
Bennett, Andrew 20, 29
Bennett, William 83
Bertram, Eva 21
Beyerchen, Alan 177
Bias, Len 81, 82
Blachman, Morris 21
black boxes: actors involved in drug business 115; and alternative explanations 73; Asian heroin entering US from Mexico 71; availability of

black boxes – *contd.*
coca paste in Colombia 116; changing patterns of drug demand 116–17; coca prices 116; covert operations by US forces and private companies 161; impact of policies on drug industry 72–3; interpretation of data, difficulty o 160; number of hectares used for coca cultivation 115, 158–9; number of planes forced or shot down or seized 114–15; number of smuggling flight prevented 115; theories undermined by 173; traffickers 71–2; trafficker anticipation of state policies 160–1
Bolivia: amount of coca cultivation 94, 97, *98,* 103, 142–3, **198**; boom in coca production 86–7; corruption in 109; defence of coca production 87; difficul implementation of anti-drug laws 153–4; drop in cocaine prices 94; ground radar installation 93; human rights abuses 203n5.6; map **197**; non-coercive programs, investment in 147–8; Operation Blast Furnace 81–2; Operation Ghost Zone 94–5; Operation Safe Haven 94; Plan Dignity 103; pressure on seen as US imperialism 87; resistance to coca eradication 153–4; results from AD investment 204n3; transportation of coca paste to Colombia 90; undermining of state by drug industry 7; verticalization of drug markets 102, 108, 116–17
Brazil, drug interdiction in 93, 202n3.6
Bresler, Fenton 71, 72
Bureau of Narcotics and Dangerous Drugs (BNDD) 38
bureaucratic turf battles as side effect of coercive drug policies 16
Burma: bilateral drug control agreement with US 55; lack of territorial control 67–8
Bush, George: coercion as solution to drug control 84; drug control as prime foreign policy interest 83
Bush, George W. 136

Cali group 111–12
Caribbean 88
Carpenter, Ted Galen 20–1, 188
causal mechanisms 3–4, 28–33, 177, 178
causality 174–6
Chavez, Demetrio Limoniel (Vaticano) 116
Cheney, Dick 83–4
Chepesiuk, Ron 20
Chernick, Marc 158
Chinese Nationalist Party *see* Kuomintang (KMT)
Chiu chau Triads: benefit from weak la enforcement 67; drug operations in Hong Kong 52; and Southeast Asian opium market 66
CIA: and drug traffickers 22–3; and th Mujahideen 60; in Southeast Asia 48–9
Clausewitz, Carl von 26, 177
Clawson, Patrick 31
Clinton, Bill 88–9, 99, 130
Clinton administration: coercive strategies priority 122–3; and military drug control 98–9; rhetorical stance on drugs 122
coca cultivation: Andean (1988–2005) *98*; Bolivia 94, 97, *98,* 103, 142–3, **198**; Colombian national parks 141; decrease in Peru 97, *98*; and fumigation in Colombia (1993–2003) **199**; fungus attacking coca plants 112; high revenues for growers 17; increase in during Plan Colombia 135; move to Colombia from Peru 101; number of hectares used for as black box 115, 158–9; reduction of in Peru 101, 103; resurgence of in Peru 150; trends in Colombia 139–40; undemanding plants 17
coca paste: availability of in Colombia 116; availability of in Colombia as black box 116; production in Peru and Bolivia 89; transportation of to Colombia 90
coca production: increases in 5
cocaine: Colombian traffickers 80; contro of as central policy objective 81; crack 81; drop in casual use 82; falling prices 81; increases in consumption 6; problems related to in US 82; production and export from Colombia 89; retail prices in US (1993–2003) **199**; usage in US 80
cocaine industry: and consumption, legalization of 179; stability of 94
coercive drug policies: aggravation of global drug problems 186; definition o coercion 200n1.3; domestic and international implications of 81–2; drug war as a habit 187; frustration as explanation for support of 188; ineffectiveness of 16–17; less effective than harm reduction 187; motives behind 13–15; as opposed to

legalization 179; perpetuated and escalated by displacement 188–9; political motivation for 187; positive results of 200n1.10; reasons for ineffectiveness of 17–19, *19*; US perceptions and politics leading to 79–89; and the US population 188; US spending on 200n1.9; *see also* side effects of coercive drug policies

Colombia: availability of coca paste in 116; "balloon effect," anticipation of by US 148; coca cultivation 139–40, 141, **198**; coca cultivation in national parks 141; cocaine traffickers 80; corruptio in 123–4; criticisms of increase in US military aid 129; de-legitimization of governmental system 155–6, 158; decertification by US 99, 123, 156 demilitarized zone 127, 138; demobilization of paramilitaries 139; displacement of coca cultivation 138, 140–1; displacement of people 134–5, 138, 147, 157; drug-related violence 84–6; effects of US drug policies 20; effects on of drug industry 5–6; extradition of traffickers from 84–5 failure of eradication program 106–7; failure to coordinate on regional basis 148–9; FARC 124–7, 132, 133, 134, 138, 139; focus of US drug policy 103; funding for neighbors 136–7; government negotiation with guerillas 124, 127; growth of smaller traffickin groups 112; guerilla presence in coca growing areas 157; guerilla retreat as tactical maneuver 139; heroin supplier to US 123; human rights abuse by paramilitaries 139; human rights violations by military 125, 129; impact on Peru by developments in 111–12; increase in coca cultivation 97, *98,* 101, 106, 108–9, 138, 145; increase in military or police presence 139; increased funding for neighboring countries 136; lack of nation-building efforts by US 157–8; Leahy Amendment 125; links between insurgents and drug trade 125–6; map **195**; negative effect of coercion 156–7; oil pipelines 124, 137–8; Operation Support Justice III 95; paramilitary forces 129–30; Plan Colombia 12; private companies in drug control efforts 128; production and export of cocaine from 89; radar stations 92; rebels and paramilitaries and the drug trade 110–11; relations with Venezuela 203n4.2; retail cocaine prices in US **199**; risks to US personnel of aerial fumigation program 127, 203n4.1; shooting down of aircraft 96; slow distribution of development aid 147; undermining of state by drug industry 7; unilateral pressure from US 85; US aid against guerillas 139; US aid to (1997–2005) **199**; US aid to police force and military 128; US funding for critical infrastructures 137–8; weak territorial control 110–11, 150–2; *see also* Plan Colombia

communism in Marseille 42

complexity: of al-Qaida after 9/11 175; and causal mechanisms 178; and criminalization 174–5; historians more able to accept 175–6; imposing limits on law-based theorizing 177; increased by state pressure 175; limits to theorizing 203n5.1; and linear causality 174; multi-causal explanations 176; sex industry in southeast Europe 175

Comprehensive Drug Abuse Prevention and Control Act 39

constructivists and side effects of foreign policy 25

contingencies 26–7, 32; border conflic between Peru and Ecuador 114; and causal mechanisms 178; Chiu chau victory over Green Gang 70; climate 70; de-legitimization of Colombian governmental system 155–6; fungus attacking coca plants 112; geography of Colombia 155; government changes 70; growth of smaller trafficking groups in Colombia 111–12; impact on Peru by developments in Colombia 111–12; imposing limits on law-based theorizing 177; insurgency and counter-insurgency in Peru 112–13; migration to US 70–1; norms 70; poverty 70; poverty in Colombia 155; socio-economic changes in Peru 113–14; Vietnam War 70

corruption: in Bolivia 109; as obstacle to drug control 109–10; of officials i Mexico 69, 87; in Peru 109; as side effect of coercive drug policies 16; in Venezuela 109–10

Cosa Nostra, use of Southeast Asian opium market 65–6

"covering laws" 26
crack cocaine 81
Craig, Richard 58
Crandall, Russell 130
Cuba 88

democratic control of military, threat to: as side effect of coercive drug policies 16
democratic stability, undermining of by drug industry 7
dependence of states on drug economy 18
displacement of the drug industry: causal mechanism of 30–3; contribution of US foreign policy 169–70; difficulty o assessing complex scenarios 173–4; explanation of **33**; flexibility of th industry 64–7, 107–9; impact of contingent factors 172–3; leading to coercive policies' perpetuation and escalation 188–9; micro perspective needed for research 173; negative consequences of 170; Plan Colombia and Andean Regional Initiative as catalysts for 165; research as hermeneutic endeavor 173; research on 20–3; selectivity of US drug policies 60–4, 104–7; social laws and flexibilit of drug industry 171–2; use of causal mechanisms to analyze 171; weak law enforcement 67–9, 109–11; *see also* alternative explanations for displacement; black boxes; contingencies
displacement theorizing 35–6
drug consumption: increases in 6; legalization of 179
drug demand: strategies for reducing *8,* 9
drug economy: dependence of states on 18; true size of 7
drug free workplace program 81
drug industry: changes in 5–7; flexibilit of 64–7; lack of data on 33–4, 71–3; legalization of 179; as "victimless crime" 17
drug supplies, effects of increase in 5–6
drug trafficking routes, extent of
drugs: ratio of weight to value of 17; strategies against 7, *8,* 9

economic interactions, changes in 19
economic security, impact of drugs on 7
Ecuador: air interdiction in 93; effect on of Plan Colombia 135; weak territorial control 152

ELN 124, 126, 127, 133
Elster, Jon 24
environment: damage to as side effect of coercive drug policies 16; impact on of drug industry 7
Epstein, Edward 38, 41
eradication, resistance to 18
Escobar, Pablo 85–6, 111
externalization of drug problems 88
extradition of traffickers from Colombi 84–5

FARC 124–7, 132, 133, 134, 138, 139
flexibility of the drug industry: enabling factors 171–2; innovative behavior of traffickers 149–50; new sources o supply 64–7; reactions to fumigation 149
Foreign Policy Analysis (FPA) 25
Forward Operating Locations (FOLs) 103
French Connection: anticipation of Turkish opium ban 65; elimination of 44–5; and motives behind US drug policies 40–2; opium supply from Southeast Asia 65; and the US–Italian Mafia 43
Friman, Richard 27
Fujimori, Alberto 99, 119
fungus attacking coca plants 112

Galán, Luis, assassination of 85
Garcia, Alan 80
Gelbard, Robert 126
George, Alexander 20, 29
Golden Triangle *see* Southeast Asia
Gooberman, Lawrence 203n5.1
government control over drug-producing regions 18
Gross, Nelson G. 68
Guzmán, Abimael 113

harm reduction: advantages to drug producing areas 180–1; alternative development (AD) 182–3; law enforcement still required 181; no use of foreign militaries for law enforcement 181–2; reducing economic inequalities 181; strategies for 179–80
Hayek, Friedrich von 24
Hellmann, Gunther 174
Hempel, Carl 26
heroin: changes in consumption patterns 37–8; increases in consumption 6; manufacturing of in Marseille 43–4
heroin industry and consumption, legalization of 179

historians and acceptance of complexity 175–6
humans: erratic behaviour of 177; as variables 177

ineffectiveness of drugs policies and side effects of 17–19, *19*
insurgency as priority to governments 18
international drug control and the UN 183–5
International Institute for Strategic Studies, The 22
International Political Economy (IPE) 27
International Relations: drugs as major topic in 6–7; laws and mechanisms in 26–30; mechanism-based theorizing 28–30; positivism in 26; research into drugs and drug policies 3; and side effects of foreign policy 24–5; social laws 26–7; structural theorists 26; under appreciation of change 27–8
Itzkowitz, Gary 28, 32

Jaffe, Jerome 39
Jelsma, Martin 182
Jervis, Robert 174, 201n1.12
Joint Air Operations Center (JAOC) 90–1

Kenney, Michael 171
Keohane, Robert 28
King, Gary 28
Krüger, Henrik 42, 66, 74
Kuomintang (KMT) 48–9
Kurki, Milja 29–30

Lamberti, Michel 72
Lamour, Catherine 72
Lansky, Meyer 44
Laos: anti-drug laws forced by US 55; CIA support of government and opium production 50; weak law enforcement 67
Latin America: drug consumption 6; *see also* names of individual countries
law-based theorizing 26–7, 28, 177, 201n1.15
Leahy Amendment 125
Ledebur, Kathryn 203n5.6
Lee, Rensselaer 20, 31
legalization of cocaine and heroin industry and consumption 179, 204n6.2
Lehder, Carlos 85
Levy, Jack 177
linear causality 174

Lockheed Martin 128
Luciano, Charles "Lucky" 43
Lupsha, Peter 58, 71–2

Manaugh, Sara 188
maps: Bolivia **197**; Colombia **195**; Mediterranean Basin **191**; Mexico **193**; Peru **196**; South America **194**; Southeast Asia **192**; world showing case study areas **190**
Marseille: communism in 42; heroin manufacturing in 43–4
Marsh, Betsy 22
Massing, Michael 80
McCaffrey, Barry 99–100, 130
McCoy, Alfred 22, 44, 48, 54, 56, 72, 186
mechanism-based theorizing 28–30, 177
Medellín group 85–6, 111
media, role in US drug crisis 82–3
Meltzer, Howard 57
Menzel, Sewall 95–6, 109–10
Merton, Robert 25
Mexico: corruption of officials 69, 87 crop eradication 57–8; drug controls applied late to 64; effects of Operation Intercept 65; eradication campaign with US 59–60; geography hampering drug control 68–9; heroin industry in 21; ineffective government drug control 66–7; lack of equipment 69; as main heroin supplier to US 58–9; map **193**; Operation Condor 69; Operation Intercept 58; opium production in 1920s and 1930s 57; poppy cultivation increase 87; relationship with US 87; smuggling of drugs by air 65; US supported cultivation during WWII 57; weak interagency coordination 69; weak law enforcement 68–9
militaries: foreign, use of for law enforcement 181; threat to democratic control of 16; US use of for drug control 10–11
Montesinos, Vladimiro 99, 119
Mora, Frank 22
Morales, Evo 153–4
Morocco 12
Morrison, Shona 23
Moynihan, Daniel Patrick 61
Müller, Harald 174
multi-causality 176
Musto, David 38

narco-guerilla paradigm 126

National Drug Control Strategy (NDCS) 83
nationalism as side effect of coercive drug policies 16
negotiation with drug industry 18
network structure of drug trafficking 31
Nicaragua 87–8
nineteenth century, drug trade in 6
Nixon, Richard: domestic motives behind foreign drugs policies 41–2; election as President 38; elimination of the French Connection 44; Operation Intercept in Mexico 58; and poppy cultivation in Turkey 45–7
non-state actors, illicit, research into 27
Noriega, Manuel 6, 11, 84, 88
norms, anti-drug 18

Office of National Drug Control Polic (ONDCP) 83
oil companies and US involvement in Colombia 128–9
Operations, drug control: Blast Furnace 81–2, 91, 202n3.1; Ghost Zone 94–5; Green Clover 99; Intercept 10, 58, 65; Just Cause 84; Laser Strike 99–100, 202n3.5, 202n3.6; Safe Haven 94; Snowcap 91–2; Support Justice III 94, 109
Opium Wars, nineteenth century 6

Painter, James 116
Pakistan 6, 60
Panama, invasion of 11, 84
paramilitaries in Colombia and the drug trade 110–11
Pastrana, Andrés 126–7, 130, 134, 138
Pentagon as pivotal drug control actor 83
personalization of drug problems 88
Peru: aerial interdiction in 94, 109; airports 110; border conflict with Ecuador 114 coca cultivation (1988–2005) **198**; coca prices 141–2; corruption in 109; decline in coca prices 101; decline in traffickin 94; decrease in coca cultivation 97, *98*; effect on of Plan Colombia 135–6, 141–2; eradication 112–13; Fujimori assumption of power 95; Fujimori election victory 99; fungus attacking coca plants 112; government control over airports 110; ground radar 92; half-hearted government drug control 86; high cost of ABDP 119; impact on by developments in Colombia 111–12; increase in US anti-drug aid 99; involvement in trafficking 116; ma **196**; Mexican traffickers in coca marke 115; non-coercive programs, investment in 147–8; Operation Green Clover 99; Operation Support Justice III 94; reduction of coca cultivation 101, 103; results from AD investment 204n3; resurgence of coca and poppy cultivation 150; rise in coffee prices 113; Shining Path (Sendero Luminoso) 6, 86, 110, 113, 152–3, 202n3.7; socio-economic changes in 113–14; suspension of aerial surveillance by US 95; trafficking groups and aircraft 92 transportation of coca paste to Colombia 90; verticalization of drug markets 102, 108; weak territorial control 152–3
Pickering, Thomas 130, 148
Plan Colombia: catalyst for displacement of drug industry 165; confusion about names of programs 203n4.3; displacement of people 134–5; drug control and anti-insurgency 133, 134; effect on neighboring countries 135–6, 141–3; effect on US drug problems 143; European criticism of 132–3; FARC response to 132; fumigation, criticisms of 132; fumigation campaign 134–5; gradual implementation of 144–6; human rights accusations 132; increase in coca cultivation 135; low priority of non-coercive elements 132; political situation in Colombia 133; push into southern Colombia 131; reaction of neighboring states 134; US contribution 131; versions of, US and Colombian 130–1; violence under 157
political representation, changes in 19
political science, attitude to complexity 175–6
Politics of Heroin, The (A. McCoy) 22, 48, 54
Popper, Karl 24
poppy cultivation: high revenues for growers 17; move from Southeast Asia 5; in Turkey 45–7
positive anti-drug strategies *8,* 9
positivism in IR 26; and complexity of change 28; limits of 173
price of drugs: decrease in 16–17; impact of source-country programs 18
process tracing 34, 36, 176–7, 203n5.7
prohibition, effects of 15

purity of drugs, increase in 17

radar stations 92–3, 99
Rattikone, Ouane 50
Reagan, Ronald: militant approach to drug control 79–80; public relations campaign against drugs 80
reform: of UN drug control policies 183–5; of US drug control policies 185–9
resistance to drug industry by states 23
Reuter, Peter 38, 58, 72, 204n6.7
Riley, Kevin 72, 116
Rockefeller, Nelson 38
Rumsfeld, Donald 189

Samper, Ernesto 123, 156
Schlegel, Kip 58, 71–2
Scott, Peter Dale 187
Seccombe, Ralph 20
security and drugs 6–7
selectivity of US drug policies: bilateral rather than multilateral relationships 148; drug controls applied late to Mexico 64; failure to coordinate ABDP activities 104–6; fighting communism a priority 61–3; focus on southern Colombia 143–4; gradual implementation of initiatives 144–7; lack of knowledge about drugs 61; political opportunism 61; preference given to coercive strategies 107, 147–8
Sendero Luminoso *see* Shining Path
sex industry in southeast Europe 175
Sharpe, Kenneth 21
Shaw, Clay 10
Shifter, Michael 148
Shining Path (Sendero Luminoso) 86, 110, 113, 152–3, 202n3.7
Sicilian Mafia and heroin manufacturing 4
Sicily, invasion of 43
side effects of coercive drug policies: bureaucratic rivalries 16; causality 27; changes in drug consumption habits 16; corruption 16; deterioration of treatment facilities 81; displacement 13; harm to other plants by fumigation 16; and ineffectiveness of policies 17–19, *19*; inflation of drug prices 15; nationalis 16; prohibition 15; restructuring of world drugs trade 56; stiffening of sanctions 81; typology of 200n1.12; undemocratic control of armed forces 16; violence 15–16; visibility of in different countries 203n5.6
side effects of foreign policy, research on 23–5
Smith, Adam 24
social laws 26–7, 174
South American drug industry: map **194**; restructuring of 101–2; *see also* names of individual countries
South Vietnam 62–3
Southeast Asia: anti-drug laws forced by US 55, 63; CIA alliances with drug traffickers 48–9, 62–3; continuation a heroin supplier 60; drug control agreements with US 55–6; expansion into global drug market 51–3; exports to Western Europe and Australia 56; heroin supply to US 202n2.11; increased exports as result of troops withdrawal 51–2; ineffective government drug control 66–7; links with the French Connection 65; map **192**; memoranda of understanding with US 55; opium dealing and consumption 201n2.4; opium production in 48; percentage of US heroin market 56; US role in wars 48–51; weak law enforcement 67–8; *see also* names of individual countries
sovereignty: as undermining anti-drug efforts 19; of US host nations, concerns about 82
Stares, Paul 21
Strange, Susan 27
strategies against drugs 7, *8*, 9
structural adjustment programs 19
structural theorists 26
supply-oriented anti-drug strategies 7, *8*, 9

technology, use by traffickers 18, 108
Thailand: common ground with US 55; cooperation with KMT 49–50; lack of territorial control 67–8
Thoumi, Francisco 155
Trafficante, Santo, Jr. 65–
Trafficante family 4
traffickers: adaptive and innovativ behavior of 107–9, 149–50; alliance with United States in Southeast Asia 48–51; anticipation of state policies as black box 160–1; and the CIA 22–3, 48–9, 62–3; Colombian cocaine 80; extradition of from Colombia 84–5; groups and aircraft in Peru 92; information on as black box 71–2; low and high tech methods of 108; Mexican, in Peruvian coca market 115; reaction of

traffickers – *contd.*
to ABDP 107–9; risks, impact on of ABDP 100; technological edge over state forces 18
trafficking routes, extent of
transportation of coca paste to Colombia 90
Tuchman, Barbara 187
Tullis, LaMond 21
Turkey 21; and the Corsican French Connection 40–1; pressure from US to stop poppy cultivation 45–7; production and use of opium 40; suspension of US aid 10

United Nations (UN): conventions, US role in 10; drug control policies, reform of 183–5
United States: alliance with drug traffickers in Southeast Asia 48–51 anti-drug budget 12–13; climate of hysteria 84; cocaine users 80; coercive nature of drug control 12; consequences of coercive drug policies 13–19; contradictions between policies 18; domestic anti-drug policies 186; domination of international drug control 9–13; drug control budget 123; drug control reform 185–9; drug problems not reduced by air interdiction 100–1; drugs as burden on economy 14–15; economic sanctions against uncooperative countries 11; energy interests as motivation 138; funding of drug control 88; heroin shortages 53–4; increased spending on international drug control 83; inefficiency of anti-dru operations 82; intelligence sharing with Colombia and Peru 92; international law enforcement 10; lifestyle changes 82; Mafia use of Southeast Asian opiu market 65–6; marijuana consumption 80; mass market for drugs, reason for 37; merging of wars on drugs, terror and insurgency 137–8; migration pressure from Colombia 126; motives behind coercive policies 13–15; Operation Intercept 10; relationship with Mexico 87; role in UN conventions 10; selectivity of drug policies 60–4; serious drug-related problems 82; support for involvement in Colombian conflict 130 suspension of aid to Turkey 10; suspension of intelligence sharing 96–7; use of military for drug control 10–11
Uribe, Alvaro 138–9

Van Raab, William 91
Van Wert, James 72
Vargas, Ricardo 106–7, 112, 116
Venezuela: corruption in 109–10; relations with Colombia 203n4.2; weak territorial control 152
Verba, Sidney 28
verticalization: of Colombian cocaine market 112; of Peruvian and Bolivian drug markets 102, 108, 116–17
Vietnam: heroin use among US military 39–40; South, involvement in drug trafficking 50–1; withdrawal of U troops from 51–2
violence: as side effect of coercive drug policies 15–16

Walsh, John 187
Walters, John 146
war restrictions, end of 19
Williams, Phil 31

Young, Stephen 15